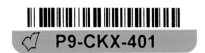

Handbook of Experimental Pharmacology

Continuation of Handbuch der experimentellen Pharmakologie

Vol. 81

Local Anesthetics

Contributors

G. R. Arthur · K. R. Courtney · B. G. Covino · J. M. Garfield
G. A. Gintant · A. J. Gissen · L. Gugino · B. F. Hoffman
S. A. Raymond · J. M. Ritchie · G. R. Strichartz · L. D. Vandam

Editor

G. R. Strichartz

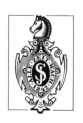

Springer-Verlag
Berlin Heidelberg New York
London Paris Tokyo

GARY R. STRICHARTZ, Ph. D., Associate Professor

Anesthesia Research Laboratories
Brigham and Women's Hospital and
Department of Pharmacology, Harvard Medical School
Boston, MA 02115, USA

With 52 Figures

ISBN 3-540-16361-1 Springer-Verlag Berlin Heidelberg New York
ISBN 0-387-16361-1 Springer-Verlag New York Berlin Heidelberg

Library of Congress Cataloging-in-Publication Data. Local anesthetics. (Handbook of experimental pharmacology; vol. 81). Includes bibliographies and index. 1. Anesthetics. 2. Local anesthesia. I. Arthur, G. R. II. Strichartz, G. R. (Gary R.), 1943– . III. Series: Handbook of experimental pharmacology; v. 81. [DNLM: 1. Anesthetics, Local – pharmacodynamics. W1 HA51L v. 81/QV 110 L811] QP905.H3 vol. 81 [RD84] 615′.1 s [617′.966] 86-20258 ISBN 0-387-16361-1 (U.S.)

© Springer-Verlag Berlin Heidelberg 1987
Printed in Germany

The use of registered names, trademarks, etc. in this publication does not imply, even in the absence of a specific statement, that such names are exempt from the relevant protective laws and regulations and therefore free for general use.

Product liability: The publisher can give no guarantee for information about drug dosage and application thereof contained in this book. In every individual case the respective user must check its accuracy by consulting other pharmaceutical literature.

Typesetting, printing and bookbinding: Brühlsche Universitätsdruckerei, Giessen
2122/3130-543210

List of Contributors

G. R. ARTHUR, Anesthesia Research Laboratories, Brigham and Women's Hospital, Harvard Medical School, 75 Francis Street, Boston, MA 02115, USA

K. R. COURTNEY, Palo Alto Medical Foundation, 860 Bryant Street, Palo Alto, CA 94301, USA

B. G. COVINO, Department of Anesthesia, Brigham and Women's Hospital, Harvard Medical School, 75 Francis Street, Boston, MA 02115, USA

J. M. GARFIELD, Department of Anesthesia, Brigham and Women's Hospital, Harvard Medical School, 75 Francis Street, Boston, MA 02145, USA

G. A. GINTANT, Masonic Medical Research Laboratory, 2150 Bleecker Street, Utica, NY 13501-1787, USA

A. J. GISSEN, Department of Anesthesia, Brigham and Women's Hospital, Harvard Medical School, 75 Francis Street, Boston, MA 02115, USA

L. GUGINO, Department of Anesthesia, Brigham and Women's Hospital, Harvard Medical School, 75 Francis Street, Boston, MA 02115, USA

B. F. HOFFMAN, Department of Pharmacology, College of Physicians and Surgeons, Columbia University, 630 168th Street, New York, NY 10032, USA

S. A. RAYMOND, Department of Anesthesia, Brigham and Women's Hospital, Harvard Medical School, 75 Francis Street, Boston, MA 02115, USA

J. M. RITCHIE, Department of Pharmacology, Yale University Medical School, 333 Cedar Street, New Haven, CT 06510, USA

G. R. STRICHARTZ, Anesthesia Research Laboratories, Brigham and Women's Hospital and Department of Pharmacology, Harvard Medical School, 75 Francis Street, Boston, MA 02115, USA

L. D. VANDAM, Department of Anesthesia, Brigham and Women's Hospital, Harvard Medical School, 75 Francis Street, Boston, MA 02115, USA

Preface

Local anesthetics are among the most widely used drugs. Their development over the past century ranges from a documented influence on Freud's *Interpretation of Dreams*[1] to the synthesis of the ubiquitously popular lidocaine, as described in Chapter 1. For surgical procedures the use of regional, epidural and intrathecal local anesthesia has increased continuously during the past decade. Local anesthetics are also applied by physicians to ameliorate unpleasant sensations and reactions to other procedures, such as tracheal intubation. The presence or the threat of cardiac arrhythmias is often countered by chronic administration of local anesthetic-like agents, such as lidocaine or procainamide. Relief of acute pain, accompanying dental manipulations, for example, and of chronic pain are also accomplished with traditional local anesthetics. And over-the-counter formulations of topical local anesthetics provide practitioners of solar indiscretion welcome relief from their otherwise unaccommodating sunburn.

In all these applications the final effect of the local anesthetic is an inhibition of electrical activity, accomplished as a reduction or total blockade of action potentials. The primary site of action is the sodium channel, a transmembrane protein which is essential for the influx of sodium ions that subserves impulse generation and propagation in nerves, skeletal muscle, and heart. The detailed mechanisms of local anesthetic action are still being investigated and Chapter 2 of this volume provides a current overview of that subject. Although there appear to be plural isozymes of sodium channels, with modestly differing pharmacological properties[2], they all seem to be susceptible to local anesthetics. The structural parameters of these drugs are related to their blocking action in Chapter 3 and to their specific role as antiarrhythmic agents in Chapter 7. Despite this signal physiological mechanism, local anesthetics do have differential effects on various tissues. The apparent ability to block impulses in certain types of nerve fibers while sparing others is critically examined in the review of Chapter 4.

In order to accomplish their clinical actions local anesthetics must distribute within and pass through numerous body compartments and tissues. Their net effectiveness arises from the dynamics of delivery and removal, the pharmacokinetics dealt with in Chapter 5. By virtue of being aromatic-linked tertiary amines, local anesthetics are amphipathic molecules; both electrically neutral and

---

[1] Freud S (1974) Cocaine papers. In: Byck R (ed) Stonehill, New York
[2] Moczydlowski E, Uehara A, Guo X, Heiny J (1986) Isochannels and blocking modes of voltage-dependent sodium channels. In: Kao CY, Levinson SR (eds) Tetrodotoxin, saxitoxin, and the molecular biology of the sodium channel. New York Acad Sci, New York

protonated species are distributed through almost all the tissues surrounding a site of injection and, indeed, throughout the body following systemic administration. Much of the clinically documented toxicity of these drugs follows their systemic distribution, producing acute responses in the cardiovascular and central nervous systems, as described in Chapters 6 and 8.

Even as their tissue distribution is relatively unlimited, the actions of local anesthetics extend beyond sodium channels of excitable cells. For example, other types of channels that respond to membrane potential, like those conducting potassium or calcium ions, are also inhibited by local anesthetics (see Chapter 2). Chemically activated ion channels, such as the postsynaptic nicotinic acetylcholine activated channel, are also susceptible to traditional local anesthetics, and other postsynaptic receptors may also be affected.

Ionic channels are not restricted to nervous tissue. Their recently discovered presence and physiological role in cells of the immune system [3] would have been considered unlikely 10 years ago. As electrophysiological techniques are applied to an increasing diversity of tissues the role of ionic channels in many physiological processes will become even more apparent. And because of their ability to circulate relatively freely and to be absorbed by almost all membranes, local anesthetics may be recognized to have broader and more subtle actions than are currently assigned.

This book considers the experimental pharmacology of local anesthetics that is pertinent to their established clinical actions. Effects on cell-to-cell interactions, such as those modifying fertility, and detailed biophysical analyses of the many, many membrane alterations rendered by local anesthetics are not included here.

Most of the contributions included here were written by 1984 and the Editor, while realizing the impossibility of publishing a completely current review of any scientific subject, does believe that these chapters represent an up-to-date compilation of this field. I wish to thank the authors for their enthusiasm and effort. My colleagues at the Brigham and Women's Hospital and Harvard Medical School have been generous in their critical interest and suggestions. Mrs. Doris Walker, of Springer-Verlag Publishers, has remained a constant and attentive devotee in the completion of this volume of the Handbook. And my secretary, Rachel Abrams, is to be credited with the good-humored patience required in dealing with the manuscripts and correspondences of a multi-authored text. Finally, I wish to acknowledge the dedication of all the investigators who study local anesthetics, for their efforts result in both the immediate excitement of things discovered and the evolution of scientific knowledge, and, more, important, in the development of safer and more secure methods of pain relief.

Boston, Massachusetts   GARY R. STRICHARTZ

---

[3] DeCoursey TE, Chandy KG, Gupta S, Cahalan MD (1984) Voltage-gated K^+ channels in human T lymphocytes: a role in mitogenesis? Nature 307:465–468

Contents

CHAPTER 5

Pharmacokinetics of Local Anesthetics
G. R. Arthur. With 5 Figures 165

CHAPTER 6

Toxicity and Systemic Effects of Local Anesthetic Agents
B. G. Covino. With 3 Figures 187

CHAPTER 7

The Role of Local Anesthetic Effects in the Actions of Antiarrhythmic Drugs

CHAPTER 8

Central Effects of Local Anesthetic Agents

CHAPTER 1

Some Aspects of the History of Local Anesthesia

L. D. VANDAM

A. Introduction

As befits its importance to the relief of suffering in man, the writings on the history of local anesthesia are extensive, as those also were in relation to its predecessor, inhalation anesthesia. Strangely, those accounts appear largely in the American literature although the first clinical application of the anesthetic properties of cocaine took place in Vienna, in 1884. Full credit, as we shall see, is now given to Koller, the perpetrator. Although his contribution was not beset with the kind of controversy that surrounded the advent of inhalation anesthesia, it might have been that local politics, Koller's aggressiveness and his religious adherence caused the event to be underemphasized abroad. Although regional anesthesia (a term reputedly coined by the American surgeon Harvey Cushing) was immediately applied clinically in America, the scientific basis and its multifold techniques were established in Germany around the turn of the century. In England, where there already existed a considerable degree of anesthetic professionalism, inhalation anesthesia continued to dominate despite decades of debate over the merits of chloroform, its mode of administration as well as adverse pharmacologic effects and toxicity. In that country to this day, regional anesthesia constitutes only a small share of practice while in America resurgence of interest in the method has occurred. Moreover, intravenous agents for induction and maintenance of general anesthesia now preoccupy practitioners both in England and on the continent. Those developments, of a certainty, relate to the intellectual environment of the times in the respective countries.

The most extensive accounts of the birth of local anesthesia reside in Hortense Koller Becker's account *Carl Koller and Cocaine* (BECKER 1963) and in Robert Byck's edited collection of *Cocaine Papers – Sigmund Freud* (BYCK 1974). Extensive coverage of the subject is to be found in T. E. Keys' *The History of Surgical Anesthesia* (KEYS 1945); in Faulconer and Keys' *Foundations of Anesthesiology* (FAULCONER and KEYS 1965); and in Fink's recent "History," an introductory chapter to a textbook on regional anesthesia (FINK 1980). A complete review of the early known pharmacology of local anesthetics was prepared by HIRSCHFELDER and BIETER (1932). In the narrative given here some of the details of the "discovery" will be treated initially because of their dramatic nature, followed by an historical background for many of the topics covered in this monograph.

B. Freud, Koller and the Early History of Cocaine

According to MORTIMER (MORTIMER et al. 1974; GAY 1976) the coca leaf was believed to be a gift to the Incan people from Manco Capac, son of the Sun God, bestowed as a token of esteem and sympathy for their suffering labors. The leaves were initially to achieve a rather narrow usage among the religious and political aristocracies of Incan society: a much broader and perhaps more sinister pattern was noted following the destruction of the Incan civilization in the sixteenth century, by Francisco Pizzaro and the invading conquistadores, as the lower classes and slaves were "paid off" in coca leaves as an effective method of increasing and prolonging their low-cost, high-output labor. In practice, coca leaves bound into a ball (cocada) with guano or cornstarch were chewed with lime or alkaline ash to release the active alkaloid.

"Thus coca served as a stimulating tonic to those working in the thin air of the Andes. Further anthropologic documentation indicated that the highly sophisticated surgical procedure of trephination was repeatedly successful in this era, as the operating surgeon allowed coca-drenched saliva to drip from his mouth onto the surgical wound, thus providing adequate (and very real) local anesthesia, and permitting the operation to proceed in relative quiet."

"Little was heard of coca as a medical entity until 1859, when the Italian physician Paolo Mantegazza declared coca leaves to be a new and exciting weapon against disease."

Then American physicians, following Mantegazza's lead, proclaimed the drug to be a panacea for almost every malady. Dr. Scherzer, an Austrian explorer and member of an expedition to South America, had brought coca leaves to Vienna. Samples were sent to Friedrich Wohler for examination, in turn given to his laboratory pupil, Albert Niemann, who then isolated the alkaloid (NIEMANN 1860). Niemann's "cocaine" crystalized in large, colorless four-to-six sided prisms, with a somewhat bitter taste and producing an anesthetic effect on mucous membranes. The crystals, which melted at 98 °C, were difficult to dissolve in water but easily soluble in alcohol and they formed salts. On heating in hydrochloric acid, benzoic acid, methyl alcohol and a little-known base, ecgonine, were formed (later on, the Merck Company gave ecgonine to Sigmund Freud, for clinical trial). Because the salts of hydrochloric or acetic acid were highly soluble they were deemed suitable for physiologic and therapeutic use.

In 1880, von Anrep published an extensive article on the physiologic and pharmacologic effects of cocaine (VON ANREP 1880). Large doses, in warm-blooded animals, produced powerful psychic agitation and excitation. Respiration and pulse were accelerated, the pupils became dilated, hyperperistalsis developed, blood pressure rose and secretions were diminished (others had already shown that the effects depended largely upon the mode of administration). Insofar as local anesthetic effects were concerned, injection under the skin as well as painting the mucous membranes brought about loss of feeling and pain. Von Anrep treated animals for 30 days with moderate doses of cocaine and detected no detrimental effects on bodily function. He clearly described the locally numbing effects on the tongue, even the dilation of the pupil upon local application, and suggested that this drug might some day become of medical importance.

According to Byck's edition of collected papers (BYCK 1974), after the introduction of cocaine in the United States, Sigmund Freud became interested in its properties. Upon reviewing the literature (Vol. IV, 1883, of the Index Catalogue of the Library of the Surgeon General's Office of the United States Army, referencing some 25 papers and ten monographs under the heading of Erythroxylin Coca) Freud wrote *Über Coca* (FREUD 1884). In this earliest of articles, Freud reviewed the history of the use of cocaine in South America, its effects on humans and animals and its many therapeutic uses. He became an enthusiastic experimenter and user, the latter in an attempt to halt the morphine addiction of a close friend, Ernst von Fleischl-Marxow, in the throes of an exquisitely painful, posttraumatic thenar neuroma. He had read Theodor Aschenbrandt's account of the prescription of cocaine for soldiers whereby their energy and capacity to endure were enhanced.

Upon receipt of a cocaine "kit" from the Merck establishment, Freud began to conduct experiments upon himself and Carl Koller, an intern in the department of ophthalmology at the Allgemeine Krankenhaus in Vienna, in an effort to define the pharmacologic properties of coca. Both swallowed cocaine (and noticed the numbing effect on the tongue) in order to test, with a dynamometer, the effect on muscle strength. However, Koller was intent on finding a drug to anesthetize the cornea and had already tried morphine sulphate and chloral bromide. He knew that Freud had relieved pain with cocaine and had read Freud's essay of 1884. In the summer of that year, after Freud had departed Vienna for a visit to Hamburg, Koller met Dr. Joseph Gartner at Stricker's Institute for Pathological Anatomy (where Koller had investigated the origins of the mesoderm in chicken embryos – an outstanding piece of work). A trace of the white powder was dissolved in distilled water and instilled into the conjunctival sac of a frog. After a minute or so "the frog allowed his cornea to be touched and he also bore injury of the cornea without a trace of reflex action or defense." Identical tests were performed on a rabbit and a dog, the results equally favorable.

Koller wrote, "one more step had now to be taken. We trickled the solution under each other's lifted eyelids. Then placed a mirror before us, took pins, and with the head tried to touch the cornea. Almost simultaneously we were able to state jubilantly: 'I can't feel anything.'" A communication on the results dated early September was read and a practical demonstration given at the Ophthalmological Congress on September 15 by Josef Brettauer, because Koller had not the means to travel to Heidelberg. Koller gave Freud full credit for the inspiration and Freud must have been more than just disappointed as he had already suggested to Leopold Konigstein the numbing properties of cocaine on the eye. The two of them had painlessly enucleated a dog's eye under the effects of cocaine, an event reported just a little bit too late, on October 17. Nevertheless, for all of the experiments beforehand and subsequently done, as well as clinical trials and his papers, Freud is considered by Byck and confreres to be the founder of psychopharmacology – the use of drugs to modify behavior and for the relief of mental illness – the forerunners of mescaline, LSD, and the amphetamines.

After Koller, James Leonard Corning, a neurologist of New York City, deserves recognition mainly for his analytical approach to regional anesthesia in man, based on prior laboratory experiments. Corning had studied abroad and received the degree of Doctor of Medicine from the University of Würzburg and then went on to practice neurology in the New York area. His textbook on local anesthesia published in 1886, was the first devoted to that subject (FAULCONER and KEYS 1965).

Having learned of Koller's report, Corning recalled that when strychnine is injected subcutaneously in the frog, the animal is thrown into violent convulsions, as a result of an effect on the functions of the spinal cord (CORNING 1885). Following laminectomy, a much smaller quantity of strychnine injected beneath the membranes of the cord produced the same effect. He assumed then, according to prior work of Hailey, that the poison could act through the mediation of the blood vessels – vascular absorption as it were. All that was necessary for the effect to take place then was to make an injection in the vicinity of the cord. Were these effects obtained via the extensive perivertebral plexus of veins, shown later by Batson to be a valveless system that acts as an accessory venous return pathway to the heart, other than the inferior vena cava?

With this line of reasoning and cognizant of the presence of the many small veins – *venae spinosa* – Corning reasoned that it might be possible to apply cocaine to therapeutic advantage. Accordingly, in a young dog, about 20 minims of a 2% solution of cocaine were injected between the spinous processes of two of the inferior processes of the dorsal vertebrae. After 5 min, incoordination of the posterior extremities developed followed by insensibility. This experimental finding was then transferred to a patient, a sufferer from spinal weakness and seminal incontinence. "To this end, I injected 30 minims of a 3% solution of the hydrochloride of cocaine into the space situated between the spinous processes of the eleventh and twelfth dorsal vertebrae." After a lapse of 6 to 8 min when nothing happened, the injection was repeated. Finally, 10 min later, anesthesia began to appear in the lower extremities and a sound could be passed through the urethra without pain. Corning concluded his report with the statement: "Whether the method will ever find application as a substitute for etherization in genito-urinary or other branches of surgery, further experience alone can show."

Corning is sometimes given credit for performance of the first spinal anesthetic but it is apparent that the cocaine must have diffused into the epidural space. Six years were to elapse before Quincke of Germany performed the first lumbar puncture, via the lateral approach, in an effort to reduce the pressure of hydrocephalus (QUINCKE 1891). Quincke gave priority to Essex Wynter who employed a Southey tube for relief of fluid pressure (WYNTER 1891).

C. Structure and Synthesis of Local Anesthetics

After Gaedicke of Germany in 1855 had isolated an alkaloid from the leaves of the coca plant and designated it as erythoxylin, and Albert Niemann had given the name cocaine to the crystalline form of the compound, Alfred Einhorn took up the cudgels when the local anesthetic properties were made evident. Einhorn must be considered among the first pharmaceutical chemists. Earlier, in Lothar Meyer's laboratory at Tübingen he had synthesized "isopropylphenylketone." According to a brief biography in FAULCONER and KEYS (1965), Einhorn's interests extended to all branches of organic chemistry, a field now referred to as biochemistry (then called iatrochemistry). He studied constitutional factors as they relate to physiologic mechanisms in the body. Not surprising, therefore, that working in Adolf von Baeyer's laboratory in Munich, he would spend many years ferreting out the chemistry of cocaine and other local anesthetics, the results reported in 1899 (EINHORN 1899). Procaine hydrochloride (Novocain) was to come later.

The 1899 paper briefly reviews the history, then notes that Koler (sic) had produced local anesthesia with cocaine. "Since that time cocaine has been used frequently despite its numerous disadvantages, namely its great toxicity, the short duration of anesthesia, the impossibility of sterilizing the solution, its high cost, and so on – all factors which stimulated chemists to seek a substitute for cocaine which is free of its disadvantages or at least possesses them to a lesser degree." No better statement of the problems associated with its use could have been made. Similar considerations influenced the synthesis of new anesthetics to this day.

Cocaine was decomposed by heating with mineral acids, to benzoic acid, methyl alcohol and nitrogen-containing ecgonine. But the interesting finding was that cocaine is closely related to atropine, for atropine when heated with acid splits into tropic acid and the nitrogen-containing tropine, with ecgonine a carbonic acid derivative of tropine. Thus atropine was synthesized from cocaine and Einhorn observed that the main effect of cocaine was to provide local anesthesia with mydriasis, a side effect (the relation of cocaine to epinephrine and norepinephrine metabolism was not known at the time); and the main effect of atropine was the production of mydriasis (its anticholinergic effects not realized then) and local anesthesia a side effect. How true the latter statement may be is a matter of conjecture but for many years atropine has been an ingredient in suppositories given for relief of rectal pain. Again Einhorn noted that when tropine was combined with tropic acid to yield mandelic acid (homatropine, employed early in ophthalmology) or benzoic acid per se, that the anesthetic effect of the three mydriatics increased when the acid structure more closely resembled that of benzoic acid.

Physiologic testing of the cocaine group showed that degradation products of cocaine, namely ecgonine, ecgonine ester and benzoyl ecgonine, had no anesthetic effect. The ecgonine molecule had to be filled to produce anesthesia. "The anesthetic capability of cocaine is therefore a function of its acid group called by Erlich the anesthesiophoric group – the most potent being the benzoyl group." With this knowledge of chemical structure, Einhorn then prepared such compounds as Eucaine, Orthoform, Nirvanine, Holocaine – all tried experimentally but clinically found wanting.

Presumably Einhorn synthesized procaine around 1904. No specific report to that effect appears in the literature so it fell to the lot of surgeon Heinrich Braun of Leipzig-Lindenau to make the report in 1905 (BRAUN 1905), along with descriptions of two other agents, Stovaine and Alypin. The chemical formulas were furnished by the Hochst Dye Works. Worth noting is that Stovaine (BRAUN 1905) was named after its French discoverer, Fourneau, which literally translates into "stove." Stovaine was popular for many years as a spinal anesthetic. Braun devoted the bulk of his paper to a description of Novocaine, which became the most widely used local anesthetic until the advent of the amide, lidocaine or lignocaine prepared by Lofgren in 1948. To this day most patients employ the term "Novocaine" as a generic term for any local anesthetic.

According to Braun's description, Novocaine is the monohydrochloride of the p-amino-benzoyl-diethyl-amino ethanol. An aqueous solution of Novocaine could be boiled without signs of decomposition, remaining clear for days in loosely closed flasks (a valuable attribute in the days when preservatives were not available). Central nervous effects were very few when average doses were given to animals. According to experiments with skin wheals made on the forearm, Braun now had a potent but short-acting local anesthetic and for the first time a nonirritating agent of ideal qualities. However, "in spite of the foregoing, the new drug in itself could not be capable of replacing cocaine" (presumably because of the short duration of action). Surprisingly, little is said of the lack of topical anesthetic activity on mucous membranes and conjunctiva other than that a 10% solution of Novocaine with epinephrine could anesthetize the nasal mucosa as rapidly and as deeply as with a 10% solution of cocaine. "This disadvantage (of short duration) can be remedied as easily by an admixture of epinephrine" (more of this subsequently). Novocaine was used in concentrations of 0.1%–0.25% always with epinephrine added, for some 150 operations, mostly procedures done on the hands and fingers (epinephrine is notably dangerous there – because of vasoconstriction and possible development of gangrene), for many dental extractions and for a variety of major operations.

The first amide type of local anesthetic, rather than an ester, was a quinoline derivative, dibucaine hydrochloride (Percaine, Nupercaine, Cinchocaine), synthesized separately by Mescher, Uhlman, and Hassner in 1929. Tetracaine hydrochloride (Pontocaine, Pantocaine), currently the most widely used anesthetic in spinal anesthesia, was first prepared in 1931, separately by Schaumann and by Ernst.

D. Epinephrine and Local Anesthesia

In no other respect have two classes of drugs been so extensively linked and used in clinical practice as have epinephrine and the local anesthetics. It is safe to say that without epinephrine the mortality from local anesthetic reactions would have been far higher than encountered. On the other hand, the addition of epinephrine to local anesthetic solutions not only delays the absorption of the anesthetic and prolongs the action, but the sometimes excessive concentrations of epinephrine or their inadvertent injection into the circulation has resulted in many a reaction and death owing to the cardiovascular actions of the catecholamine, particularly in dental practice. Indeed, many a so-called local anesthetic reaction is the result of the pharmacologic properties of epinephrine used mainly in the treatment of asthmatic crises, anaphylactoid reactions and for cardiovascular resuscitation.

John Jacob Abel, the first professor of pharmacology at the newly created John Hopkin Hospital Medical School and the first professor in America of that discipline, was also the first to isolate a hormone of any variety – epinephrine, in 1897 (ABEL 1957). His other accomplishments included the founding of three journals: The *Journal of Experimental Medicine*, the *Journal of Biological Chemistry* and the *Journal of Pharmacology and Experimental Therapeutics*, all extant today. Later, he was the first to crystalize insulin, subsequently, the originator of plasmapheresis, and innovator in the use of extracorporeal dialysis with Rowntree and Turner – using collodion membranes in the treatment of drug intoxication. He also is regarded as the discoverer of hirudin, an extract of the leech head once used for anticoagulation; and, finally, the synthesizer of the phthaleins subsequently so extensively applied in the evaluation of hepatic and renal function.

In the article on the "Blood Pressure Raising Constituent of the Suprarenal Capsule," ABEL (1897) reviewed the history: how Schafer and Oliver in 1894 had raised the blood pressure to a great height above normal with a small amount of aqueous extract of the gland; that Gottleib could revive a heart that had stopped beating as a result of chloral hydrate poisoning; and that Bates in 1896 had shown that an aqueous solution applied to the eye produced vasoconstriction, prevented hemorrhage and prolonged, indefinitely, the action of cocaine. However, the extract was a powerful poison leading to fatal effects when injected directly into the circulation.

In 1856, Vulpian had treated an extract of the adrenal gland with ferric chloride to retrieve a chromagen of emerald green color, which in turn when treated with iodine, gave a beautiful rose carmine. Employing a modification of Vulpian's method, Abel produced a benzoyl compound which he classed with the pyrrols, piperidine bases or alcohols – a powerful blood pressure-raising constituent. For all his expertise, Abel did not obtain the pure product, even in subsequent experiments, and it remained for Takamine, a one-time worker in his laboratory, to accomplish that goal – engendering much controversy over the priority for isolation.

E. K. Marshall, later the Professor of Pharmacology at the Hopkins, gives this graphic account of the consequences of Abel's achievement: "Scarcely a night passes in the accident room of any large hospital that patients suffering from asthma are not given an injection of epinephrine which gives dramatic relief to those sufferers in the course of a few minutes. Many individuals covered with urticaria (hives) obtain complete relief from this troublesome condition by an injection of epinephrine. Due to the fact that this substance causes a marked constriction of blood vessels – it is used thousands of times every day in the connection with local anesthetics. Every time a tooth is extracted, every time a minor surgical operation is performed, this substance is used in connection with the local anesthetic" (ABEL 1957).

It is worth noting that Abel and the others obtained their products from the suprarenal capsule, as we know now that epinephrine is secreted in man only in the adrenal medulla by the chromaffin cells. The presence of the latter helps to explain why such vivid chromagen effects were obtained with extracts. Indeed a neoplasm arising from the adrenal medulla and other chromaffin bodies of the sympathetic nervous system is known as phaeochromocytoma, *phaeo* being a combining form from the Greek meaning dun-colored (any of several colors varying from red to yellow). Further, any extract from the adrenal cortex unless purified would yield a variety of steroids among them aldosterone, a mineralocorticoid, an excess of which causes hypertension.

As noted above, Heinrich Braun popularized the use of epinephrine in conjunction with procaine after the former had already been used with cocaine. Braun was a remarkable man, as were all of the other pioneers (FAULCONER and

KEYS 1965). At Strassburg, in 1881, as a medical student he gave chloroform anesthesia for the surgeon Karl Thiersch. Later, himself a surgeon, he devised an anesthesia machine which for a long time was one of the standard models in Germany. In the field of local anesthesia, he discovered the local anesthetic action of quinine derivatives, introduced nerve conduction blocks and popularized the combination of cocaine with epinephrine, a substitute for the tourniquet previously used to keep the local anesthetic from being too rapidly absorbed. Dental nerve blocks were his forte as well as a technic for injecting the trigeminal nerve (in the treatment of tic doloureux). These accomplishments were presented in his textbook, *The Scientific Foundations and the Practical Application of Local Anesthesia* (FAULCONER and KEYS 1965).

In an 1903 article, BRAUN (1903) discussed the practical importance of epinephrine in local anesthesia, especially in inducing anemia of the mucosa in rhinolaryngology and urology, thereby allowing one to lower the concentration of cocaine, and diminishing the danger of intoxication – toxic effects of the epinephrine were not discovered. Directions for the preparation of various epinephrine concentrations in conjunction with cocaine were given, along with the kind of epinephrine preparation used. For example: anesthesia of a finger is produced after 5 to 10 min when 1 cc of a 1% or 1.5 to 2 cc of a 0.5% solution of cocaine with epinephrine (3 drops = 1:1000 in one cc) is injected at the base of the finger in the usual manner, without the use of a tourniquet. Further examples of clinical application are given throughout the text.

BIETER (1936) and LESER (1940) later, in using skin wheals on the forearm or animal dermis, provided tables describing the degree of prolongation of anesthetic effect achieved. Bieter's data are shown as follows:

Table 1. Bieter's data

0.2 cc, 0.125%	Epinephrine content				
Solution	0 min	1:500 000 min	1:200 000 min	1:100 000 min	1:500 000 min
Procaine HCl	16.6	65.4	89.2	87.2	83.0
Metycaine	18.5	54.8	68.5	59.5	71.9
Cocaine HCl	20.3	59.9	88.2	85.3	88.1
Panithesine	20.6	84.2	125.1	111.8	94.2

Both Bieter and Leser found that concentrations of epinephrine stronger than 1:500,000 provided little further prolongation of anesthesia and parenthetically, a higher incidence of central cardiovascular effects owing to the epinephrine.

Over the years other methods of prolonging local anesthesia have been tried. The use of the basic form of the anesthetic as in "cocaine milk" or procaine base was essayed according to the belief that the higher lipid solubility of the base would provide better anesthesia as well as its prolongation. The problem of solubility of these bases in aqueous or other media (polyethylene glycol), however, created practical difficulties. Similarly, local anesthetics dissolved in an oily base (olive oil, peanut oil) were thought to act as repositories from which the anesthetic would be slowly released, thereby prolonging anesthesia. However, any prolongation obtained was found to be the result of destruction of the smaller nerve fibers caused by a neurolytic agent in the menstruum, benzyl alcohol (DUNCAN 1943).

Thus far in this section we have focused on the properties of epinephrine when added to solutions of local anesthetics. However, it has always been known that topically applied cocaine alone yields a considerable degree of vasoconstriction in its own right, thus enhancing its usefulness in operations involving mucous membranes. Indeed the combination of epinephrine with cocaine, although producing the desired local anemia, has sometimes resulted in greater cardiovascular toxicity. An explanation for the vasoconstrictive action of cocaine was not forthcoming until TRENDELENBURG (1958) showed that the injection of increasing amounts of cocaine enhanced the response of the nictitating membrane of a spinal cat preparation to preganglionic stimulation and to injections of norepinephrine. The volume change in the size of the spleen was also increased, and so was the blood pressure response, as cocaine was found to add to the effect of injected norepinephrine, and also to the concentration of circulating norepinephrine. Cocaine thus prolonged the half-life of injected norepinephrine (NE) causing supersensitivity to it by delaying its inactivation. These observations were corroborated later when the metabolism of labeled norepinephrine, after its release from postganglionic sympathetic nerve endings, could be quantified. Uptake, the more prominent means of limiting the duration of action of NE, was delayed. Interestingly, Chen in 1928 had observed that cocaine could diminish the blood pressure raising effects of ephedrine. That observation probably related to the fact that ephedrine acts indirectly through the release of norepinephrine, and cocaine would already have diminished the stores of NE at the nerve ending.

The foregoing observations of the effect of cocaine on endogenous norepinephrine kinetics and dynamics help to explain the psychotomimetic properties of the local anesthetic as well as its addictive properties. An accumulation or delay in the metabolism of NE in brain could be a factor, a phenomenon very much in line with modern concepts of psychopharmacology and the use of drugs that effect the dynamics of epinephrine, norepinephrine, and serotonin, in treatment of both depressive and manic psychoses.

E. Toxicity of Local Anesthetics

Early on, the signs of acute cocaine poisoning in man were readily apparent and that is why considerable efforts were made to reduce the dosages used and why epinephrine was employed with the anesthetic solutions (actually a dangerous combination with cocaine, from the standpoint of catecholamine toxicity) and also one of the reasons why Novocaine eventually replaced cocaine for the majority of nerve blocks performed.

EGGLESTON and HATCHER (1919) in several papers were able to document, experimentally, the dynamics of the toxicity clinically observed. In their 1919 report all of the information necessary for the prevention and treatment of local anesthetic reactions was presented. As a prelude, they noted that Matteson in Medical and Surgical Reports for 1891 had presented abstracts of a large number of acute, fatal, and nonfatal cases of cocaine poisoning: also a comprehensive bibliography of cocaine poisoning was to be found in a communication by Wildenroth in 1911. In a previous paper, the authors had cited the fact that deaths had been recorded following such small doses of cocaine as 16, 40, and 60 mg, respectively, while survival after 1.25 g subcutaneously had occurred. Typical symptoms and the course of a nonfatal intoxication (lodge) were as follows.

A 40 year old healthy man was given a subcutaneous injection of 20 minims of a 2% solution of cocaine – no more than 13 mg of drug. In 2 to 3 min, the patient became nervous with heightened reflexes, rapid pulse, deepened respiration, vertigo, and flickering before his eyes. Nausea developed in about 10 min, followed by vomiting. At the end of about 1 h after injection, toxic symptoms were at their height, when the following were noted: pulse 120, respirations deepened, the inspiratory time probably increased to four times the length of the exspiratory time, reflexes greatly increased, clonic spasms of all muscles of the limbs, arms and inferior maxillary – pupils markedly dilated – muscles of the lower jaw were in tonic contraction. (The patient recovered in about 2 h after the injection.)

Similar reactions had been observed with beta-eucane, Stovaine, alypin, and Novocaine. As a result, the Therapeutic Research Committee of the Council on Pharmacy and Chemistry made a plea for the reporting of all accidents of the kind. Consequently, Eggleston and Hatcher were impelled to carry out their experimental studies; a summary of their conclusions is as follows:

1. A close similarity exists between the symptoms produced in man and in lower animals, especially the cat.
2. The several different local anesthetics are shown to be mutually and quantitatively synergistic, so far as their fatal actions are concerned.
3. The capacity of the cat to withstand the intravenous injection of several times the fatal dose of any of the local anesthetics, except cocaine and holocaine, has been shown by repeated injections of large doses, or the continuous injection of relatively dilute solutions.
4. The toxicity of the local anesthetics for the cat, after subcutaneous injection, has been shown to depend upon the ratio between the rate of absorption and that of elimination, and the local anesthetics can be divided into two classes with reference to that ratio.
5. The simultaneous, subcutaneous injection of epinephrine with the local anesthetics materially reduces the toxicity of the latter, by delay in the rate of their absorption but this reduction is much less marked in the cases of cocaine and holocaine.
6. The absorption of several of the local anesthetics from the mucous membranes of the nose and pharynx of the cat has been shown to be no more rapid than from the subcutaneous tissues.
7. The elimination of the local anesthetics in the cat had been demonstrated to be due to their rapid destruction by the liver and this takes place in the excised, perfused organ as well as in the liver of the intact animal.
8. Various efforts have been made to influence the toxicity of the local anesthetics for the cat, and severe acute hemorrhage and narcosis by chloral hydrate alone seem not to have any material influence. Both of these measures tend to increase the cat's susceptibility to the toxic actions of the local anesthetics, probably by diminishing the rate of their destruction.

9. All of the local anesthetics have been shown to be synergistic with epinephrine on the blood pressure, in a manner analagous to cocaine.
10. The employment of artificial respiration, combined with stimulation of the heart by the intravenous injection of epinephrine, is capable of saving cats from death following the intravenous injection of as much as twice the average fatal dose of the local anesthetics.
11. Stimulation of the heart by the previous injection of ouabain permits the cat to recover from intravenous injections of nearly twice the average fatal dose of the local anesthetics, when the temporary paralysis of the respiratory center is combated by the use of artificial respiration.
12. The success of the last two measures depends upon the rapid destruction of the local anesthetics by the liver.

Since publication of that report, very little has been added to our knowledge of toxic reactions to the local anesthetics. Puzzling was their failure to discern that absorption of local anesthetics from mucous membranes is much more rapid than from subcutaneous tissues. Any deviations from fact today relate to a lack of information on pharmacokinetics at the time: for instance, that the ester compounds depend to a large extent for their metabolism on hydrolysis mediated by circulating pseudocholinesterase. Probably the use of an agent such as thiopental to terminate the convulsions may carry a disadvantage in the way of myocardial depression as suggested by the experimental effects of chloral hydrate. Since the publication of the above findings, several investigators have confirmed the lethality of local anesthetics according to the site of injection and the vascularity of the region (FOLDES et al. 1960).

Tatum, Atkinson, and Collins (TATUM et al. 1925) enlarged upon Hatcher and Eggleston's precepts by pointing out that: artificial respiration alone is sufficient to raise the minimal fatal dose of cocaine in the rabbit (this does not apply to the dog or cat); the prophylactic administration of barbital sodium and paraldehyde to the dog produces a condition in which a fourfold increase in tolerance to a toxic dose occurs; convulsions are completely and practically instantaneously controlled by an intravenous injection of the barbital-paraldehyde mixture; and, the likelihood of recovery from acute intoxication by cocaine in the dog is roughly inversely proportioned to the time convulsions are permitted to continue. For a long time these findings have dictated prophylactic and therapeutic approaches to the treatment of local anesthetic convulsions in man. Whether the current use of diazepam rather than a barbiturate to prevent or terminate convulsions is any better remains to be established (MUNSON and WAGMAN 1972; deJONG and BONIN 1982). From the standpoint of prophylaxis, however, it has been shown that a narcotic dose of a barbiturate, rather than mere sedation, is necessary to forestall central stimulation and convulsions.

Two other major contributions to the understanding and treatment of local anesthetic reactions stand out. The first was TANAKA and YAMASAKI's report (TANAKA and YAMASAKI 1966) on the selective blocking of cortical inhibitory synapses by lidocaine, with the excitatory synapses more resistant to the drug. And the second was ENGLESSON's (1974) finding based on the observance of seizure activity in the cortical EEG and amygdala following the intravenous infusion of several different local anesthetics in the cat. A fall in $PaCO_2$ or hydrogen ion activity was found to decrease local anesthetic toxicity, in disagreement with the well-known observation that hyperventilation in man is an epileptiform-inducing maneuver. A current review of local anesthetic toxicity is COVINO's contribution to this volume, Chap. 6.

F. The Nervous Impulse and the Action of Local Anesthetics

At the time of the first clinical demonstration of local anesthetic activity in the 1880's, the neurosciences were in the formative state. KANDEL (1982), in an essay on the origins of modern neuroscience, noted that at the turn of the century the field consisted of several distinct and isolated disciplines; neuroanatomy as typified by the studies of Ramon y Cajal; physiology as evidenced by the investigations of Sherrington and Adrian; pharmacological studies begun by Langley; and the behavioral field led by Pavlov and Freud. The gradual interaction among workers in these fields plus their relation to other areas of biology had important scientific influences on the development of local anesthesia. While only several of the major advances can be considered here, a broader insight can be had by perusing Hodgkin's monograph on *The Conduction of the Nervous Impulse* (HODGKIN 1964) and Adrian's earlier treatise on *The Mechanisms of Nervous Action* (ADRIAN 1932). It is also worth noting that Overton's and Meyer's independent observations on the lipid solubility of inhalation anesthetics, around the turn of the century, leading to the lipid solubility theory of narcosis, are quite relevant to modern concepts of the mode of action of local anesthetics.

A major step forward occurred in the 1930's. According to COLE (1982), electrochemistry had its origins in Galvani's investigations of electrical nerve excitability with his frog leg experiments, and the controversy with Volta. For a long time the nerve muscle preparation remained the experimental preparation even as it was once used by Claude Bernard to define the locus of action of curare, and today for similar studies on neuromuscular pharmacology.

Insofar as experimental preparations are concerned William's monograph on the anatomy of the squid WILLIAMS (1909) attracted little notice until YOUNG (1936) delivered a paper on the structure of nerve fibers and synapses in invertebrates before a group of neuroscientists of one of the Cold Spring Harbor Symposia. After a discussion of the characteristics and methods of determining the nature of nerve sheaths, Young described the ventral nerve cord of the annelid worms, containing segmented fibers – these fibers having already been studied for electrical conductivity and subsequently figuring prominently as experimental tools. He then went on to picture the nerves of the decapod cephalopods, such as in the squid, *Loligo*, or the cuttlefish, *Sepia* – the largest being found in a large Atlantic squid, *Loligo pealii*. Each fiber consists of a mass of axoplasm surrounded by a sheath which stains like vertebrate connective tissue, that is, collagenous material interspersed with nuclei. If the individual axon is cut in such a way that the end is not closed off, then the contents pour out in a stream. Young implied that there was need for further neurohistological work in order to clarify some aspects of neuronal physiology.

In regard to Young's revelations, COLE (1982) remarks that, "this was a most dramatic passing on of the baton, from an anatomist to a biophysicist." "Young was clearly the pivotal character who turned axon research from the poorly specified terms to the clearly defined physical and electrical axon properties." Subsequently, most if not all of the essential studies on the conduction of the nervous impulse and the first of those on the mode of action of local anesthetics were carried out on invertebrate nerve fibers as described by Young. The action potential in nerve was found to be accomplished by a dramatic increase in the resting conductance of the nerve membrane, and the "ionic hypotheses" arose because it was found that the nerve membrane became very leaky to ions during the peak of the action potential – without a detectable fundamental change in the structure of the membrane. Hodgkin and Huxley and Curtis and Cole (CURTIS and COLE 1938; COLE and HODGKIN 1939) then demonstrated that the action potential did not simply short-circuit the resting potential to zero as hitherto predicted, but that the resting potential is overshot and reversed by some 50 mV. This was then shown to be the result of a sudden inrush of Na $+$ ions down its concentration gradient (see Chap. 2).

A second catalyst to research in the field was the introduction of the voltage clamp technique by George MARMONT (1949), later modified by electrophysiologists and employed extensively to this day. Marmont pointed out that the Curtis, Cole, and Hodgkin studies had been productive because of the ability to introduce an electrode into the axoplasm of the giant squid axon. However, those electrodes were small and incapable of passing currents across the membrane. Prior studies on membrane excitability, impedance and so on requiring passage of current, had always utilized external electrodes. Marmont listed the unsatisfactory aspects of such external techniques: nonuniformity of current density requiring tedious calculations – often uncertain: when the current was large enough to render the membrane "active," not merely passive, the magnitude of a subsequent current could not be controlled.

What the voltage clamp method does is to allow direct measurement of a current of uniform density passing through the membrane, as well as the potential across it – in a known area of the membrane. One is able to control current density, or the potential drop across the membrane or some other parameter such as the rate of change of potential drop, regardless of whether the membrane becomes active or not. Thus, the effects of propagation are removed from the experiment, for the area of membrane under investigation will tend to react at all points in the same manner at a given instant.

HODGKIN (1964) said of the voltage clamp that, in essence, instead of having to deal with a cable, the nerve can be treated as an isolated patch of membrane and the operator, by controlling the voltage across the membrane, can do with it what he wants.

With a background of these techniques, Ritchie et al. (RITCHIE and GREENGARD 1966) addressed the concept long held that the uncharged form of a local anesthetic is the active moiety in producing blockade. As noted earlier, (cocaine milk, etc.) this idea was based on experimental findings that local anesthetics are more effective in alkaline solutions in which the base predominates, than in neutral or acidic solutions. As those experiments were usually carried out on the cornea in vivo or on intact sheathed nerves, penetration through considerable thicknesses of tissue were involved. Therefore they argued that, "the greater effectiveness at alkaline pH simply resulted from a more effective rate of penetration through periaxonal tissues, for two factors probably determine the effectiveness of a local anesthetic: a) the penetration from site of application to site of action and, b) the actual anesthetic action at the receptor site." Consequently, they attempted to resolve the matter by employing desheathed nerve preparations which would minimize the effect of penetration. In contrast to findings in the sheathed nerves, it was found that local anesthetics are more effective in neutral than in alkaline solutions. The results were confirmed on single, myelinated fibers of the frog, and in order to explain any experimental discrepancies from other studies, on desheathed rabbit vagus nerves on the sciatic nerve of the frog. In all types of fiber – mammalian myelinated, mammalian non-myelinated and amphibian myelinated – alkaline anesthetic solutions were more effective in sheathed preparations and neutral solutions more effective in desheathed preparations. Thus the cation is the more active form of the local anesthetic and the uncharged molecule important only for penetration. Subsequent studies with lidocaine and dibucaine reemphasized the importance of the cation for inducing anesthesia. However, experiments with Novocaine and benzocaine suggest that both forms of the molecule may be active. In the case of procaine, the uncharged form would seem to be relatively more active than the cationic form. "True local anesthetic activity resides in the aromatic, lipophilic part of the local anesthetic: and, the presence of a charged, cationic head to the molecule, intensifies the activity but is not absolutely required" (RITCHIE and GREENGARD 1966).

The physiology of peripheral nerve fibers, myelinated and unmyelinated, in relation to their size has always been important in local anesthesia, with regard to their susceptibility to block, and in relation to conduction velocity and duration of action potential. GASSER and ERLANGER (1929), employing a quantitative neurophysiological technique – which permitted study of the conducted action potential –, seemed to settle one of the issues for the time being. The effects of compression on nerve are important from the standpoint of understanding injuries. According to Gasser, as early as 1881, Luederlitz, on the basis of clinical impression, found that upon compression of the sciatic nerve of the rabbit, that mobility is more affected than sensation. In 1885, Herzen had shown that pressure on nerves blocks the sensation of contact and cold before those of warmth and pain, which was later confirmed by Goldscheider. As the electrical axon potentials are the same in individual fibers in all medullated fibers larger then 5 microns and only the threshold of excitation and velocity of conduction vary, it would seem that fiber size is important in resistance of nerves to compression block.

After the introduction of local anesthesia, Goldscheider observed temperature to disappear before pain in the distribution of a cocainized nerve branch. Subsequent observations of this kind employing other local anesthetics failed to provide the reason for the differential effect although differences in chemical constitution and corresponding differences in affinities were invoked. Gasser and Erlanger reasoned that the solution to the problem of the mechanism of the differential susceptibility of nerve fibers was to be found in some quality of nerves which varies from fiber to fiber. Thus, local anesthetic blocks were applied to a short section of nerve, the nerve stimulated at one end and the action potential recorded from the other by means of the cathode ray oscillograph. With pressure, as expected, the larger fibers were the first to be blocked. On the other hand, results obtained with cocaine were not as uniform. On the whole, however, "a differential action was visible in every mammalian nerve studied: and wherever it occurred, in nerves of all species, it was the same in kind; small fibers were blocked before large ones." In Chap. 4 of this volume RAYMOND and GISSEN provide a thorough review of differential loss of sensation by nerve blocking procedures.

G. Pharmacokinetics of Local Anesthetics

The original studies on the metabolism of cocaine were largely devoted to studies of urinary excretion and cumulative toxicity. Those investigations yielded no traces of urinary excretion of cocaine in the rabbit, so it was concluded that the rabbit is capable of detoxifying cocaine at a rapid rate (rabbit liver also contains an atropinase which rapidly hydrolyzes that drug rendering that species immune to poisoning by *Datura stramonium*, an atropine-containing weed). With the availability for the first time of a quantitative method for estimating cocaine, WOODS et al. (1951) studied plasma levels, tissue distribution and urinary excretion of cocaine in the dog and rabbit. Plasma levels could be depicted graphically after the dog had received cocaine orally, subcutaneously and intravenously, and in the rabbit after subcutaneous administration. The conclusions reached in that study, the first of its kind, were predictive of the pharmacokinetics later found with drugs of all kinds. In the dog, intravenous injection was followed by a rapid initial rise then fall in plasma concentration, the subsequent gradual decrease probably the result of tissue metabolism and to a small extent, urinary excretion (missing here is the explanation based on redistribution in extracellular fluids and tissues as well as the factor of protein binding in plasma and tissues). Peak plasma levels were lower following subcutaneous injection but sustained longer, while oral administration gave low plasma levels of short duration. As 1%–12% of the administered cocaine was excreted in urine over a 24-h period, 88%–99% was assumed to be metabolized. After subcutaneous injection in the rabbit, much lower plasma concentrations developed than in the dog, and only traces (less than one percent) appeared in urine. Thirty minutes after intravenous injection, the concentrations in spleen and kidney were higher than in any other tissues, about three times higher than in liver, but only 30% higher than in cerebral cortex, suggesting that, "cocaine has a much greater affinity for tissues than for plasma." Finally, the convulsive plasma level in the dog ranged from 3.3 to 6.9 µg per ml.

Insofar as procaine is concerned, THIEULIN (1921) showed that the actual decomposition of procaine into para-aminobenzoic acid and diethyl-aminoethanol takes place in plasma. Subsequently, in order to demonstrate the site of metabolism for procaine and other local anesthetics, liver damage was deliberately induced so that it could be shown that the cat was thereby made much more susceptible to toxic reactions upon injection with cocaine, procaine, and tutocaine. In 1935, DUNLOP further elaborated on the fate of procaine in the dog. In the normal healthy dog, procaine was rapidly converted into non-toxic end products, procaine as such disappearing entirely from the circulating blood. The end products were eliminated more slowly by the kidneys, and in the absence of the kidneys traces were found in blood so long as the animal survived. Then came a strange statement, that blood alone has an effect upon procaine, and while the liver is not essential in the detoxification, that organ detoxifies procaine much more rapidly than do other tissues. Thus the fundamental processes in the metabolism of procaine were outlined.

The mechanisms began to be unraveled when KISCH et al. (1943) described a "procaine esterase." They found that human plasma and serum could hydrolyze procaine into the product p-aminobenzoic acid. The effects of incubation time, incubation temperature, pH, concentration of procaine, concentration of enzyme and age of serum upon the activity of the hydrolyzing agent were defined. The responsible agent was called "the procaine esterase," its activity expressed in terms of the percent of added procaine hydrolyzed. Inactivation experiments provided additional evidence that the agent was indeed an enzyme, with serum much more efficient in the hydrolysis than plasma, while the liver definitely showed a higher enzymatic activity than other organs. Human spinal fluid showed only 1/100 to 1/170 of the procaine-hydrolyzing effect of serum in the same human subject. It was believed that the procaine esterase was different from such known enzymes as lipase, cholinesterase, and tropine esterase. The last two conclusions are interesting, indeed, as later these investigators reported that incubation of serum with prostigmine or eserine increased the inhibitory effect. Then, BRODIE et al. (1948), using quantitative methods, confirmed the fate of procaine in man following its administration intravenously and showed that hydrolysis into diethyl-aminoethanol and p-aminobenzoic acid took place with unusual rapidity, with further transformation of the diethyl-aminoethanol into unknown products. Subsequently it was shown that halogen substitution in the procaine molecule (e. g. 2-Cl-procaine) markedly increased the rate of hydrolysis in human plasma, about four to five times (FOLDES et al. 1956).

In the meantime, an interesting observation was made by GREIG and her collaborators (GREIG et al. 1950). Procaine, orthoxine, and mesidicaine, which do not ordinarily produce local anesthesia when applied to the surface of the cornea (rabbit, for example), may be made to do so by previous or simultaneous application of a physostigmine solution. The effect may have been the result of a change in permeability of the cornea via inhibition of cholinesterase activity. Nupercaine, butyn, and pyrrolocaine, all topical or surface anesthetics, inhibited cholinesterase activity in minute concentrations.

By the time the use of lidocaine, an amide, became established in practice, methods for studying its metabolism were much more advanced so that the properties of the enzyme system responsible for its oxidative metabolism in hepatic microsomal enzymes could be quantified, the amide-hydrolyzing enzyme solubilized and purified (HOLLUNGER 1960). And it became possible to use a two-compartment open model to evaluate the kinetic parameters governing the distribution and elimination of lidocaine, most essential knowledge not only for regional anesthesia but also when the drug came to be infused for treatment of ventricular arrhythmias in man (BOYES et al. 1971).

H. Summary and Conclusions

Rather than a chronological listing of topical events, this compilation focuses on some of the elemental scientific contributions that comprise the foundation of local anesthetic practice. The individuals responsible, except for the prime movers, are depicted not so much as discoverers but in the context of their environments, the influence of forebears and the current pace of scientific progress. Strong parallels exist among the origins of inhalation, regional and intravenous anesthesia, listed in the order in which they achieved clinical importance. With the exception of the intravenous route, effective agents were available as early as the sixteenth century: various soporific sponges for inhalation, diethyl ether prepared by Valerius Cordus and given to chickens in their feed by Paracelsus, and the use of localized pressure or cold for local anesthesia. Similarly, the numbing effect of cocaine on the tongue was already apparent to the Incas. Injections had been made intravenously in animals in mid-seventeenth century, but the agents were nonspecific and not designed to produce unconsciousness. In each instance, however, the initial practical demonstrations in man fell to the lot of persons prepared by motivation and their environments to become innovators.

In a real sense the discovery of local anesthesia, as well as inhalation and intravenous anesthesia, falls into the pattern of "multiples," in the language of Robert MERTON (1961). Owsei TEMKIN (1971) added that, "Sociologists of science have cited in evidence for social causation the multiple appearance of the same discovery. The independent use of anesthesia by Long, Wells, and Morton is a well-known example." So it was with the advent of local anesthesia in the contributions of Freud, Koller, and Corning. For inhalation anesthesia, Humphry Davy predicted its clinical utility and von Anrep was just as prescient with regard to local anesthesia.

All of the medical disciplines which were visible around the turn of the century had to await those developments in the basic sciences that would give each a sound footing, a process that continues to this day. None of the three anesthetic techniques achieved that status until well into the fourth decade as suggested in this review. Toward the end of the nineteenth century medical science was nascent. It is said that the first laboratory for the study of pharmacology was established in Strassburg in 1878, at the termination of the Franco-Prussian War. In the United States, E. S. Minot of the newly created department of physiology at Harvard University commented as follows on the phenomenon of development of fatigue in muscle: "This is the first time, so far as I am aware, that so extended a physiological research requiring the use of physical methods has been carried out in America." It was only in the first decade of the twentieth century that the Western Hemisphere began to establish chairs of pharmacology at major universities and medical schools. In his 1909 presidential address before the American Society for the Advancement of Clinical Investigation, S. J. Meltzer depicted the need for a differentiation of medicine into science and practice. And those days were the stirrings of science as related to local anesthesia.

To recapitulate, in the words of CAWS (1969): "The development of science is a stepwise process; nobody starts from scratch and nobody gets far ahead of the rest. At any point in history there is a range of possible discovery; the trailing edge is defined by everything known at the time, and the leading edge is a function of what is already known, together with variables representing available instrumentation, the capacity of brains, and so on."

References

Abel JJ (1957), Investigator, teacher, prophet. 1857–1938. Williams and Wilkins, Baltimore

Abel JJ, Crawford AC (1897) On the blood pressure-raising constituent of the suprarenal capsule. Bull Johns Hopkins Hosp 8:151–156

Adrian ED (1932) The mechanism of nervous action. Oxford Press, London

Anrep, VK von (1880) Über die physiologische Wirkung des Cocain. Arch Ges Physiol 21:38–77

Becker HK (1963) Carl Koller and cocaine. Psychoanal Quart 32:309:373

Bieter RN (1936) Applied pharmacology of local anesthetics. Am J Surg 34:500–510

Boyes RN, Scott DB, Jebson PJ, Godman MJ, Julian DG (1971) Pharmacokinetics of lidocaine in man. Clin Pharmacol Ther 12:105:116

Braun H (1903) Über den Einfluß der Vitalität der Gewebe auf die örtlichen und allgemeinen Giftwirkungen lokaler anästhesierender Mittel und über die Bedeutung des Adrenalins für die Localanästhesie. Arch Klin Chir 69:541–591

Braun H (1905) Über einige neue örtliche Anästhetika (Stovain, Alypin, Novocain). Dtsch Med Wochenschr 2:1667–1671

Brodie BB, Lief, PA, Poet R (1948) The fate of procaine in man following its intravenous administration and methods for the estimation of procaine and diethyl-aminoethanol. J Pharmacol Exp Ther 94:359–366

Byck R (1974) Cocaine papers. Sigmund Freud. New American Library, New York

Caws P (1969) The structure of discovery. Scientific discovery is no less logical than deduction. Science 166:1375–1380

Cole KS (1982) Squid axon membrane. Impedance decrease to voltage clamp. Annu Rev Neurosci 3:303–323

Cole KS, Hodgkin AL (1939) Membrane and protoplasmic resistance in the squid giant axon. J Gen Physiol 22:671–678

Corning JL (1885) Spinal anaesthesia and local medication of the cord. NY Med J 42:183–185

Curtis HJ, Cole KS (1938) Transverse impedance of the giant squid axon. J Gen Physiol 21:757–765

deJong RH, Bonin JD (1981) Benzodiazepines protect mice from local anesthetic convulsions and death. Anesth Analg 60:385–389

Duncan D, Jarvis WH (1943) Comparison of the actions on nerve fibers of certain anesthetic mixtures and substances in oil. Anesthesiology 4:465–474

Dunlop JG (1935) Fate of procaine in the dog. J Pharmacol Exp Ther 55:464–481

Eggleston C, Hatcher RA (1919) A further contribution to the pharmacology of the local anesthetics. J Pharmacol Exp Ther 13:433–487

Einhorn A (1899) On the chemistry of local anesthetics. MMW 46:1218–1220

Englesson S (1974) The influence of acid-base changes on central nervous system toxicity of local anaesthetic agents. I. Acta Anaesth Scand 18:79–87

Faulconer A, Keys TE (1965) Foundations of anesthesiology. Thomas, Springfield, IL

Fink BR (1980) History of local anesthesia. In: Cousins MJ, Bridenbaugh PO (eds) Neural blockade in clinical anesthesia and management of pain, chap 1. Lippincott, Philadelphia

Foldes FF, Davis DL, Plekss OJ (1956) Influence of halogen substitution on enzymatic hydrolysis. Anesthesiology 17:187–195

Foldes FF, Molloy R, McNail PG, Koukal LR (1960) Comparison of toxicity of intravenously given local anesthetic agents in man. JAMA 172:1493–1498

Freud S (1884) Über Coca. Zentralbl Ges Ther 2:289–314

Gasser HS, Erlanger JA (1929) The role of fiber size in the establishment of a nerve block by pressure or cocaine. Am J Physiol 88:581–591

Gay GR, Inaba DS, Rappolt TR Sr, Gushue GF Jr, Perkner JJ (1976) "An' ho, ho, baby, take a whiff on me": La Dama Blanca. Cocaine in current perspective. Anesth Analg 55:582–587

Greig ME, Holland WC, Lindvig PE (1950) The anesthetization of the rabbit's cornea by non-surface anesthetics. Br J Pharmacol Chemother 5:461–464

Hatcher RA, Eggleston C (1916) A contribution to the pharmacology of novocaine. J Pharmacol Exp Ther 8:385–405

Hirschfelder AD, Bieter RN (1932) Local anesthetics. Physiol Rev 12:190–282

Hodgkin AL (1964) The conduction of the nervous impulse. Thomas, Springfield, IL

Hollunger H (1960) On the metabolism of lidocaine. Acta Pharmacol Toxicol 17:356–389

Kandel E (1982) The origins of modern neuroscience. Annu Rev Neurosci 5:299–303

Keys TE (1945) The history of surgical anesthesia. Schuman's, New York

Kisch B, Koster H, Strauss E (1943) The procaine esterase. Exp Med Surg 1:51–64

Leser AJ (1940) Duration of local anesthesia in relation to concentrations of procaine and epinephrine. Anesthesiology 1:205–207

Marmont G (1949) Studies on the axon mambrane. J Cell Comp Physiol 34:351–382

Merton RK (1961) Singletons and multiples in scientific discovery. A chapter in the sociology of science. Proc Am Phil Soc 105:470–486

Mortimer WG (1974) History of coca, the "divine plant" of the Incas. AND/OR Press, San Francisco

Munson ES, Wagman IH (1972) Diazepam treatment of local anesthetic-induced seizures. Anesthesiology 37:523–528

Niemann A (1860) Sur l'alcoloide de coca. J Pharmacol 34:474–475

Quincke H (1891) Die Lumbalpunction des Hydrozephalus. Berl Klin Wochenschr 28:929–933

Ritchie JM, Greengard P (1966) On the mode of action of local anesthetics. Annu Rev Pharmacol 6:405–430

Tanaka K, Yamasaki M (1966) Blocking of cortical inhibitory synapses by intravenous lidocaine. Nature 209:207–208

Tatum AL, Atkinson AJ, Collins KH (1925) Acute cocaine poisoning, its prophylaxis and treatment in laboratory animals. J Pharmacol Exp Ther 26:325–335

Temkin O (1971) The historiography of ideas in medicine. Chapter I. In: Clarke E (ed) Modern methods in the history of medicine. Athlone, London

Thieulin J (1921) Urinary elimination of procaine. Chem Abstr 15:1167

Trendelenburg U (1958) The supersensitivity caused by cocaine. J Pharmacol Exp Ther 125:55–65

Williams LW (1909) The anatomy of the common squid, Loligo pealii. Leseur, Leiden

Wöhler P (1860) Über eine organische Base in der Coca. Ann Chemie du Pharmac 114:213

Woods LA, McMahon FG, Seevers MH (1951) Distribution and metabolism of cocaine in the dog. J Pharmacol Exp Ther 101:200–204

Wynter WE (1891) Four cases of tuberculous meningitis in which paracentesis of the theca vertebralis was performed for the relief of fluid pressure. Lancet I:981–982

Young JZ (1936) Structure of nerve fibres and synapses in some invertebrates. Cold Spring Harbor Symp Quant Biol 4:1–12

CHAPTER 2

The Action of Local Anesthetics on Ion Channels of Excitable Tissues

G. R. STRICHARTZ and J. M. RITCHIE

A. Introduction

Local anesthetics are chemicals that reversibly block action potentials in excitable membranes. The generation and propagation of action potentials depend on the opening and closing of ionic sodium, and usually also of potassium, channels that span excitable nerve and muscle membranes (HODGKIN and HUXLEY 1952; HILLE 1970). Both the shape of individual action potentials and the frequency of bursts of impulses are determined by the kinetic properties of these ion channels which, in turn, are controlled by the membrane potential of the cell. Local anesthetic molecules interfere with the function of these ion channels in such a way as to block the generation and conduction of action potentials (TAYLOR 1959; HILLE 1966).

The aim of this chapter is to describe briefly the physiology of impulse transmission and then to detail the mechanism whereby local anesthetics block ion channels. We will present a current view of anesthetic action trying to reveal areas of ignorance and controversy, thereby providing a framework for the experimental questions that should be addressed in the coming years.

B. Physiological Basis of Generation of the Action Potential

I. Role of Ion Channels

Action potentials are transient membrane depolarizations that result from a brief increase of the sodium (P_{Na}), and usually also from a delayed increase of the potassium (P_K), permeabilities of the membrane. The rapid increase in P_{Na} permits a flow of sodium ions into the cell, thus depolarizing the membrane. The action potential is then terminated upon membrane repolarization caused by the extinction ("inactivation") of this increase in P_{Na} together, in many cells, with the help of a slower, subsequent increase in P_K which allows an efflux of potassium ions, thus repolarizing the membrane more rapidly (Fig. 1a). Both P_{Na} and P_K increase because they depend intrinsically on the membrane potential. Local anesthetics selectively inhibit peak P_{Na}, whose value is normally about 5–6 times greater than the minimum required for impulse conduction, i. e., there is a safety factor of conduction of about 5–6 (see CHIU and RITCHIE 1984). Local anesthetics reduce this safety factor, decreasing both the rate of rise of the action potential and its conduction velocity. When the safety factor falls below unity, conduction fails and

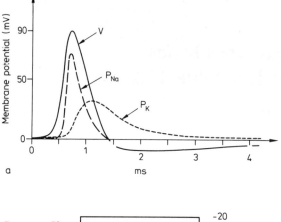

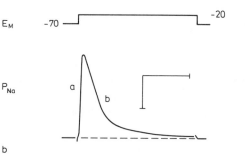

Fig. 1. a The time course of an action potential (V) and the underlying sodium (P_{Na}) and potassium (P_K) permeabilities. For this computed propagating action potential the initial rise in V precedes the increase in local P_{Na} and is due to local circuit current flowing from an adjacent excited region of membrane. After HODGKIN and HUXLEY (1952). **b** The time course of sodium permeability change during a step-voltage depolarization from -70 to -20 mV. Phase a shows the increase in permeability caused by channel activation, phase b the decline due to channel inactivation. Data from frog myelinated axon under voltage clamp, T = 10 °C. Calibrations: *horizontal,* 5 ms; *vertical,* 10^{-9} cm$^3\cdot$s^{-1}.

block occurs. The reduction of P_{Na} (or the closely related sodium conductance, g_{Na}) is thus the major effect of local anesthetics involved in conduction block.

II. Kinetic Properties of Sodium Channels

Discrete aqueous pores through the excitable membrane, called sodium channels, are the molecular structures that mediate its sodium permeability (HILLE 1970). These sodium channels open and close as they switch between several different molecular configurations governed by voltage-dependent kinetics. Channel "gating" kinetics can be studied with voltage-clamp methods, in which the membrane potential is held at constant values for controlled time intervals. An adequately voltage-clamped membrane has no current flowing parallel to the membrane (longitudinal current) and, therefore, the membrane potential is spatially uniform, and, except during the very brief periods during which the potential is being changed, the transmembrane current has little capacitive component. As a consequence of these restrictions, membrane currents under voltage clamp are composed exclusively of ionic currents. Under these conditions the ionic sodium currents flowing across the membrane is proportional to P_{Na} and, thus, to the number of open ion-conducting sodium channels.

The time course of sodium current during a short depolarizing voltage clamp pulse is shown in Fig. 1b. A rapid increase in the current, produced by the fast

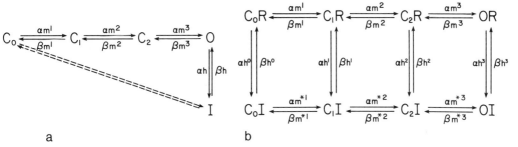

a   b

Fig. 2. a A linear gating scheme to model sodium channel kinetics. States C are closed, O is open, I inactivated. Rate constans α and β are intrinsically voltage-dependent; αs increase with depolarization, βs increase with hyperpolarization. An equilibrium between C_0 and I can be reached without passing through the conducting state, as represented by the dashed lines. After ARMSTRONG and BEZANILLA (1977). **b** A two dimensional scheme for channel gating which elaborates on Fig. 2a. Channel states are defined by C_0 or O states and by R or I states. Rate constants α and β depend on membrane voltage as in 2a, but "m" dimension reactions (*horizontal:* activation) are faster (5–10 ×) than "h" dimension reactions (*vertical:* inactivation). The only ion conducting state is OR and inactivation processes can occur from any of the R substates

activation of channels to an open, conducting state, is followed by a slower decline whose time course of decay has one or more exponential components corresponding to *inactivation* of channels to nonconducting states.

The inactivation of sodium channels is not the reversal of the activation reaction (which is termed "deactivation"), rather inactivation temporarily converts channels to a state (or states) from which they cannot open in response to depolarization. These inactivated states are slowly converted back to the closed, resting form when the membrane is repolarized. One simple scheme that describes these kinetics is shown in Fig. 2a (after BEZANILLA and ARMSTRONG 1977). At the normal resting potential (i. e., about -70 mV), most channels are in closed states, denoted as $C_0 - C_2$. Upon depolarization the channels change configuration, first changing to an open, ion-conducting state O, and then to an inactive non-conducting state I. Although both C and I states correspond to nonconducting channels, they differ in that depolarization can recruit channels to the conducting O state from C, but not from I.

All these conversions among channel states occur because the rate constants that determine the forward and reverse rates of the activation conformational transitions, α_m and β_m, are themselves determined by the membrane potential (HODGKIN and HUXLEY 1952). Channel gating is voltage-dependent because channel macromolecules appear to have a charged or dipolar moiety which translates or rotates in response to changes in the membrane electric field, thereby producing the changes among the various conformational states. This, in turn, means that there are small displacement currents that are direct consequences of such translational or rotational changes. Such currents originate from charge movement restricted to within the membrane and not from ionic current flowing through the membrane. These displacement currents, known as *gating currents*, have been used to investigate the molecular details of channel opening and inactivation (ARMSTRONG and BEZANILLA 1974; KEYNES and ROJAS 1974), and they are dealt with in more detail below.

The membrane must be repolarized before channels in the I state can return to the C states, a process that can occur without going through the open state, as indicated by the dashed line in Fig. 2a. In fact, even at negative resting potentials there is an equilibrium between the C_0 and I states. At -70 mV about 60% of the channels are in C_0 and 40% in I, although the quantitative distribution between these states depends on the particular nerve being studied as well as the temperature, pH, and ionic conditions. Still, in all cases more negative resting potentials lead to a shift in the equilibrium towards C_0 and more positive potentials towards I; at -120 mV essentially all the channels are in the C_0, and at -40 mV nearly all are in I.

The distribution of channels between the C_0 and I states is an important determinant of excitability. After the depolarization of the action potential, many sodium channels are in the I states and cannot immediately be opened by subsequent depolarizing stimuli. This phenomenon contributes largely to the refractory behavior of nerve membranes. For in order for the normal impulse threshold to be restored, the channels must return to their resting C_0-I equilibrium, a process that takes 1–5 msec in frog myelinated nerve at room temperature (HILLE 1970) but much less time in mammalian myelinated nerve at 37 °C (CHIU et al. 1979). Therefore, circumstances that shift the C_0-I reaction to the inactivated state, or that slow the rate of recovery of channels from inactivated to closed conformations, will elevate the threshold for firing a single impulse and lower the maximum frequency of bursts of impulses, perhaps stopping repetitive firing altogether.

The kinetic scheme of Fig. 2a is a simplified model, useful for introducing the basic concepts of sodium channel kinetics. A more general scheme is shown in Fig. 2b, which differs from Fig. 2a in that both closed and open channels can be converted directly to inactive forms (NONNER 1980; BEZANILLA and ARMSTRONG 1977; HORN et al. 1981). If the rate constants for inactivation, α_h and β_h, are the same for every activation state, then this scheme degenerates to that of HODGKIN and HUXLEY (1952).

An alternative explanation for the time course of P_{Na} has been proposed recently by ALDRICH et al. (1983). These authors found that once single sodium channels in cultured excitable cells opened, they then closed at the same rate, regardless of membrane potential and that the apparently slower inactivation of macroscopic currents was due to the delayed opening of a fraction of sodium channels. Although this concept differs markedly from the more traditional kinetic models, the same general interpretations of local anesthetic action will apply for most of the observations presented here regardless of this difference. The exact kinetic scheme for sodium channel gating is still unknown and may well differ in detail among different membranes, but the essential steps shown in Fig. 2a are sufficient to explain most of the effects of local anesthetics described here.

III. Gating Currents

When the charged or dipolar portion of the channel moves in response to changes in the intra-membrane electric field, a small current across the membrane is created. This displacement current differs from the ionic currents carried by sodium and potassium ions; rather it resembles the transient current that charges or discharges the membrane capacitance when the membrane potential is changed. These socalled "gating currents" have been measured during changes from closed to open states and during the reverse reaction (ARMSTRONG and BEZANILLA 1974; KEYNES and ROJAS 1974). Gating currents corresponding to transitions to and from inactivated states have not yet been detected. When more sodium channels are shifted into the I state (by long-term depolarization of the membrane) both the ionic sodium currents and the gating currents are reduced proportionately (TAYLOR and BEZANILLA 1983). Furthermore, the gating currents that flow when a membrane is repolarized after a short test depolarization, and which reflect the return of open channels to closed states, become increasingly smaller with longer and larger test depolarizations, i.e., during conditions that favor the conversion of channels to the inactivated form (ARMSTRONG and BEZANILLA 1977; NONNER 1980). Such results suggest that the conversion of channels to inactivated states is accompanied by a degree of *immobilization* of the gating charge: in this condition an inactivated channel cannot, it seems, undergo the conformational changes required to reach the open state. Although all of the ionic current inactivates, not all of the gating charge can be immobilized, showing either that part of the charged channel components can still move without yielding an open channel or that a portion of the gating charge does not come from sodium channels. The nature of sodium channel inactivation is important because local anesthetics appear to bind selectively to inactive forms of the channel, so stabilizing them as will be described below.

IV. Pharmacological Dimensions of the Sodium Channel

Results of pharmacological and biochemical experiments provide some information about the structure of the sodium channel. The channel seems to be a lipoglycoprotein firmly situated in the membrane. It consists of an aqueous pore spanning the membrane, which is narrow enough at at least one point to discriminate between sodium and other ions; for example, sodium ions pass through about twelve times more easily than do potassium ions (HILLE 1972). The channel also includes a portion that changes configuration in response to changes in membrane potential, thereby gating the passage of ions through the pore. Ion selectivity is conferred by structures well within the pore, for it is not altered by modifications of the outer (SPALDING 1980) or inner (ARMSTRONG et al. 1973) openings of the channel. At least part of the gating structure is located near the axoplasmic opening of the channel, judged from its susceptibility to modification by drugs and proteolytic enzymes applied internally (NONNER et al. 1980; ARMSTRONG et al. 1973; OXFORD et al. 1978; EATON et al. 1978); but gating kinetics also can be modified by drugs and toxins that act from within the hydrophobic region of the membrane (KHODOROV 1978; STRICHARTZ et al. 1978) and at the external surface (ADAM et al. 1976; CAHALAN 1975; WANG and STRICHARTZ 1983; WANG 1984).

Certain non-proteinaceous toxins that block sodium channels without changing their kinetics, such as tetrodotoxin (TTX) and saxitoxin (STX), act at the outer opening of the channels. Physiological studies show that these toxins block sodium channels with 1:1 stoichiometry (HILLE 1968); and measurements of the binding of these toxins have permitted the direct determination of channel densities in a number of excitable membranes (RITCHIE and ROGART 1977). These densities range from $35 \mu m^{-2}$ in small nonmyelinated nerve fibers to $20,000 \mu m^{-2}$ at the node of Ranvier of myelinated nerves. On an average length basis, there are relatively few sodium channels in nonmyelinated nerve membranes; in garfish olfactory nerve, for example, the ratio of sodium channels to phospholipid molecules is 1:60,000 and corresponds with a mean distance between the sodium channels (if arranged in a regular square array) of about $0.2 \mu m$ (STRICHARTZ 1977; RITCHIE 1978, 1979). In the densely packed node of Ranvier the channels are separated by only 70 A, on average, but despite their close proximity they appear to open and close independently of one another. These channels, although they are extremely sparse, can, however, be readily studied both electrophysiologically, because they mediate large ionic currents, and biochemically, because many ligands bind to the channels with high affinity, having equilibrium dissociation constants of 1–10 nM (RITCHIE 1978; CATTERALL 1980; STRICHARTZ 1981; BARHANIN et al. 1983). Application of these high affinity ligands has permitted the isolation and purification of sodium channels which are pharmacologically activatable when reconstituted in lipid bilayer vesicles (AGNEW et al. 1978; HARTSHORNE et al. 1980; BENESKI and CATTERALL 1980; BARCHI et al. 1980; ROSENBERG et al. 1984a). This detergent-solubilized macromolecule is a glyco-protein of 250–300,000 daltons molecular weight, which may or may not include a smaller 40,000 dalton protein (MILLER et al. 1983). Recent reports describe reconstitution of voltage-activated single channel events in phospholipid bilayers containing single polypeptides purified from eel electroplax (ROSENBERG et al. 1984b), demonstrating that a single macromolecule from this organ is sufficient to regenerate molecular sodium permeability.

C. The Action of Local Anesthetics on Sodium Channels

Two general theories have been proposed to explain the action of local anesthetics on sodium channels; one considers the general perturbation of the bulk membrane structure by anesthetics and its consequences for channel function; (SEEMAN 1972; LEE 1976) and the other proposes a direct binding of local anesthetic molecules to specific receptors on the sodium channel (STRICHARTZ 1973). During the past decade much evidence has accumulated to support the latter specific receptor hypothesis (see HILLE 1980). Nevertheless, general membrane perturbation may still provide part of the explanation for anesthetic actions, and it is doubtful that local anesthetic action can be accounted for solely in terms of an action at a classical receptor site.

I. Distribution of Local Anesthetics and the Mechanism of Their Blocking Action

The classical tertiary amine anesthetics, being lipid-soluble, are distributed throughout all the nerve compartments at equilibrium. Depending on the lipid solubility of both the cation and free base forms, and on the intracellular and extracellular pH, anesthetic molecules will be found as both cationic and neutral species in the aqueous interstitial and axoplasmic compartments, and primarily as the uncharged base within the membrane lipid (UEDA et al. 1980). The distribution in the latter will depend on the lipid solubility of the anesthetic, which is usually expressed in terms of the oil:water or octanol:water partition coefficient (although, it should be noted, biological membranes have structural and chemical features that are significantly different from those of bulk hydrocarbons). Normally, the neutral form of tertiary (3°) amine local anesthetics can pass relatively easily across the nerve membrane. However, it has been possible to restrict these molecules to only one side of the nerve membrane by using quaternary (4°) amine derivatives, which are essentially impermeant and so remain on the side of application.

The results of many experiments on 4° amine anesthetics show that sodium (and potassium) channels are blocked only by these drugs when present in the axoplasmic phase, and not by drugs present in the extracellular solution (FRAZIER et al. 1970; STRICHARTZ 1973; HILLE et al. 1975; CAHALAN 1978). These findings are consistent with results of other experiments in which both the intracellular and extracellular pH were varied in perfused squid giant axons and the degree of block from externally applied 3° amine anesthetics measured (NARAHASHI et al. 1970). The cationic form of these anesthetics appears to be much more potent than the uncharged base, and to exert its blocking activity from the axoplasmic surface of the membrane.

However, the channel blocking activity of neutral anesthetic molecules is not absent. Benzocaine, which has no 3° amine group, and the alcohols, the barbiturates and other general anesthetics also block sodium channels; many of the specific features of block of 3° and 4° amine anesthetics are manifested by these neutral compounds (RITCHIE and RITCHIE 1968; COURTNEY 1975; HILLE 1977 a, b; MROSE and RITCHIE 1978; SWENSON and OXFORD 1980; BEAN et al. 1981; KENDIG 1981; HAYDON and URBAN 1983 a–c). Indeed, it was the observation of the wide structural variety of agents showing "local anesthetic" action on sodium channels that first raised the question of whether there was just a single specific receptor for mediating local anesthesia, and it provided some support for the idea that there is more than one mechanism (or site) of action, as will be discussed in more detail below.

One aspect of the blocking action of local anesthetics strongly suggests a direct and specific interaction between anesthetic molecules and sodium channels. During repetitive brief membrane depolarizations the degree of anesthetic block is increased; when the membrane is returned to the resting condition, the degree of block returns to its original level. This phenomenon, called "use-dependence" (COURTNEY 1975), is a characteristic feature of channel blockade by local anesthetics of the 4° and 3° amine type, and it is also found in block by many drugs not normally considered as local anesthetics (YEH and NARAHASHI 1977; SHAPIRO 1977; SWENSON and OXFORD 1980; STRICHARTZ 1980).

Voltage-clamp experiments reveal two components of anesthetic action that underlie use-dependent block. First, channels are blocked more effectively by charged anesthetics when a particular, well-defined, pattern of changes in membrane potential which sequentially opens and closes the sodium channels is used (Strichartz 1973, 1975; Hille et al. 1975; Courtney et al. 1978). Once a channel has been opened, an anesthetic molecule appears to "enter" it and prevents the passage of a sodium ion through it. The channel, however, can "close" with the anesthetic still bound within it. In this case a charged anesthetic dissociates only very slowly from the "closed" channel. But if the channel is re-opened, the charged anesthetic may then leave quite rapidly. Uncharged anesthetic molecules may gain access to the receptor site from the membrane interior, bypassing the channel gates (Hille 1977b). Thus, from early experiments it appeared that use-dependence occurs because anesthetics gain access and bind to sites when the channels are "open," and dissociate only slowly from them when they are "closed." By contrast, uncharged anesthetics may dissociate rapidly from closed channels since their exit is not restricted to the aqueous portion of the channel, so such molecules produce considerably less use-dependent blockade (Hille 1977b; Schwarz et al. 1977; Courtney and Etter 1983).

The second feature of anesthetic block that demonstrates direct interaction with sodium channels is a change in the sodium inactivation process (Courtney 1975; Hille 1977a). When a membrane has been treated by local anesthetics, larger membrane hyperpolarizations are required to remove the apparent inactivation, in other words, to shift the channels from the I to the C_0 state (see Fig. 2). This apparent shift in the C_0-I equilibrium increases with increased use-dependent block (Courtney 1975). From these results it appears that local anesthetics bind more strongly to inactivated forms of the channel and hence stabilize the non-conducting configurations (Hille 1980; Shapiro 1977). But the complete description is more complicated.

When normal inactivation is abolished by the enzyme mixture pronase, acting intracellularly, use-dependent block by many lidocaine derivatives is no longer detected (Cahalan 1978; Yeh 1978). But if channel inactivation is prevented instead by the presence of certain polypeptide toxins or by treatment with selective oxidizing reagents, then use-dependent block still persists (Shepley et al. 1983; Wang and Strichartz 1984). Thus, use-dependence may arise from the binding of anesthetic molecules to a part of the molecule that is essential for inactivation; and when this segment is enzymatically degraded, anesthetic binding is also removed. The modifications of inactivation by external treatments do not modify this anesthetic binding site. In addition, the inhibition of channels by local anesthetics in unstimulated membranes is not altered by either of these treatments. Perhaps block of resting channels occurs through a different receptor or involves different binding kinetics than that for use-dependent block (Yeh 1980; Strichartz 1985; Strichartz and Wang 1985).

II. The Modulated Receptor Hypothesis: Past and Present Formulations

These phenomena have led to a model of the sodium channel, part of which forms a local anesthetic binding site whose affinity for the drug is modified by membrane potential. This latter process involves a voltage-dependent conformational change as well as a direct effect of voltage on the binding reaction per se (STRI-CHARTZ 1973). The *modulated-receptor* hypothesis proposed by HILLE (1977b), which explains many of the experimental observations, is illustrated in Fig. 3a. Channel gating is simplified by consideration of only three states, resting, open, and inactivated. Anesthetic molecules, denoted by asterisks, bind with higher af-

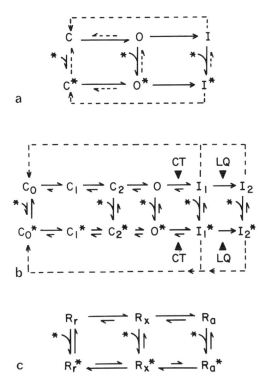

Fig. 3. a The modulated receptor hypothesis as presented by HILLE (1977b), after the scheme of COURTNEY (1974, 1975). Drug molecules (*) interact more readily with open (*O*) and inactivated (*I*) channel states than with closed resting (*C*) states, and channel activation kinetics are not modified by anesthetics. Solid lines indicate the net direction of reactions during depolarizations, broken ones the relaxations after repolarization. Inhibition corresponds to the selective affinity for and stabilization of the inactivated state by anesthetic molecules. **b** Expanded modulated-receptor scheme. Unlike 3a, the anesthetics (*) combine with "less closed" channel states (C_2) as well as with several inactivated states (I_1, I_2). "CT" and "LQ" refer to reaction steps affected by chloramine-T and α-scorpion toxin treatments which inhibit normal channel inactivation (see text). Some activation steps are modified by anesthetic binding, accounting for changes in gating current kinetics. **c** A generalized kinetic scheme for local anesthetic action. Receptor state R_r predominates at rest and has lower anesthetic affinity than either state R_x or R_a, both of which are populated by depolarization. Receptor states are not identified explicitly with the gating states postulated in Fig. 2; 2 gating states may have the same affinity or 1 gating state might encompass two different receptor conformations. The transitions between receptor states are modulated by anesthetic binding. The kinetics of binding reactions differ among various drugs accounting for the range of potencies for relative tonic and use-dependent inhibition. From STRICHARTZ and WANG 1985)

finity to the *I* state, which is populated during a depolarization. Reversal of this binding reaction during the period between depolarizing pulses is slow, leading to an accumulation of channels in *I**, and thus modelling use-dependence (HILLE 1978; SCHWARZ et al. 1977).

The original model should be modified to indicate that use-dependent inhibition can occur in the absence of the normal fast sodium channel inactivation (CAHALAN 1978; SHEPLEY et al. 1983; WANG and STRICHARTZ 1984a). In studies with dyes containing amino groups (ARMSTRONG and CROOP 1982), the kinetics of block of Pronase-modified sodium currents could be accounted for quantitatively by postulating that channels in the kinetic sequence between open and closed conformations as well as open channels would bind the blocking drugs. Recent experiments with quite polar 3° amine local anesthetics on myelinated nerve show that full use-dependent block can be achieved by depolarizing pulses which are too brief to open most of the channels, but long enough to put them all in "less closed" states (WANG and STRICHARTZ 1984; STRICHARTZ and WANG 1986a). These observations suggest a modification of the original modulated-receptor hypothesis, as shown in Fig. 3b.

The rates at which an anesthetic molecule can bind to, and dissociate from, open and closed channels determine the time-course of the development of use-dependent block. Molecules that bind very rapidly to open channels and dissociate slowly from closed channels will reach equilibrium block conditions after only a few channel-opening pulses; molecules that associate slowly with open channels will require many more pulses to permit the blocking reaction to reach its equilibrium. For drugs that dissociate rapidly from closed channels, use-dependent block will "accumulate" when the time between depolarizing pulses is short compared to the time required for the dissociation reaction (COURTNEY 1980; COURTNEY and ETTER 1983). Furthermore, drugs that rapidly enter and rapidly leave both closed and open channels will show little use-dependence. Small, lipophilic drugs do behave this way. Benzocaine or octanol action shows little dependence on stimulus pulse frequency, yet the inactivation process of sodium channels is also modified by both drugs, at rest and after stimulation (HILLE 1977b; SWENSON and OXFORD 1980; HAYDON and URBAN 1983b).

Two types of explanations account for these observations. In the first, there is only one common receptor for charged and neutral local anesthetics located in the aqueous pore of the channel. It is accessible to charged drug molecules only by passage through the gated "hydrophilic" pore of the channel; but it can also be reached by neutral molecules passing from the membrane lipid interior by a "hydrophobic" pathway in the channel pore. Anesthetics at the binding site can be protonated from the external solution, but not from the axoplasmic solution, implying that the receptor lies close to the outer end of the channel (SCHWARZ et al. 1977). Thus, lowering the extracellular pH "locks" 3° amine anesthetic molecules into the receptor site, limiting their dissociation route to the hydrophilic pathway. The hydrophilic pathway suggested for charged molecules restricts drug diffusion and results in slow rates of anesthetic binding and dissociation; and there is thus a clear use-dependence at low stimulus frequencies. In contrast, the hydrophobic pathway, accessible only to uncharged molecules, is relatively easily traversed and the binding reaction equilibrates rapidly.

The second explanation for these phenomena postulates that there are separate and distinct modes of action of neutral and charged drugs, and that these have corresponding separate sites. Neutral drugs may distribute in the membrane interior and disrupt channel function through some "generalized perturbation" which does not require actual binding to the channel, in addition to any specific, site-mediated action. As a consequence channels are less likely to open during a depolarization, but can be recruited to an "activatable" closed state by large hyperpolarizations. In this manner they appear to be "inactivated." Charged drugs act at a specific site on the channel, where their binding produces changes which can be very similar to those accompanying normal channel inactivation, or can be quite different (CAHALAN et al. 1980). These two models differ in detail, but they both contain a component in which channel gating leads to modified anesthetic binding and such binding acts reciprocally to modulate channel gating. This is a concept of wide general application, probably extending to the actions of many drugs which affect ion channels.

Another modification of the generalized modulated receptor hypothesis should be kept in mind. In the past, different conformations of the local anesthetic receptor were identified with different "states" of the channel, states that were hypothesized in order to account for the observed gating phenomena. But we now know of several voltage-dependent changes of drug affinities which have no correlation with any observed channel gating (MOCZYDLOWSKI et al. 1984; STRICHARTZ and WANG 1986 b) and it is probable that several conformations of a receptor occur within a single gating "state" of the sodium channel.

At this time it seems appropriate to restate the modulated receptor hypothesis in a most general form and to re-examine the specific interpretations of the original model. A receptor for local anesthetics should show voltage-dependent changes in drug affinity, but not necessarily be identified with gating conformations; a general scheme of this type is shown in Fig. 3 c. In addition to this more general kinetic model, the physical interpretation bears reconsideration. Since "open" channels may not be required for use-dependent inhibition, anesthetic molecules may not necessarily bind in the channel pore to exert their action. The term "block" evokes a specific image of drug action for many readers, yet local anesthetics may not always act by *occluding* the channel (see D. III. 6, p. 31). By considering alternative interpretations of local anesthetic actions, investigators will be able to expand the modulated receptor hypothesis in new, imaginative directions.

Although its details are not proven, the modulated receptor model has great appeal, and its general consequences are considerable. The apparent potency of local anesthetics must depend on the conditions of testing. For example, the resting membrane potential, the internal and external pH, the nature of the buffer, the frequency and size of depolarizing pulses, and the temperature of the preparation, which may have differing effects on drugs with hydrophobic or hydrophilic access to the receptor(s), will all be important (HILLE 1977 a, b; COURTNEY 1980; SCHWARZ et al. 1977; BRADLEY and RICHARDS 1984). Anesthetics with higher lipid solubilities would be expected to be more potent both because they would be more concentrated in the nerve membrane and because of their increased access to the sodium channel receptor. On the other hand, their binding affinity for a receptor located in an aqueous pore would be expected to be less than that of more polar compounds. Although some of these parameters have been experimentally approached (COURTNEY 1980), much remains to be studied (cf. Chap. 3, p. 54).

D. Current Questions in Local Anesthetic Action

The various experimental results presented above permit us to refine some of the basic questions concerning local anesthetic action: (1) What is the location of the site(s) in the sodium channel at which anesthetic molecules bind? (2) How many sites are there? (3) What factors control anesthetic binding to these site? (4) Do channel blockade and modification of inactivation occur as a result of the same single process? and, finally, (5) Is there indeed a single mechanism of action? Some of these questions have been addressed by recent experiments and will be reviewed briefly below. Clearly, these questions can only be answered completely when we fully understand the structural details underlying channel function. Studies of local anesthetic action have provided part of our understanding of this latter function, which means that the two sets of questions, and the very concepts involved, are to some degree complementary.

I. Location of Local Anesthetic Binding Site(s) in the Sodium Channel

Regions of the sodium channel have been identified by their susceptibility to various biochemical and pharmacological treatments rather than by any true molecular dimensions. The channel is viewed as a large protein, glycosylated on its external-facing portions (COHEN and BARCHI 1981) and, when it is "open," it provides a relatively hydrophilic pathway for ions to traverse the membrane. Toxins such as tetrodotoxin and saxitoxin totally occlude the channel, seemingly by binding at or near the outer opening of the channel in a manner that is independent of voltage or stimulation frequency (NARAHASHI et al. 1967; HILLE 1968; ULBRICHT and WAGNER 1975; ALMERS and LEVINSON 1975; KRUEGER et al. 1979). [However, in BTX-modified sodium channels studied in lipid bilayers there is a clear voltage-dependent change in TTX affinity at potentials beyond $0 \, mV$ (KRUEGER et al. 1983; MOCZYDLOWSKI et al. 1984). Whether this also occurs in BTX-free channels has not yet been shown.] Evidence from electrophysiology (WAGNER and ULBRICHT 1976) and radio-labelled tetrodotoxin and saxitoxin binding (COLQUHOUN et al. 1972; HENDERSON et al. 1973) shows that there is no direct interaction between local anesthetics and this part of the channel.

In contrast, conditions that decrease the passage of ions through the channel potentiate the block by local anesthetics. For example, when the extracellular sodium ions are replaced by impermeant $Tris^+$ ions, the use-dependent block of outward currents by $4°$ local anesthetics is enhanced (SHAPIRO 1977; CAHALAN and ALMERS 1979 b); and when a nerve already blocked by $4°$ anesthetic is further treated with TTX, (which prevents external sodium ions from entering the channel pore), the use-dependent reduction of the on-gating current is abolished.

Under such conditions the on-gating current is always as small as it is after use-dependent block has reached its steady-state (CAHALAN and ALMERS 1979a). One conclusion from these studies is that sodium ions in the channel compete with local anesthetic molecules for a common binding site. But another interpretation is that the presence of sodium ions in the channel prevents the binding of local anesthetics to the inactivated form by some indirect effect, and not by direct competition.

Drugs that activate sodium channels at rest and inhibit their subsequent inactivation include veratridine, aconitine, and batrachotoxin (BTX) (see CATTERALL 1980; STRICHARTZ 1981). The permeability of BTX-modified channels has been studied in two ways: by voltage-clamp (KHODOROV 1978), and by ion-flux studies both in axons (HENDERSON and STRICHARTZ 1974) and neuroblastoma and muscle cells in culture (CATTERALL 1975; STALLCUP 1977). Results of both types of experiments show an apparent competition between BTX and local anesthetics. The activator drugs are highly lipophilic molecules, and it is most unlikely that they bind in the aqueous channel pore. Therefore, the apparent competition between BTX and local anesthetics requires either that the anesthetic bind to a site at the hydrophilic regions of the channel, perhaps at the protein-lipid interface of the macromolecule, or that the interaction is by some indirect, allosteric mechanism. The latter possibility could result from reciprocal effects of the drugs on sodium channel inactivation. Local anesthetics selectively stabilize an inactivated configuration and BTX stabilizes a non-inactivating channel, so the action of one drug could preclude that of the other without a requirement for direct competition. Indeed, local anesthetic molecules inhibit the binding of radio-labelled BTX to rat brain synaptosomes, and with the same order as their potency for blocking sodium conductance (POSTMA and CATTERALL 1984). Kinetic analysis shows that this inhibition is due, at least in part, to allosteric interactions; both the rate constants for binding and for dissociation of BTX are modified by local anesthetics. The antagonism between local anesthetics and BTX reveals a telling aspect when examined under voltage clamp. The ion selectivity of BTX-modified channels is different from that of normal channels; larger ions become relatively more permeant. Alone, local anesthetics produce no change in ion selectivity. But when the action of BTX is reversed by local anesthetics, the ion selectivity of the membrane becomes more like that of normal channels. These results imply that ions can permeate channels that are binding local anesthetics, which would make it unlikely that the binding site is in the channel pore. The question remains unsettled for the moment: Is the site where anesthetics antagonize BTX action also a normal channel-blocking site?

II. Factors that Determine Rates of Action and Potencies of Local Anesthetics

The ability of any particular local anesthetic to produce tonic and use-dependent blockade of channels depends on how that anesthetic gains access to the binding site(s), which in turn depends on the size, shape, and lipid solubility of the anesthetic. COURTNEY (1980) has studied a series of 12 compounds with local anesthetic activity and related the parameters that describe their tonic and use-dependent block with calculated "lipid solubilities." He found that smaller molecules had faster rates for blocking and dissociating from open sodium channels, and thus produced a relatively smaller use-dependent block. The more lipid-soluble anesthetic molecules produced a greater tonic block and a relatively smaller use-dependent block corresponding to a preferred block of closed channels. The findings on lipophilic drugs agree with the results on the effects of extracellular pH on the action of lidocaine (SCHWARZ et al. 1977), which show that neutral molecules enter and leave a binding site rapidly, regardless of the configuration of the channel, but that protonated molecules can depart from the site only when the channel is "open". The higher resting block observed with more lipophilic molecules could result from two phenomena: there is either a hydrophobic region at the actual binding site that increases the affinity of the anesthetic for the binding site, or there is a higher concentration of anesthetic in the membrane that equilibrates rapidly with the binding site(s) of the sodium channel. These two explanations are not easily discriminated from each other experimentally, since it is impossible to measure directly either the free anesthetic concentration in the membrane near the binding site or (since the sodium channels are so sparsely distributed) that of the bound anesthetic.

COURTNEY's (1980) results are consistent with the general observation, that the more lipophilic molecules in a homologous series are more potent anesthetics (BUCHI and PERLIA 1971; BOKESCH et al. 1986). Undoubtedly, part of this agreement arises because the preparations tested had numerous tissue diffusion barriers between the bathing solution and the nerve membrane-barriers, and these barriers are penetrated best by lipophilic compounds. A second reason for agreement is that the low stimulation frequencies at which most anesthetics were tested reveal only the closed channel block, which is relatively larger for the more lipophilic compounds (COURTNEY 1980; COURTNEY and ETTER 1983). Drug stereoisomers having the same hydrophobicity parameters produce large differences in use-dependent inhibition but are equipotent for resting block, implying structural discrimination by at least one specific receptor (YEH 1980). A similar stereospecificity has been reported for the inhibition of BTX binding by local anesthetics (POSTMA and CATTERALL 1984) suggesting that this activity corresponds more to the stimulated than to the resting anesthetic receptor conformation.

III. The Number and Nature of Local Anesthetic Binding Sites

1. Tonic and Use-Dependent Block

It is questionable whether all the effects of local anesthetics can be explained in terms of a single anesthetic binding site. Thus, a study of the anesthetic concentration-dependence both of "tonic" block (measured at very low depolarization pulse frequencies) and of "use-dependent" block strongly suggests that anesthetic molecules are bound to two distinct binding sites mediating each of these processes. The affinities of these two sites for the anesthetic differ, sometimes by a factor of more than 10 (KHODOROV et al. 1976). For example, when quaternary local anesthetics are perfused inside squid giant axons, one enantiomer produces both a tonic and a use-dependent block, while its optical isomer produces only a tonic block (YEH 1980). This observation is consistent with an earlier analysis of 4°-amine local anesthetic action, which modeled block by two binding steps in sequence, the first being independent of repetitive channel opening and the second requiring channel opening and hence showing use-dependence (STRICHARTZ 1973). In contrast, experiments studying the tonic and use-dependent block of P_{Na} by mixtures of procaine and benzocaine or lidocaine gave results consistent with only one common binding site for these three anesthetics (RIMMEL et al. 1978; SCHMIDTMAYER and ULBRICHT 1980). This site appears to bind only one anesthetic molecule of either neutral or amine type; and the different anesthetics bind in a mutually exclusive manner.

One could argue that the apparent observation of two affinities, documented above, is nevertheless compatible with the modulated-receptor model. For the higher affinity could correspond to anesthetic binding to inactivated channels and the lower affinity binding to non-inactivated channels; only one binding site would be in each channel and only one anesthetic could bind at any one time. However, when the inactivation function of the channel is irreversibly inhibited (perhaps even removed) by treatment with protease(s) at the axoplasmic membrane surface, the use-dependent block is inhibited with little change in the tonic blockade (CAHALAN 1978; YEH 1980). And when procaine is present exclusively at the inside surface of the node of Ranvier only a tonic depression of P_{Na} occurs, with no use-dependence (KHODOROV et al. 1976), although external application does produce a use-dependent block (COURTNEY 1980). Both findings suggest the presence of at least two separate modes of local anesthetic action. These modes could correlate with two separate receptor sites, or with a combination of a specific receptor and non-specific membrane perturbant action. Many agents not usually classified as local anesthetics inhibit sodium channel function. Alcohols, hydrocarbons, and volatile inhalational anesthetics, all electrically uncharged, depress P_{Na} in squid giant axons (SWENSON and OXFORD 1980; BEAN et al. 1981; HAYDON and URBAN 1983 a–c). Although the detailed actions of these agents are not identical and none of them show use-dependent effects at low frequencies (KENDIG et al. 1979; STRICHARTZ 1980), their overall effects are similar to those of tonic block by traditional local anesthetics. It is hard to imagine a single specific receptor for all these various agents, and far more likely that they act, at least in part, through some non-specific membrane perturbation. In this regard, it is interesting to note that the thermodynamic activity of the aqueous concentration of benzocaine for conduction block is of the same order as that found for many of the general anesthetic agents (MULLINS 1954; MILLER 1981). We are drawn therefore, to speculate that benzocaine (and indeed all local anesthetics in their uncharged form) share with general anesthetics the ability to block nerve conduction by a mechanism, as yet unknown, that does not involve a specific receptor site of the kind required in the modulated-receptor hypothesis. This mechanism does not require only that anesthetic molecules dissolve in the lipid bilayer, for the blocking effect of a given neutral anesthetic increases as the temperature is lowered, whereas its solubility and membrane uptake are decreased by cooling (BRADLEY and RICHARDS 1984).

2. Gating Currents

Studies on sodium channel gating currents in the presence of local anesthetic also suggest two binding sites (CAHALAN et al. 1980). When quaternary amine anesthetics, or other related compounds, are present inside axons they produce a use-dependent change of gating current as well as of ionic current (CAHALAN and ALMERS 1979 a; GUSELNIKOVA et al. 1979; KHODOROV et al. 1979). Recall that gating currents reflect a transition of sodium channels from closed to open configurations and back. The closed-open step produces "on-gating" currents and the reverse step produces "off-gating" currents. During repeated depolarization of anesthetic-treated axons the on-gating currents become smaller in a use-dependent way similar to that of the ionic sodium currents (CAHALAN and ALMERS 1979 a, b; REVENKO et al. 1982). This suggests that sodium currents are reduced because fewer channels can open in the presence of the anesthetics. After a long depolarization the off-gating currents are reduced in drug-free nerves, indicating that sodium channels that have become inactivated cannot undergo the transition from open to closed states (ARMSTRONG and BEZANILLA 1977). This so-called off-gating charge "immobilization" is affected in either of two ways by local anesthetics: after a long depolarization the degree of charge immobilization can be smaller, or larger, than that in the drug-free condition indicating that the anesthetic is either potentiating or antagonizing, respectively, the normal inactivation mechanism (CAHALAN and ALMERS 1979 a; CAHALAN et al. 1980; NEUMCKE et al. 1981; REVENKO et al. 1982). Anesthetic molecules thus appear to interact with channels to produce charge immobilization, either by supporting endogenous inactivation mechanisms or by providing a new inactivation function and interfering with the normal one (YEH and ARMSTRONG 1978). These apparently different mechanisms, in effect, may be a consequence of having different anesthetics binding at different sites on the channel.

Earlier we noted that there is a component of the gating current that is not subject to immobilization; see B. III, p. 25). This component also is not sensitive to local anesthetic (benzocaine and QX314) in concentrations that markedly reduce the other component, which does exhibit immobilization (CAHALAN and ALMERS 1979 a, b; BEKKERS et al. 1984). But even though the non-immobilized gating charge is not affected by local anesthetics, it may still arise from an electrically charged portion of the channel, because this remaining charge has faster kinetics than the immobilized charge and may well represent only the first step in the transitions of the activation.

3. The Different Molecular Forms of Local Anesthetics

The experiments described above showing the separability of tonic and use-dependent block (YEH 1980) strongly suggest that there may be more than one kind of site at which the amine local anesthetics bind to block conduction. A different approach to the question of whether there is a single, unique site of action of local anesthetic drugs comes from considering the fact that the amine local anesthetics can exist either as charged or uncharged molecules depending on the environmental pH. Early experiments strongly suggested that most of the local anesthetic activity of lidocaine, for example, resided in the cationic form. This conclusion was

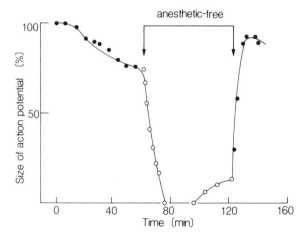

Fig. 4. The amplitude of the action potential of the nonmyelinated fibers of the rabbit vagus nerve in a preparation exposed either to 5 μM dibucaine at pH 9.2 (●) or to anesthetic-free Locke solution at pH 7.2 (○). Note the paradoxical marked intensification of block in the anesthetic-free solution and the substantial recovery on again bathing the nerve in the anesthetic-containing solution

based on experiments in desheathed nerve (Fig. 4) where it was found that during a period that nerve fibres were being loaded with anesthetic in the neutral form (by applying the drug in alkaline solution), conduction continued relatively normally in spite of the relatively high, progressively increasing, concentration of neutral local anesthetic present. However, when the anesthetic was then washed out of the preparation on switching to anesthetic-free solution, but at pH 7.0 when much of the trapped drug was converted to the cationic form, a prompt and complete block of conduction ensued (RITCHIE et al. 1965).

This experiment clearly showed (at least for the particular anesthetic used, dibucaine) that the cationic molecule was much more potent than the uncharged molecule. However, the uncharged molecule cannot be devoid of local anesthetic activity; for benzocaine, which lacks the terminal amino group and hence can never exist in the cationic form, nevertheless produces effective local anesthesia (RITCHIE and RITCHIE 1968) and reduces both ionic sodium currents and gating currents (HILLE 1977a; NEUMCKE et al. 1981). These considerations again raise the question whether both forms of the drug bind to the same site but with different efficacy, or whether there is more than one site of action of the local anesthetic molecules?

4. Inactivation and Local Anesthetic Action

Examining the question of whether amine local anesthetics and neutral analogs act by common or by different mechanisms HILLE (1977b) concluded that all the inhibitory actions of these drugs can be attributed to binding to a single receptor in the membrane. This was an important conclusion, for until then it had been assumed that the charged cationic terminal of the amine anesthetics was necessary for local anesthetic action (see, for example, RITCHIE 1975). On that basis benzocaine could not act by binding to the same site, but had to work by some other mechanism (not necessarily involving binding to a specific site).

Hille's conclusion was based largely on his finding that benzocaine produces the same kind of large shift of the sodium inactivation curve, in the hyperpolarizing direction along the voltage axis, as does lidocaine. This argument, however, became considerably weakened by the demonstration that the volatile anesthetics (SHRIVASTAV et al. 1976; BEAN et al. 1981; HAYDON and URBAN 1983 b), hydrocarbons (HAYDON and KIMURA 1981; HAYDON and URBAN 1983 a) and octanol (SWENSON and OXFORD 1980) all produce similar voltage shifts in the steady-state inactivation curve. These diverse agents might also act at this same single site, but this seems unlikely, for DUBOIS and KHODOROV (1982) have shown that the "protection" from amine local anesthetics afforded by BTX treatment does not occur when n-butanol blocks the channel. This may be an example of terminology and phenomenology obscuring the details of mechanism. "Inactivation" is a general description of the unavailability of channels for voltage-gated opening; it is not indicative of one specific change of state of the channel brought about by operation of a particular physico-chemical mechanism.

5. Competition Between Local Anesthetics

Although discussion of the various experiments described above centered around the question of whether or not the various agents all competed with each other for the same single receptor, it was strange that no actual experiments were conducted to examine the question of competition directly until 1978. Then MROSE and RITCHIE (1978) determined the concentrations of two amine local anesthetics (lidocaine and mepivacaine) and of two neutral agents (benzocaine and benzyl alcohol) that separately produced equal degrees of depression of the compound action potential of a nerve trunk. They then applied 1:1 mixtures of various pairs (i. e. the final concentrations of the two individual drugs were halved). The results were clearcut; mixtures of similar pairs (the two amines or the two neutral agents) were equipotent with the two primary solutions whereas mixtures of dissimilar pairs (an amine and a neutral agent) produced a markedly different degree of block of conduction compared with the block produced by either of the two primary solutions alone. For example, with lidocaine and benzocaine solutions that separately produced the same reduction in action potential size, a 1:1 mixture of the two solutions produced a 70% greater reduction. In mammalian nerve the discrepancy between the enhanced response to the mixture and the responses to either drug alone is less marked, being only 15%–20% (RITCHIE, unpublished observations); nevertheless the deviation is still statistically significant $(0.02 < P < 0.01, n = 7)$. These findings are incompatible with the hypothesis of two agonists competing at equilibrium for the same receptor site.

Support for the idea that there is more than one site of action comes from experiments on drug competition carried out by HUANG and EHRENSTEIN (1981) on quite a different system. They studied the interaction of benzocaine and a quaternary lidocaine analog (QX572) on the uptake of sodium through batrachotoxin-activated sodium channels in cultured neuroblastoma cells. Their experimental protocol was simple. Studying the rate of uptake of radioactive sodium as a function of anesthetic concentration, they determined the equilibrium dissociation constants for inhibition of sodium uptake for each drug separately, and then the equilibrium dissociation constant of the one drug in the presence of a fixed concentration of the other. (The inhibition arises from an apparent competition be-

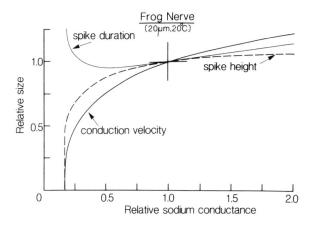

Fig. 5. The dependence on the sodium conductance (expressed relative to its normal value) of both the computed action potential amplitude and conduction velocity

tween the anesthetics and BTX; see D. I., p. 33.) Classical theory requires that if simple competition exists between the two at a single site, the value of the equilibrium dissociation constant under this circumstance should be increased; in this event, it was found actually to decrease. This result, like that of MROSE and RITCHIE (1978), is totally incompatible with a simple system in which the two drugs compete for the same BTX receptor site.

In light of the above it is interesting that more recently SCHMIDTMAYER and ULBRICHT (1980), looking at the responses of single myelinated fibers of the frog to mixtures of lidocaine and benzocaine, have arrived at quite a different conclusion from that of HUANG and EHRENSTEIN (1981) and MROSE and RITCHIE (1978). Measuring the effects of local anesthetics on the sodium current under voltage clamp, they showed that in a system where 0.25 mM lidocaine produced a fractional block of sodium current of 0.71, and 0.5 mM benzocaine produced a fractional block of 0.76, the 1 : 1 mixture (i.e., 0.125 mM lidocaine plus 0.25 mM benzocaine) produced a fractional block of 0.73 $\pm$ 0.03 (SEM), which, as they point out, is consistent with the idea that both drugs act at a single receptor.

However, the findings of SCHMIDTMAYER and ULBRICHT (1980) though *consistent* with the hypothesis of a single site, cannot negate findings, such as those of MROSE and RITCHIE (1978) or of HUANG and EHRENSTEIN (1981), that are clearly inconsistent with this hypothesis. In terms of logic, only a single inconsistent finding is required to upset an argument based on any number of consistent findings, but the process cannot be used in reverse.

The apparent discrepancy in the results might just reflect differences in the experimental indices of local anesthesia used. The advantages of using the action potential (as in MROSE and RITCHIE 1978) is that it involves the use of a sensitive detector of small deviations from a null point. As seen in Fig. 5 simple computer simulations of the type described by RITCHIE and STAGG (1982) show that when 70%–80% of the channel receptors are occupied (and the action potential has fallen to about half its normal value), a small percentage change in receptor occupancy produces a very large change in action potential height. On the other hand, the use of voltage-clamped single myelinated fibers, which has the advantage that the fall in sodium conductance gives a direct linear measure of the binding of an anesthetic molecule to the receptor, has the disadvantage of a loss of sensitivity. For example, suppose there is indeed just one site, with lidocaine and benzocaine having equilibrium dissociation constants of interaction with this site of 0.05 mM and 0.125 mM respectively. Then solutions of 0.1 mM lidocaine and 0.25 mM benzocaine will each separately produce a fractional block of 0.67, and when mixed together will produce the same block of 0.67. This hypothetical case more or less conforms with the case studied experimentally by Schmidtmayer and Ulbricht (1980). Suppose, however, that there are two independent binding sites: a first site that binds both lidocaine and benzocaine with equilibrium dissociation constants of 0.05 mM and 0.25 mM, respectively; and a second that binds only benzocaine with an equilibrium dissociation constant of 0.50 mM. Then the same standard solutions, 0.1 mM lidocaine and 0.25 mM benzocaine, will each separately produce a block of 0.67; however, an equal mixture of the two will produce a somewhat greater block of 0.68. The determination whether there are one or two sites thus depends on distinguishing these two predictions of the single-site and double-site hypothesis (0.67 and 0.68 respectively) from each other, which would not be easy.

The above example was taken for the sake of illustration, and there are many other possible variants. Indeed, if one allows the two primary responses of the standard solutions to differ greatly (letting the fractional block by the one solution be 0.7 and the block by the other to be 0.3, and if one again assumes that lidocaine (or benzocaine) interacts with only one of the receptors whereas benzocaine (or lidocaine) interacts with both receptors, one can readily choose values of the equilibrium dissociation constants such that the response to equal mixtures of the two solutions is greater than, the same as, or even less than that predicted on the basis of a single site of action.

6. Specific and Nonspecific Mechanisms of Action of Local Anesthetics

In this previous discussion, the values of anesthetic potency were confined to those producing the tonic or resting block. Further experiments on voltage-clamped axons provide support for competition between different anesthetics during use-dependent block. Benzocaine has some component of action which favors an "inactivated-like" state of sodium channels, but cannot be fully expressed when channels are inhibited by procaine (Rimmel et al. 1978) or by lidocaine (Schmidtmayer and Ulbricht 1980). One simple explanation for these observations is that charged and neutral local anesthetics can bind, with mutual exclusion, to the same site on the channel; their relative rates of binding and dissociation from this receptor as the channel changes conformation produce the observed changes in use-dependent block. But another explanation is that there are in fact separate sites for the binding of neutral and charged anesthetics, and that the binding of one type favors a conformation of the channel which has little or no affinity for the other (Almers and Cahalan 1982). This involves a more general model than the first proposition, and it could readily account for the apparent discrepancy between the results from use-dependent block (Schmidtmayer and Ulbricht 1980; Rimmel et al. 1978; Pichon et al. 1981) and those from the "tonic block" assays of Mrose and Ritchie (1978) and Huang and Ehrenstein

(1981). For use-dependent blockade will test the nonequilibrium inhibition by anesthetics apparently competing for several voltage-modulated channel states, whereas tonic inhibition results from the equilibrium binding of anesthetics to the channel states in the resting membrane, and there is no reason, a priori, to expect these two assays to agree, unless there is only one receptor with a single affinity for any anesthetic, regardless of channel state. Indeed, ZABOROVSKAYA and KHODOROV (1982) have shown that a charged anesthetic has a higher affinitiy for normal, resting sodium channels than for batrachotoxin-modified channels, whereas neutral benzocaine blocks the two forms identically. One exclusive anesthetic receptor cannot explain this result.

There is no doubt concerning the general validity of the modulated receptor hypothesis for local anesthetic action, namely that there is in the sodium channel of excitable membranes a site to which local anesthetics bind in a manner that depends on the conformation of the channel. Clearly, the hypothesis would gain in elegance if it could be shown to be the *exclusive* mechanism of local anesthetic action. Unfortunately, as discussed in the previous section, there is at the moment neither theoretical nor experimental basis for this assumption. A single binding site for local anesthetics just cannot easily account for the diversity of experimental findings in studies on tonic and use-dependent block on gating currents, on the potency of different molecular forms, and on the competition between charged and uncharged molecules. Whether this means that there are two distinct binding sites for which lidocaine or benzocaine each have a different affinity, or whether there is a large number of different sites for which each drug has a different spectrum of affinities, or whether there is more than one kind of mechanism of action (for example, a modulated receptor and another non-receptor mechanism of action analogous to that involved in anesthesia with alcohol) remains open at the present time.

Granted that there is a specific binding site in the sodium channel to which local anesthetics bind, what other possible sites or mechanism of action exist? One possibility suggested by RITCHIE (1975) is that the lipophilic portion of the local anesthetic molecule enters the lipid axolemmal membrane leaving its cationic head exposed on the external face. There is thus an increase in the density of the fixed positive charges in the membrane, an effective increase in the true transmembranal potential and hence a decrease in excitability. Studies of ionophoric conductances in artificial lipid bilayers show that local anesthetics can change the electric potential by adsorbing at the membrane surface (MCLAUGHLIN 1975). However, such a mechanism would be expected to change the voltage-dependence of sodium channel activation and also to be accomplished by the $4°$ amine anesthetics, which do modify the conductances in bilayers. Neither of these occurs in nerves and a more likely hypothesis is that local anesthetics act in their uncharged form more like general anesthetics to produce conduction block, (RITCHIE and RITCHIE 1968; RITCHIE 1975) and this possibility is discussed below.

General anesthesia can be produced by a large number of substances of quite diverse and unrelated chemical structure. The concentrations of the different agents required to produce general anesthesia vary, on a molar basis, by several orders of magnitude (see MILLER 1981). However, when expressed in terms of thermodynamic activity (FERGUSON 1939; see also MULLINS 1954; MILLER 1981)

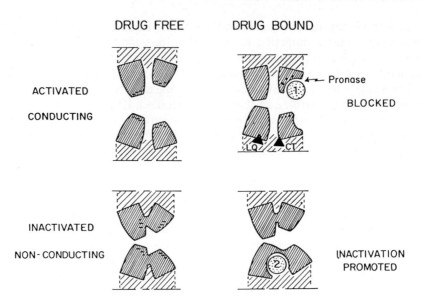

Fig. 6. A highly schematic diagram of sodium channel inhibition by local anesthetics. Two distinct sites for anesthetic binding are shown, located near the cytoplasmic entrance to the hydrophilic pore (*1*) and at the macromolecule's protein:lipid interface (*2*). Site 1 is exposed during activation and is sensitive to digestion by exogenous cytoplasmic proteases. Polar and charged anesthetics bind preferably at site 1: uncharged lipophilic anesthetics act at site 2, as might alcohols, inhalational anesthetics, and various hydrocarbons. The filled triangles indicate proposed sites for the action of α-scorpion toxins (*LQ*) and chloramine-T (*CT*), agents that inhibit normal channel inactivation but have minimal effects on use-dependent block

their potencies become remarkably constant. Thus, taking the thermodynamic activity of a saturated solution as unity, one finds that all the agents produce general anesthesia in a thermodynamic concentration of 0.02–0.04. For the few such agents that have also been tested for local anesthetic potency, the concentrations required have been up to 5 times greater. It is interesting, therefore, in this context to note that: first, the aqueous solubility of benzocaine (and of the uncharged forms of local anesthetics) is quite low (less than 5 mM); and secondly the thermodynamic activity of the concentration required to produce nerve block (0.25–1 mM) is of the same order (0.05–0.20 mM) as that found for the other general anesthetic agents studied. We are drawn, therefore, to speculate that benzocaine (and indeed all local anesthetics in their uncharged form) shares with general anesthetics the ability to block nerve conduction by a mechanism, as yet unknown, that does not involve a specific receptor site of the kind required in the modulated receptor hypothesis.

Two probable loci for local anesthetic action are designated in the schematic of Fig. 6. One site lies near the channel pore at the axoplasmic opening, although not necessarily "within" the pore. The other site exists at the protein:lipid interface of the channel macromolecule. The first site (1) selctively binds the more polar and the charged local anesthetics, with an affinity that is increased by depolarizing voltage pulses, accounting for much use-dependent inhibition; binding here is quite susceptible to channel exposure to internal proteolytic enzymes. The second site (2) selectively binds the more lipophilic anesthetics. Channels appear to be functionally more inactivated by drugs bound at this site, which has much weaker specificity than site 1. Proteolytic enzymes do not affect binding at this locus, which is probably also the site where the alcohols and the volatile general anesthetics act. Site 1 and 2 can be occupied simultaneously by their corresponding ligands, although there may be some interactions between the two sites.

E. New Kinds of Local Anesthetic Agents

With the exception of benzocaine, all the local anesthetics in general use today are of the amino type (such as lidocaine and procaine). In their cationic form the evidence is now strong that these amino local anesthetics block conduction because they interact with a binding site on the sodium channel macromolecule to prevent complete channel activation. The various amino local anesthetics seem to compete with each other in a simple manner, although the detailed consequences of their specific actions may vary.

However, as has been suggested above, interaction with this site may not be the only mechanism for blocking the sodium channel and hence nerve conduction. For example, barbiturates and various volatile general anesthetics are known to block conduction (see NEUMAN and FRANK 1977; KENDIG 1981; STRICHARTZ 1980) by some as yet unidentified mechanism. Presumably benzocaine, and possibly the uncharged forms of the amino local anesthetics, also act in this way. In addition there are a variety of pharmacological agents and toxins that interact quite specifically with the sodium channel at sites other than that at which the amino local anesthetics interact (see RITCHIE 1979; STRICHARTZ 1980). Two such agents are tetrodotoxin (TTX), which is produced by various pufferfish, sunfish, salamanders, octopi, and frogs, and saxitoxin (STX), which is produced by certain marine dinoflagellates. These toxins, which are chemically different from each other (and totally distinct from the amino local anesthetics in general), have only one known pharmacological action: they specifically block sodium channels in excitable tissues by combining with a site at the outer opening of the sodium channel and which is accessible from the external but not from the internal side of the plasmalemma. Both act in the identical way in nanomolar concentrations; and on removal of the toxins recovery of conduction is complete and rapid. Although these toxins, because of their cationic charge at physiological pH, do not readily penetrate cellular membranes, and so are unlikely to be clinically effective as local anesthetics, they do raise the possibility that a new class of local anesthetics may be developed, perhaps based on modifications of the original toxin molecules. The importance of these two toxins lies in the fact that their site of action seems to be quite different from the site of action of the amino local anesthetics. Thus their spectrum of toxic reactions may be quite different from those in current use. Furthermore, the possibility is raised of producing alkylating analogs, which having been directed to the site of action, namely the sodium channel, by the high pharmacological specificity for a binding site, may by subsequent alkylation produce local anesthesia of extremely long duration of action – analogous to the long-lasting blockade of adrenergic receptors by the alkylating agent dibenzylene.

A local anesthetic agent that acted at a site different from that of the conventional amino local anesthetic would be extremely valuable on quite different grounds (see EHRENSTEIN and HUANG 1981). For example, consider the case of two blocking agents A and B in concentrations C_A and C_B respectively, whose equilibrium dissociation constants with the appropriate binding site(s) are K_A and K_B respectively. Since the safety factor for conduction in these fibres is about 5.5 (CHIU and RITCHIE 1984), the minimum concentration required to block conduction would be such that $C_A/K_A = 4.5$. If A and B were two amino local anesthetics acting at the same modulated receptor site, a 1 : 1 mixture of the two solutions (i. e. containing 0.5 C_A plus 0.5 C_B) would again be just minimally effective, being equal in potency to each of the original two solutions; and the toxicity of the mixture would not differ greatly from that of the original solutions. However, if they acted at two quite independent sites, they would be much more effective; and indeed the concentrations of each in the mixture could be reduced by a further factor to produce a mixture containing 0.3 C_A and 0.3 C_B (the remaining sodium conductance being $(1 + 0.3 \times 4.5)^{-2}$, i.e., virtually equal to $(1 + 4.5)^{-1}$ obtaining in the case of each of the single drugs). If as is sometimes the case with drugs of completely different structure, the toxicities of the two molecules were different, this reduction in the total amount of drug present might be of great significance clinically. Indeed, the beneficial effect from the use of two agents acting at different sites would be even greater if one used, as is likely clinically, concentrations in excess of the minimal blocking concentration. For example, if C_A and C_B were each twice the minimal blocking concentration, a 1 : 1 mixture of the two solutions would be 3.4 times the minimal blocking concentration of that mixture. This would therefore produce a degree of block that was both more intense and more longlasting, without increasing the toxicity; indeed since each drug is present in half the concentration present in the two original solutions, the toxicity may even be considerably less.

It is because of these considerations that a local anesthetic agent acting at some different site from that of the amino local anesthetics would be desirable. Tetrodotoxin and saxitoxin have indeed been tested in this regard; and it has been found that when mixed with conventional local anesthetics, they produce a rapid onset of block characteristic of the amino local anesthetics but with a much longer duration of action. This potential for enhancement of blocking activity by the use of mixture of agents has been demonstrated in isolated nerves in vitro by STAIMAN and SEEMAN (1975) who found in frog sciatic nerve that the duration of conduction block produced by mixtures of saxitoxin and local anesthetic agents was markedly longer, and more intense, than with either saxitoxin or the local anesthetic agents alone. It has also been studied extensively by ADAMS et al. (1976) who examined the local anesthetic activity of mixtures of saxitoxin with procaine, lidocaine, dibucaine, mepivacaine, and cocaine when used to produce sciatic nerve block in the rat and epidural anesthesia in the dog. They found that the duration of block with an saxitoxin-bupivacaine mixture was at least 1.5–2 times longer than with either agent alone, and the block with other mixtures 4–8 times longer.

F. Effects of Local Anesthetics on Potassium Channels

Local anesthetics are able to block potassium channels, but at higher concentrations than those required to block sodium channels. The predominant effect according to TAYLOR (1959) is simply a reduction in the potassium permeability of the membrane by a factor that is independent of membrane potential. The susceptibility of K^+ channels to local anesthetics, relative to that of Na^+ channels, depends on the particular anesthetics and, perhaps to a lesser extent, on the membrane under study. For example, TAYLOR (1959) found that in the squid axon treated with procaine K^+ currents were reduced by 13% when Na currents were 60% blocked. The more lipophilic anesthetic dibucaine inhibited Na^+ current almost completely with no detectable effect on K^+ currents (GILLY and ARMSTRONG 1980). In amphibian node of Ranvier, amine-type local anesthetics are also much more active in blocking sodium channels, but have some effect on potassium channels. HILLE (1966) recorded about a 15% reduction of I_K with lidocaine and a smaller decrease but pronounced slowing of current activation with procaine in frog nodes treated with 3.5 mM anesthetic, sufficient to block I_{Na} totally. ARHEM and FRANKENHAEUSER (1974) showed that the relative blocking potencies of lidocaine, procaine, and benzocaine to produce a given reduction in $P_{Na}:P_K$ in toad axons were 8.5, 47, and 7.3, respectively. In theory the ability of anesthetics to block impulses by inhibiting inward sodium currents will be compromised by any action of anesthetics in reducing the outward potassium currents. Any blocking effect on the potassium channels, however, is unlikely to be important clinically as far as conduction block of very rapidly conducting fibers is concerned. The potassium conductance grows too slowly compared to the large, rapid sodium conductance to affect the initial generation of the nerve impulse, (although it does clearly affect the falling phase of the action potential). Indeed, as far as conduction velocity is concerned, computer simulations similar to those carried out by RITCHIE and STAGG (RITCHIE and STAGG 1982; see also FRANKENHAUSER and HUXLEY 1964; GOLDMAN and ALBUS 1968; HUTCHINSON et al. 1970) confirm the slightness of this effect. As Fig. 7 shows, when the relative sodium conductance (in the computation) is decreased there is a progressive fall

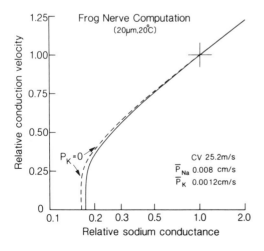

Fig. 7. The computed effect of completely blocking the potassium conductance (i.e. with $P_K = 0$) on the minimum sodium conductance at which conduction is just possible

in conduction velocity; and conduction fails when the relative conductance has fallen to a value of about 0.175 (i. e. the safety factor is about 5.6). When the same simulation is performed but in the absence of a voltage-dependent potassium conductance, the conduction velocity is scarcely affected except near block when the relative sodium conductance can be decreased by a further slight amount (about 6%) before conduction block occurs. This would correspond with an increase in the amount of local anesthetic required to produce block of only 7%.

In contrast, for slower conducting fibers where sodium channels are more sparse and the action potential rises more slowly, effects of anesthetics on potassium channels may strongly reduce their potency. By example, simulations of membrane action potentials of a Hodgkin-Huxley squid axon at 6 °C showed that 7–8 times as much anesthetic was needed to block impulse generation when the potassium channels as well as the sodium channels were inhibited by the drug (at half the affinity) (STRICHARTZ 1985). Indeed, one source of differential anesthetic fiber blockade could be the densities of sodium and potassium channels in various axons.

G. Conclusion

The amino local anesthetics block conduction by inhibiting normal activation of the sodium channel, hence preventing the influx of sodium ions and so causing conduction block. The balance of experimental evidence is not in favor of just one single mechanism of local anesthetic action. One mechanism – possibly the major mechanism involved with the commonly used amino local anesthetics – seems to involve a specific, voltage-dependent, modulated receptor, to which the local anesthetic molecule specifically binds to inhibit the channel. There also seems to be another mechanism, which may be similar to the mechanism by which general anesthetics block conduction, that is particularly relevant in the case of the uncharged forms of local anesthetics. The actions of drugs which represent both classes are characterized by a reduction of macroscopic membrane permeability paralleled by a decrease in the gating current, which arises from some of the conformational changes a channel undergoes during the opening process. From this decrease in gating current and from the altered voltage-dependence of certain gating functions, it appears that an anesthetized channel is in an "inactivated" state. However, channels which do not inactivate rapidly can also be inhibited by local anesthetics in both tonic and use-dependent modes. The inhibitory mechanism may involve conversions to "slowly inactivated" conformations with greater affinity for anesthetics. Since the use-dependent inhibition by some, but not all, local anesthetics is removed after exposure to proteolytic enzymes in the axoplasm, the anesthetic binding site itself or some kinetic modulator of that site is located towards the inner surface of the channel. The fact that actions of only some anesthetics are lessened by enzyme digestion could mean that their kinetic schemes differ from those of the drugs that show altered activity and not necessarily that they involve separate binding sites (STARMER et al. 1984). For all the mechanistic interpretations of local anesthetic action, the assignment of channel states derived from gating studies to anesthetic receptor conformations with different affinities must be justified on the basis of current experimental evidence rather than loose agreements in kinetics and voltage-dependence.

The possibility of blocking conduction in yet other ways is currently being explored. New kinds of local anesthetics, acting by still different mechanisms, would be important if they had a different spectrum of toxicities from the amino local anesthetics currently used. Furthermore, by using combinations of nerve blocking drugs that acted independently at different sites, more intense, longer-lasting, blockade is in principle possible while at the same time reducing toxicity.

Acknowledgements. The authors thank Dr. John F. Butterworth for thoughtful comments on the manuscript. During the period over which this chapter was written, financial support was provided by the US Public Health Service in the form of research awards to JMR (NS 08304 and NS 12327) and to GRS (GM/NS 30160 and GM 15904).

References

Adam KR, Schmidt H, Stampfli R, Weiss C (1976) The effect of scorpion venom on single myelinated nerve fibers of the frog. Br J Pharmacol 26:666–677

Adams HJ, Blair MR Jr., Takman BH (1976) The local anesthetic activity of tetrodotoxin alone and in combinations with vasoconstrictors and local anesthetics. Anesth Analg 55:568–573

Agnew WS, Levinson SR, Brabson JS, Raferty Ma (1978) Purification of the tetrodotoxin binding component associated with the voltage-sensitive sodium channel from *Electrophorus electricus* electroplax membranes. Proc Natl Acad Sci USA 75:2606–2610

Aldrich RW, Corey DP, Stephens CF (1983) A reinterpretation of mammalian sodium channel gating based on single channel recording. Nature 306:436–441

Almers W, Cahalan MD (1982) Block of sodium channels by internally applied drugs: two receptors for tertiary and quaternary amine compounds? In: Salanki J (ed) Adv Physiol Sci, Pergamon Press

Almers W, Levinson SR (1975) Tetrodotoxin binding to normal and depolarized frog muscle and the conductance of a single sodium channel. J Physiol (Lond) 247:483–509

Arhem P, Frankenhaeuser B (1974) Local anesthetics: effects on permeability properties of nodal membrane in myelinated nerve fibres from Xenopus. Potential clamp experiments. Acta Physiol Scand 91:11–21

Armstrong CM, Bezanilla F (1974) Charge movement associated with the opening and closing of the activation gates of the Na channels. J Gen Physiol 63:533–552

Armstrong CM, Bezanilla F (1977) Inactivation of the sodium channel. II. Gating current experiments. J Gen Physiol 70:567–590

Armstrong CM, Croop RS (1982) Simulation of Na channel inactivation by thiazin dyes. J Gen Physiol 80:641–662

Armstrong CM, Bezanilla F, Rojas E (1973) Destruction of sodium conductance inactivation in squid axons perfused with pronase. J Gen Physiol 62:375–391

Barchi RL, Cohen SA, Murphy LE (1980) Purification from rat sarcolemma of the saxitoxin-binding component of the excitable membrane sodium channel. Proc Natl Acad Sci USA 77:1306–1310

Barhanin J, Pauron D, Lombet A, Norman RI, Vijverberg HPM, Giglio JR, Lazdunski, M (1983) Electrophysiological characterization, solubilization and purification of the *Tityus* γ toxin receptor associated with the gating component of the Na$^+$ channel from rat brain. EMBO J 2:915–920

Bean BP, Shrager P, Goldstein DA (1981) Modification of sodium and potassium channel gating kinetics by ether and halothane. J Gen Physiol 77:233–253

Bekkers JM, Greeff NG, Keynes RD, Neumcke B (1984) The effect of local anaesthetics on the components of the asymmetry current in the squid giant axon. J Physiol (Lond) 352:653–668

Beneski DA, Catterall WA (1980) Covalent labeling of protein components of the sodium channel with a photoactivable derivative of scorpion toxin. Proc Natl Acad Sci USA 77:639–643

Bezanilla R, Armstrong CM (1977) Inactivation of sodium channel: I. Sodium current experiments. J Gen Physiol 70:547–566

Bokesch PM, Post C, Strichartz GR (1986) Structure-activity relationship of lidocaine homologues on tonic and frequency-dependent impulse blockade in nerve. J Pharmacol Exp Ther 237:773–781

Bradley DJ, Richards CD (1984) Temperature-dependence of the action of nerve blocking agents and its relationship to membrane-buffer partition coefficients: thermodynamic implications for the site of action of local anaesthetics. Br J Pharmacol 81:161–167

Buchi J, Perlia X (1971) Structure-activity relations and physicochemical properties of local anesthetics. In: Lajtha A (ed) International Encyclopedia of Pharmacology and Therapeutics 8. Pergamon, London, pp 39–129

Cahalan M (1975) Modification of sodium channel gating in frog myelinated nerve fibers by *Centruroides sculpturatus* scorpion venom. J Physiol (Lond) 244:511–534

Cahalan M (1978) Local anesthetic block of sodium channels in normal and pronase-treated squid giant axons. Biophys J 23:285–311

Cahalan MD, Almers W (1979 a) Interactions between quaternary lidocaine, the sodium channel gates and tetrodotoxin. Biophys J 27:39–56

Cahalan MD, Almers W (1979 b) Block of sodium conductance and gating current in squid gian axons poisoned with quaternary strychnine. Biophys J 27:57–74

Cahalan M, Shapiro BI, Almers W (1980) Relations between inactivation of sodium channels and block by quaternary derivatives of local anesthetics and other compounds. In: Fink BR (ed) Molecular mechanism of anesthesia. Raven, New York, Progress in Anesthesiology, vol 2

Catterall WA (1975) Cooperative activation of action potential Na$^+$ ionophore by neurotoxins. Proc Natl Acad Sci USA 72:1782–1786

Catterall WA (1980) Neurotoxins that act on voltage-sensitive sodium channels in excitable membranes. Ann Rev Pharmacol Toxicol 20:15–43

Chiu SY, Ritchie JM (1984) On the physiological role of internodal potassium channels and the security of conduction in myelinated nerve fibers. Proc R Soc Lond (Biol) 220:415–422

Chiu SY, Mrose HE, Ritchie JM (1979) Anomalous temperature dependence of the sodium conductance in rabbit nerve compared with frog nerve. Nature 279:327–328

Cohen SA, Barchi RL (1981) Glycoprotein characteristics of the sodium channel saxitoxin-binding component from mammalian sarcolemma. Biochim Biophys Acta 645:253–261

Coluhoun D, Henderson R, Ritchie JM (1972) The binding of labelled tetrodotoxin to non-myelinatet nerve fibers. J Physiol (Lond) 227:95–126

Courtney KR (1974) Frequency-dependent inhibition of sodium currents in frog myelinated nerve by GEA 968, a new lidocaine derivative. PhD thesis, Dept. of Physiology and Biophysics, University of Washington

Courtney KR (1975) Mechanism of frequency-dependent inhibition of sodium currents in frog myelinated nerve by the lidocaine derivative GEA-968. J Pharmacol Exp Ther 195:225–236

Courtney KR (1980) Structure-activity relations for frequency-dependent sodium channel block in nerve by local anesthetics. J Pharmacol Exp Ther 213:114–119

Courtney KR, Etter EF (1983) Modulated anticonvulsant block of sodium channels in nerve and muscle. Eur J Pharmacol 88:1–9

Courtney KR, Kendig JJ, Cohen EN (1978) The rates of interaction of local anesthetics with sodium channels in nerve. J Pharmacol Exp Ther 207:594–604

Dubois JM, Khodorov BI (1982) Batrachotoxin protects sodium channels from the blocking action of oenanthotoxin. Pflugers Arch 395:55–58

Eaton DC, Brodwick MS, Oxford GS, Rudy B (1978) Arginine-specific reagents remove sodium channel inactivation. Nature 271:473–475

Ehrenstein G, Huang LYM (1981) Synergism based on binding of drugs to separate but equivalent binding sites. Science 214:1365–1366

Ferguson J (1939) The use of chemical potentials as indices of toxicity. Proc R Soc Lond (Biol) 127:387–404

Frankenhauser B, Huxley AF (1964) The action potential in the myelinated fibre of *Xenopus laevis* as computed on the basis of voltage clamp data. J Physiol (Lond) 171:302–325

Frazier DT, Narahashi T, Yamada M (1970) The site of action and active form of local anesthetics. II. Experiments with quaternary compounds. J Pharmacol Exp Ther 171:45–51

Gilly WF, Armstrong CM (1980) Gating current and potassium channels in the giant axon of the squid. Biophys J 29:485–492

Goldman L, Albus JS (1968) Computation of impulse conduction in myelinated fibres; theoretical basis of the velocity-diameter relation. Biophys J 8:596–607

Guselnikova G, Peganov E, Khodorov B (1979) Blockage of the gating current in the node of Ranvier by the quaternary lidocaine derivative QX-572. Dok Akad Nauk SSSR 224:1492–1495

Hartshorne RP, Catterall WA (1981) Purification of the saxitoxin receptor of the sodium channel from rat brain. Proc Natl Acad Sci USA 78:4620–4624

Haydon DA, Kimura JE (1981) Some effects of n-pentane on the sodium and potassium currents of the squid giant axon. J Physiol (Lond) 312:57–70

Haydon DA, Urban BW (1983a) The action of hydrocarbons and carbon tetrachloride on the sodium current of the squid giant axon. J Physiol (Lond) 338:435–450

Haydon DA, Urban BW (1983b) The action of alcohols and other non-ionic surface active substances on the sodium current of the squid giant axon. J Physiol (Lond) 341:411–427

Haydong DA, Urban BW (1983c) The effects of some inhalation anaesthetics on the sodium current of the squid giant axon. J Physiol (Lond) 341:429–439

Henderson R, Strichartz G (1974) Ion fluxes through the sodium channels of garfish olfactory nerve membranes. J Physiol (Lond) 238:329–342

Henderson R, Ritchie JM, Strichartz GR (1973) The binding of labelled saxitoxin to the sodium channels in nerve membranes. J Physiol (Lond) 235:783–804

Hille B (1966) The common mode of action of three agents that decrease the transient change in sodium permeability in nerves. Nature 210:1220–1222

Hille B (1968) Pharmacological modifications of the sodium channel of frog nerve. J Gen Physiol 51:199–219

Hille B (1970) Ionic channels in nerve membranes. Prog Biophys Mol Biol 21:1–32

Hille B (1972) The permeability of the sodium channel to metal cations in myelinated nerve. J Gen Physiol 59:637–658

Hille B (1977a) The pH-dependent rate of action of local anesthetics on the node of Ranvier. J Gen Physiol 69:475–496

Hille B (1977b) Local anesthetics: hydrophilic and hydrophobic pathways for the drug-receptor reaction. J Gen Physiol 69:497–575

Hille B (1978) Local anesthetic action on inactivation of the Na Channel in nerve and skeletal muscle: possible mechanisms for antiarrhythmic agents. In: Morad M (ed) Biophysical aspects of cardiac muscle. Academic, New York

Hille B (1980) Theories of anesthesia: general perturbations versus specific receptors. Prog Anesthesiol 2:1–6

Hille N, Courtney K, Dum R (1975) Rate and site of action of local anesthetics in myelinated nerve fibers. Prog Anesthesiol 1:13–20

Hodgkin AL, Huxley AE (1952) A quantitative description of membrane current and its application to conduction and excitation in nerve. J Physiol (Lond) 117:500–544

Horn R, Patlak J, Stevens CF (1981) Sodium channels need not open before they inactivate. Nature 291:426–427

Huang L-Y M, Ehrenstein G (1981) Local anesthetics QX572 and benzocaine act at separate sites on the batrachotoxin-activated sodium channel. J Gen Physiol 77:155–176

Hutchinson NA, Koles ZJ, Smith RS (1970) Conduction velocity in myelinated nerve fibres of *Xenopus laevis*. J Physiol (Lond) 208:279–289

Kendig J (1981) Barbiturates: active form and site of action at node of Ranvier sodium channels. J Pharmacol Exp Ther 218:175–181

Kendig JJ, Courtney KR, Cohen EN (1979) Anesthetics: molecular correlates of voltage- and frequency-dependent sodium channel block in nerve. J Pharmacol Exp Ther 210:446–452

Keynes RD, Rojas (1974) Kinetics and steady-state properties of the charged system controlling sodium conductance in the squid giant axon. J Physiol (Lond) 239:393–434

Khodorov BI (1978) Chemicals as tools to study nerve fiber sodium channels: effects of batrachotoxin and some local anesthetics. In: Tosteson DC, Ovchinnikov YA, Latorre R (eds) Raven, New York

Khodorov B, Shishkova L, Peganov E, Revenko S (1976) Inhibition of sodium currents in frog Ranvier node treated with local anesthetics. Role of slow sodium inactivation. Biochim Biophys Acta 433:409–435

Khodorov B, Goselnikova G, Peganov E (1979) Effect of benzocaine of Na^+ and gating currents in the node of Ranvier. Dokl Akad Nauk SSSR 244:1251–1255

Krueger BK, Ratzlaff RW, Strichartz GR, Blaustein MP (1979) Saxitoxin binding to synaptosomes, membranes and solubilized binding sites from rat brain. J Membr Biol 50:287–310

Krueger BK, Worley JF, French RJ (1983) Single sodium channels from rat brain incorporated into planar lipid bilayer membranes. Nature 303:172–175

Lee AG (1976) Model for action of local anesthetics. Nature 262:545–548

McLaughlin S (1975) Local anesthetics and the electrical properties of phospholipid bilayer membranes. In: Fink BR (ed) Molecular mechanisms of anesthesia. Raven, New York, pp 193–220

Miller JA, Agnew WS, Levinson SR (1983) Principle glycopeptide of the tetrodotoxin/saxitoxin binding protein from Electrophorus electricus: isolation and partial chemical and physical characterization. Biochemistry 22:462–470

Miller KW (1981) General anesthetics. In: Wolf M (ed) Burger's medicinal chemistry, 4th ed. Wiley, New York, pp 623–644

Moczydlowski E, Hall S, Garber SS, Strichartz GR, Miller C (1984) Voltage-dependent blockade of muscle Na^+ channels by quanidinium toxins. Effect of toxin charge. J Gen Physiol 84:687–704

Mrose HE, Ritchie JM (1978) Local anesthetics: do benozcaine and lidocaine act at the same single site? J Gen Physiol 71:223–225

Mullins LJ (1954) Some physical mechanisms in narcosis. Chem Rev 54:289–323

Narahashi T, Haas HG, Therrien EF (1967) Saxitoxin and tetrodotoxin: comparison of nerve blocking mechanism. Science 157:1441–1442

Narahashi T, Frazier D, Yamada M (1970) The site of action and active form of local anesthetics. I. Theory and pH experiments with tertiary compounds. J Pharmacol Exp Ther 171:32–44

Neuman RS, Frank GB (1977) Effects of diphenylhydantoin and phenobarbital on voltage-clamped myelinated nerve. Can J Physiol Pharmacol 55:42–47

Neumcke B, Schwarz W, Stampfli R (1981) Block of Na channels in the membrane of myelinated nerve by benzocaine. Pflugers Arch 390:230–236

Nonner W (1980) Relations between the inactivation of sodium channels and the immobilization of gating charge in frog myelinated nerve. J Physiol (Lond) 299:573–603

Nonner W, Spalding BC, Hille B (1980) Low intracellular pH and chemical agents slow inactivation gating in sodium channels of muscle. Nature 284:360–363

Oxford GS, Wu CH, Narahashi T (1978) Removal of sodium channel inactivation in squid giant axons by N-bromoacetamide. J Gen Physiol 71:227–247

Pichon Y, Schmidtmayer J, Ulbricht W (1981) Mutually exclusive blockage of sodium channels of myelinated frog nerve fibres by benzocaine and the indole alkaloid ervatamine. Neurosci Lett 22:325–330

Postma SW, Catterall WA (1984) Inhibition of binding of H-Batrachotoxin A 20-α-Benzoate to sodium channels by local anesthetics. Mol Pharmacol 25:219–227

Revenko SV, Khodorov BI, Shapovalova LM (1982) The effect of yohimbine on sodium and gating currents in frog Ranvier node membrane. Neuroscience 7:1377–1387

Rimmel C, Walle A, Kesler H, Ulbricht W (1978) Rates of block by procaine and benzocaine and the procaine-benzocaine interaction at the node of Ranvier. Pflugers Arch 376:105–118

Ritchie JM (1975) Mechanism of action of local anesthetic agents and biotoxins. Br J Anaesth 47:191–198

Ritchie JM (1978) Sodium channel as a drug receptor. In: Straub RW, Bolis L (eds) Cell membrane receptors for drugs and hormones. A multidisciplinary approach. Raven, New York, pp 242–277

Ritchie JM (1979) A pharmacological approach to the structure of sodium channels in myelinated axons. Annu Rev Neurosci 2:341–362

Ritchie JM, Ritchie B (1968) Local anesthetics: effect of pH on activity. Science 162:1394–1395

Ritchie JM, Rogart RB (1977) The binding of saxitoxin and tetrodotoxin to excitable membranes. Rev Physiol Biochem Pharmacol 79:1–50

Ritchie JM, Stagg D (1982) A note on the effects of potassium conductance (g_k) on conduction velocity in myelinated fibres. J Physiol (Lond) 328:32–33 P

Ritchie JM, Ritchie BR, Greengard P (1965) The active structure of local anesthetics. J Pharmacol Exp Ther 150:152–159

Rosenberg RL, Tomika, SA, Agnew WS (1984 a) Reconstitution of neurotoxin-modulated ion transport by the voltage-regulated sodium channel isolated from the electroplax of *Electrophorus electricus*. Proc Natl Acad Sci USA 81:1239–1243

Rosenberg RL, Tomiko SA, Agnew WS (1984 b) Single-channel properties of the reconstituted voltage-regulated Na channel isolated from the electroplax of *Electrophorus electricus*. Proc Natl Acad Sci USA 81:5594–5598

Schmidtmayer J, Ulbricht N (1980) Interaction of lidocaine and benzocaine in blocking sodium channels. Pflugers Arch 387:47–54

Schwarz W, Palade PT, Hille B (1977) Local anesthetics: effect of pH on use-dependent block of sodium channels in frog muscle. Biophys J 20:343–368

Seeman P (1972) The membrane actions of anesthetics and tranquilizers. Pharmacol Rev 24:583–655

Shapiro BI (1977) Effect of strychnine on the sodium conductance of the frog node of Ranvier. J Gen Physiol 69:915–920

Shepley MP, Strichartz GR, Wang GK (1983) Local anesthetics block non-inactivating sodium channels in a use-dependent manner in amphibian myelinated axons. J Physiol (Lond) 341:62 P

Shrivastav BB, Narahashi T, Kitz RJ, Roberts JD (1976) Mode of action of trichloroethylene on squid axon membranes. J Pharmacol Exp Ther 199:179–188

Spalding BC (1980) Properties of toxin-resistant sodium channels produced by chemical modification in frog skeletal muscle. J Physiol (Lond) 305:485–500

Staiman AL, Seeman P (1975) Different sites of membrane action for tetrodotoxin and lipid-soluble anaesthetics. Can J Physiol Pharmacol 53:513–524

Stallcup W (1977) Comparative pharmacology of voltage-dependent sodium channels. Brain Res 135:37–53

Starmer CF, Grant AO, Strauss H (1984) Mechanisms of use-dependent block of sodium channels in excitable membranes by local anesthetics. Biophys J 46:15–28

Strichartz GR (1973) The inhibition of sodium currents in myelinated nerve by quaternary derivatives of lidocaine. J Gen Physiol 62:37–57

Strichartz GR (1975) Inhibition of ionic currents in myelinated nerves by quaternary derivatives of lidocaine. In: Fink BR (ed) Molecular mechanism of anesthesia. Raven, New York, pp 1–11

Strichartz GR (1977) The composition and structure of excitable nerve membrane. In: Jamieson GA, Robinson DM (eds) Mammalian cell membranes, vol 3. Butterworths, London, pp 172–205

Strichartz GR (1980) Use-dependent conduction block produced by volatile general anesthetic agents. Acta Anesthesiol Scand 24:402–406

Strichartz GR (1981) Pharmacological properties of sodium channels in nerve membranes. In: Waxman SG, Ritchie JM (eds) Demyelinating disease: basic and clinical electrophysiology. Raven, New York

Strichartz GR (1985) Interactions of local anesthetics with neuronal sodium channels. In: Covino B, Fozzard HA, Rehder K, Strichartz GR (eds) Effects of anesthesia. Clinical physiology series. American Physiological Society, Bethesda, MD pp 39–52

Strichartz G, Wang GK (1986a) The kinetic basis for phasic local anesthetic blockade of neuronal sodium channels. In: Miller KW, Roth S (eds) Molecular and cellular mechanisms of anesthetics. Plenum Publishing Corp, New York, pp 217–226

Strichartz G, Wang GK (1986b) Rapid voltage-dependent dissociation of scorpion α-toxins coupled to Na channel inactivation in amphibian myelinated nerve. J Gen Physiol (in press)

Strichartz GR, Chiu SY, Ritchie JM (1978) The effect of Δ^9-tetrahydrocannabinol on the activation of sodium conductance in the node of Ranvier. J Pharmacol Exp Ther 207:801–809

Swenson RP, Oxford GS (1980) Modification of sodium channel gating by long chain alcohols: ionic and gating current measurements. Prog Anesthesiol 2:7–16

Taylor RE (1959) Effect of procaine on electrical properties of squid axon membrane. Am J Physiol 196:1071–1078

Taylor RE, Bezanilla F (1983) Sodium and gating current time shifts resulting from changes in initial conditions. J Gen Physiol 81:773–784

Ueda I, Yasuhara H, Shieh DD, Lin HC, Lin SH, Eyring H (1980) Physical chemistry of the interaction of local anesthetics with model and natural membranes. Prog Anesthesiol 2:285–294

Ulbricht W, Wagner HH (1975) The influence of pH on the rate of tetrodotoxin action on myelinated nerve fibres. J Physiol (Lond) 252:185–202

Wagner HH, Ulbricht W (1976) Saxitoxin and procaine act independently on separate sites of the sodium channel. Pflugers Arch 364:65–70

Wang GK (1984) Irreversible modification of sodium channel inactivation in toad myelinated nerve fibres by the oxidant chloramine-T. J Physiol (Lond) 346:127–141

Wang GK (1984b) Modification of sodium channel inactivation in single myelinated nerve fibres by methionine-reactive chemicals. Biophys J 46:121–124

Wang GK, Strichartz GR (1983) Purification and physiological characterization of neurotoxins from venoms of the scorpions *Centruroides sculpturatus* and *Leiurus quinquestriatus*. Mol Pharmacol 23:519–533

Wang GR, Strichartz GR (1984) Local anesthetics produce phasic block of sodium channels during activation. Biophys J 45:286a

Yeh JZ (1978) Sodium inactivation mechanism modulates QX314 block of sodium channels in squid axons. Biophys J 24:569–574

Yeh JZ (1980) Blockage of sodium channels by stereoisomers of local anesthetics. Prog Anesthesiol 2:35–44

Yeh JZ, Armstrong CM (1978) Immobilization of gating charge by a substance that simulates inactivation. Nature 273:387–389

Yeh JZ, Narahashi T (1977) Kinetic analysis of pancuronium interaction with sodium channels in squid axon membranes. J Gen Physiol 69, 293–323

Zaborovskaya LD, Khodorov BI (1982) Reversible blockage of batrachotoxin-modified sodium channels by amine compounds and benzocaine in frog node of Ranvier. Gen Physiol Biophys 1:283–285

CHAPTER 3

Structural Elements
which Determine Local Anesthetic Activity

K. R. COURTNEY and G. R. STRICHARTZ

A. Introduction

I. Scope of Review and Methodology

The potency of local anesthetics can be evaluated in a variety of preparations which span a broad range of organizational levels. At the clinical level the ability of a drug to provide relief of pain is the essential measure of potency, be it acute pain from immediate trauma or chronic pain from more protracted or historical courses. At the other extreme, the inhibition of ion channels in excitable membranes is a direct measure of the molecular action of drugs on their target sites. In this chapter we direct our attention primarily towards the responses of microscopic systems, for the consequences of local anesthetics for pain relief almost certainly derive from their basic action on excitable membranes. The more complex measurements of potency are not ignored, however, for many analyses of local anesthetic action, both past and present, have relied on the reactions of whole animals or complex systems in vitro, and the results deserve review.

Our goal is to evaluate the contributions of different structural elements of traditional local anesthetic molecules to their potency. Since local anesthetics produce complex changes, even on isolated excitable membranes and their ion channels when resolved under closely controlled conditions, the meaning of potency depends on the method of measurement. The chapter begins, therefore, with a brief description of the tissue preparations and modes of assessing anesthetic action. We then review briefly the measurement and meaning of the physico-chemical attributes of local anesthetics in Sect. B. Properties of these drugs in solution as well as in membranes are discussed. In Sect. C the results of modern electrophysiological investigations on the actions of local anesthetics are reviewed and analyzed with regard to the contributing roles of different regions of the local anesthetic molecule. Section D provides an assessment of the comparative pharmacology of local anesthetics as impulse blockers and anti-arrhythmics. Finally, in Sect. E, we review critically the current kinetic schemes and the physical chemical models proposed to explain the molecular mechanisms of local anesthetic action.

II. Measurements of Anesthetic Action

1. In Vivo Studies

Studies of the potency of local anesthetics in vivo provide two advantages. First, they closely resemble the circumstances of clinical administration of the drugs, and second, and not unrelated, they provide the ability to detect any toxic reactions that may accompany their preferred effect. Blockade of electrical impulse conduction in vivo depends on multiple factors, including the concentration, volume and locus and mode of delivery of anesthetic, local circulation, pH, pCO_2, the size as well as the species of animal, the particular nerve being blocked, the assay for impulse activity and its inhibition, and, finally on the physico-chemical characteristics of the blocking agent. Because the molecular properties of an anesthetic molecule define the manner in which all the foregoing factors influence its distribution and action, it is not possible to derive precise information about anesthetic: receptor interactions alone from in vivo studies.

Despite the complexities of in vivo measurements, a few general conclusions about structure and action can be made. Larger, more hydrophobic anesthetics are generally more potent; less drug is required for complete block of physiological and electrical activity and the block endures for a larger time (Covino and Vassallo 1976). Local anesthetics with higher pK_a values have a slower onset of block than those with lower pK_a values, all other properties being similar. Both of these general observations are indicative of the distribution of anesthetic molecules through the nerve and reflect the rate of penetration across the epineurium of the peripheral nerve and the subsequent partitioning among the axons within. Oftentimes similar structural factors govern penetration of the epineurium and the access to the actual site of action in the axon membrane, resulting in parallel potencies determined by complex in vivo measurements and quite direct, in vitro assays, such as those described in the following section (A. II. 2). But these similarities should not be taken as justification for using in vivo measurements to assess anesthetic-receptor interactions. Since the objective of this chapter is to describe the molecular correlates between structure and the blockade of impulses and ion channels, we will not discuss results of in vivo studies further. Our final statement is a caveat against making conclusions about local anesthetic potencies in vivo from a comparison of separate reports which, invariably, use different animals, nerves, or solutions. Such comparisons are almost certain to be confused by the variations in factors essential for the measurement of neuronal blockade. Indeed, the most consistently controlled situations for providing behavioral data are the many regional, epidural and spinal procedures conducted daily in hospitals throughout the world. The average results of these procedures on anesthetic potency agree quite well among many different clinics.

2. In Vitro Systems

The analgesic action of local anesthetics relies directly on their ability to block nerve impulses. This effect, in turn, results from their interaction with the ion channels that carry the ionic currents across the excitable plasma membrane. Local anesthetics interact with several types of ion channel (see Chap. 2), but impulse blockade occurs because of their inhibition of voltage-dependent sodium channels and that is the activity on which our molecular analysis eventually will focus. The following passages describe the methods of assessing local anesthetic potency on isolated tissues.

a) Isolated Nerve

Compound action potentials can be recorded easily from isolated peripheral nerve, and more papers are probably published on the action of local anesthetics on this preparation than on any other. The shape of the compound action potential depends on the composition of fibers in the nerve and on the method of recording. Differential recordings with extracellular bipolar electrodes measure the currents which flow outside the nerve during the propagation of impulses in the conducting individual axons (action currents: Fig. 1). Since conduction velocities

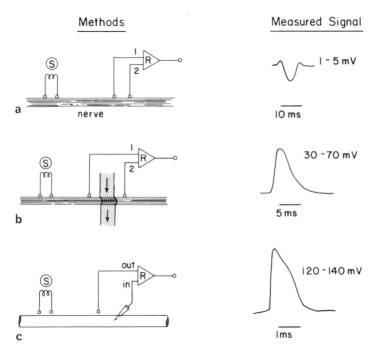

Fig. 1 a–c. Methods for recording neuronal impulse activity. **a** Extracellular recording of the compound action potential (APc). The stimulating source (s) passes currents between electrodes near the nerve. Propagated impulses are measured by amplifier R as the difference in voltage between electrodes 1 and 2, a voltage due to extracellular flow of the action current. The measured signal is a relatively small, triphasic wave. **b** Sucrose-gap system for recording compound action potentials. The solutions containing the two extracellular recording electrodes are separated by a volume ("gap") of flowing isotonic sucrose (stippled band). The impulse does not propagate past the sucrose-gap, producing a monophasic measured APc of larger amplitude than in **a**, and which is added to the "compound resting potential". **c** Intracellular recording of an impulse in a single axon is accomplished by a microelectrode that penetrates the axon membrane and permits a direct measurement of both the true resting potential and the absolute amplitude of the propagating impulse

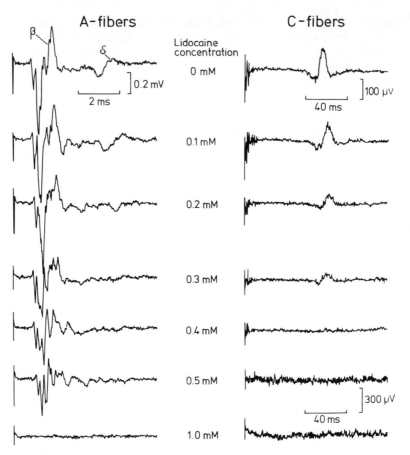

Fig. 2. The differential inhibition of separate elevations of a compound action potential by increasing concentrations of lidocaine. Extracellular impulses (as in Fig. a) were recorded from the sural nerve of the cat under barbiturate anesthesia. A desheathed length of nerve of 8 mm was exposed to flowing drug solutions at 33 °C and pH 7.4. The signal from slower A δ fibers disappeared at the lower drug concentrations, followed by the loss of the unmyelinated, C-fiber signal and, finally, the abolition of activity in the larger, A β fibers. Traces show steady-state results, reached after 10–12 min of continuous perfusion. From STRICHARTZ and ZIMMERMANN (1983)

differ among different fibers, the net effect of the action currents from all fibers is the interactive sum of the dispersed signals from nerve fibers distributed throughout the nerve. The electrical properties of axons near the surface probably distort the time course of the currents from fibers located more deeply in the nerve. As the individual action potentials are inhibited, by local anesthetics for example, the conduction time between the two recording electrodes changes and their voltage difference reflects this change as well as the absolute reduction of the integrated action currents (Fig. 2). In fact, the difference in peak-to-trough amplitude of a biphasically recorded action potential could change little as the impulse begins to decrement because of the contrary effects of conduction slowing on the difference signal. This is an extreme example, but one of several reasons why the amplitude of such biphasically recorded signals is sometimes not a valid measure of the inhibition of nerve impulses. For similar reasons, the area under such signals can not be used either.

When the intact epineurial sheath is not removed from the nerve, extracellular biphasic recordings are the only measurements possible. Although the presence of this sheath presents a major barrier to the diffusion of local anesthetics (RITCHIE et al. 1965b; CATCHLOVE 1972), and the ensheathed nerve better represents the clinical situation than its desheathed counterpart, its inclusion removes the response of impulse blockade to the applied drug one step further from the primary action of the drug. Treatments that accelerate drug penetration of the sheath, such as elevated CO_2 (see below), almost always influence the impulse blocking potency in other ways and do not help to clarify the basic mechanism of action.

Monophasic recording of action potentials avoids some of the problems noted above. Impulse propagation to the second, reference electrode is usually prevented by either of two means: mechanical or pharmacological interruption (e. g. nerve crush or nerve block), or removal of conducting ions (e. g. sucrose gap). However, even with monophasic methods the recorded action potential is the interactive sum of the individual axon signals dispersed in time. Thus, reductions of the peak amplitude or the area of such compound action potentials will arise from several factors: reduction in amplitude of impulses in individual axons, failure of propagation in individual axons, and differential slowing causing dispersive broadening within the compound signal.

One advantage of the sucrose-gap method on multi-axon preparations is the ability to measure the average resting potential Fig. 1 B). The electrical continuity of the conducting axoplasm passing through the sucrose-gap, from which extracellular ions have been removed, provides a resistive "lead" to the insides of the fibers lying proximal to the gap. Thus the effect of drugs on resting potentials as well as action potentials can be assayed. A major qualification on this method is that the flow of sucrose solutions per se appears to hyperpolarize the nerve membranes adjacent to the gap (JULIAN et al. 1962; POOLER and VALENSENO 1983). As we will show later, resting membrane potential often strongly modulates local anesthetic action, so the potency of agents measured in sucrose-gap is truly less than their potency measured without sucrose (COURTNEY et al. 1978a).

b) Single Cells

To measure membrane (E_m) potentials accurately requires placing intracellular electrodes in single cells or electrical syncytia preparations (e.g. cardiac muscle): Fig. 1 C. Then the recorded rates of change of the membrane potential during a nerve impulse are approximately proportional to the toal ionic current crossing the cell membrane (depending on the fraction of that current which flows longitudinally within the cell to subserve impulse propagation: JACK et al. 1975). However, even if the time derivative of E_m can be measured, and the impulse depolarizes the tissue uniformly, the rate of change is not a direct measure of the action of channel-blocking drugs. Ionic channels which are opened by depolarizations, in turn influence the membrane potential through the ionic currents they conduct

(HODGKIN et al. 1952). This accounts for the regenerative nature of the action potential and prevents any simple relationship, in general, between the effect of a local anesthetic and the rate of rise of an action potential (COHEN et al. 1981).

In order to overcome all of these artifacts and to measure directly the inhibition of ion channels, voltage-clamp methods must be used. Accurate results require the control of the membrane potential spatially over the entire membrane area that contributes current and at a rate which is fast compared to the kinetics of the signal being measured. The permeability changes ascribed to the different kinds of ion channels contained in one membrane can usually be studied separately by using the proper sequence of potential steps, replacing permeant ions by impermeant substitutes, or using specific pharmacological agents. An example of the last is the addition of tetraethylammonium ions (TEA$^+$) to solutions bathing an amphibian myelinated nerve to specifically block the voltage-dependent potassium channels. This permits the study of ion currents resulting from permeability changes due exclusively to voltage-dependent sodium channels (Na$^+$ channels). It is these Na$^+$ channels that are the targets of local anesthetics causing impulse blockade, and to which our attention now turns.

c) Properties of Na$^+$ Channels

Two electrical signals associated with the functioning of Na$^+$ channels can be measured by voltage clamp. Ionic Na$^+$ currents flowing through conducting channels show the time course and voltage dependence of the permeability change directly.

Much smaller, asymmetric, capacitive currents, called "gating currents" result from the motion of the electrically charged channel molecules as they undergo the conformational changes leading to opening (activation) and subsequent closing (inactivation) in response to membrane depolarization. In the following paragraphs a brief description of Na$^+$ channels dynamics is presented. A more detailed treatment appears in Chap. 2.

When a typical nerve membrane is rapidly depolarized from the resting potential (ca. -70 mV) to -20 mV and held there, the sodium permeability follows the time course for I_{Na} shown in Fig. 3. An inital, rapid rise in the permeability, called "activation," is followed by a slower, spontaneous decline, called "inactivation." As the size of the depolarizing test pulse is increased, both the peak transient sodium permeability and the rate of activation increase. Finally, at potentials beyond about $+20$ mV, the peak permeability reaches its maximum value and is not changed by larger depolarizing steps. The molecular interpretation of this behavior is that the membrane contains a finite number of Na$^+$ channels that mediate the flow of sodium ions, and that both the probability of channel opening and the rate of opening, or activation rate, are greater for larger membrane depolarizations. However, for a sufficiently large depolarization a limiting fraction of channels will be opened and the maximum permeability will be reached.

Further, sodium channels will eventually spontaneously close during depolarization, by an "inactivation" reaction, resulting in only a transient peak sodium permeability. Activation and inactivation appear to represent sequential, interacting events in the voltage-dependent opening of sodium channels. At least part of the multi-step activation process must transpire before inactivation can begin.

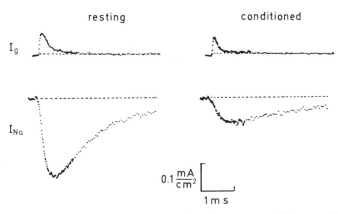

Fig. 3. Ionic sodium currents (I_{Na}) and asymmetric gating currents (I_g) in a squid axon. Note how the gating current occurs during the rapid activation phase of increasing sodium current. Both currents are already reduced at rest by intracellular perfusion with the lidocaine derivative QX-314 (*"resting"*), and are reduced still further, and to the same extent, by a train of depolarizing *"conditioning"* pulses. This result demonstrates the parallel, reversible loss of recruitable sodium channels (I_{Na}) and the associated conformational transitions reflected in the gating current (I_g). From CAHALAN and ALMERS (1979)

A simple kinetic scheme describes the gating of sodium channels. As depicted in Fig. 4, it shows separable activation and inactivation processes (the vertical transitions). Inactivation occurs more rapidly (and less reversibly) from activated states selectively populated by depolarization than from the resting, closed state. These activated states include the open state and, probably, closed states preceding the open state. At the end of this chapter, we will return to this scheme to model the kinetic effects of local anesthetics.

Macroscopic sodium currents can be simulated by different behaviors of the underlying microscopic events, the opening and closing of individual sodium channels. Channels in normal membranes abruptly open to a single conductance value some time after membrane depolarization and then abruptly close after a characteristic "open time" (SIGWORTH and NEHER 1980). One view proposes that relatively brief channel openings occur dispersed throughout the period of measurable conductance and the falling phase of macroscopic currents occurs because fewer channels open later (ALDRICH et al. 1983). An alternative view is that most channels open in the period before the peak current is reached and that the decline in current reflects the slow closing of these opened channels. Two points of further dispute concern the voltage-dependent nature of the inactivation processes and whether channels once closed can ever open again during the same depolarization step (VANDENBERG and HORN 1984). For the purposes of this chapter it is sufficient to know that channels open and close rapidly to single conductance values.

Changes in channel distribution among the various states in response to depolarization occur because the individual rate constants for activation and, perhaps, for inactivation, are themselves intrinsically voltage-dependent (Fig. 4). For example, at -70 mV, β_m exceeds α_m and very few channels are converted to O, the

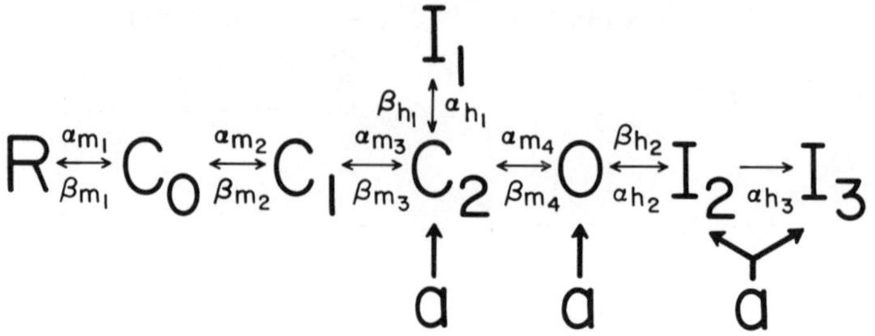

$$R \underset{\beta_{m_1}}{\overset{\alpha_{m_1}}{\rightleftarrows}} C_0 \underset{\beta_{m_2}}{\overset{\alpha_{m_2}}{\rightleftarrows}} C_1 \underset{\beta_{m_3}}{\overset{\alpha_{m_3}}{\rightleftarrows}} C_2 \underset{\beta_{m_4}}{\overset{\alpha_{m_4}}{\rightleftarrows}} O \underset{\alpha_{h_2}}{\overset{\beta_{h_2}}{\rightleftarrows}} I_2 \underset{\alpha_{h_3}}{\overset{}{\rightleftarrows}} I_3$$

Fig. 4. A linear kinetic scheme to describe gating of sodium channels. Resting channels (R) undergo transitions through a series of closed intermediate states (C_0, C_1, C_2) before opening to conducting conformations (O). Channels can be stabilized in non-conducting, non-recruitable inactivated (I) states via transitions from open or intermediate states. Local anesthetic molecules (a) may interact selectively with intermediate, open or inactivated states of the channel, depending on the particular drug in use (also see Fig. 12). After ARMSTRONG and BEZANILLA (1977); ARMSTRONG and CROOP (1982)

open state. At -20 mV, α_m is greater than β_m, the equilibrium of the activation reactions is suddenly shifted toward O, and the channels relax to this new equilibrium state. However, at -20 mV, α_h also exceeds β_h; thus O or C states relax in turn to the I states. The rate constants, α_m and β_m, are classically considered to be 3–5 times faster than α_h and β_h, resulting in more rapid activation and slower inactivation. However, in the analysis of ALDRICH et al. (1983) channel closing is as fast or faster than channel opening.

Another aspect of inactivation is important for local anesthetic action. Transitions between closed and inactivated channels can occur near the resting potential without requiring that the channel pass through an open state. The equilibrium between R and I states is specified by the resting potential and has been defined, classically by the parameter h, the fraction of the maximum peak current that can be recruited by a standard test depolarization: $h = R/(R+I)$ (HODGKIN and HUXLEY 1952; ARMSTRONG and BEZANILLA 1977). At more negative potentials the channels are mostly in R and can be recruited to the O state during subsequent depolarization, but at less negative resting potentials, channels tend more to the I state from which they cannot open upon depolarization. In myelinated nerves, about 70% of the channels are in R at the resting potential ($h = 0.7$) but the exact value depends on how the parameter is tested and thus demonstrates that the relationship between sodium activation and inactivation can be altered in a complex way by the voltage conditions preceding a test depolarization (HAHIN and GOLDMAN 1978). Following a transient depolarization, produced under voltage clamp or as an action potential, channels in the I state will relax back to R with a time course that depends on the level of the afterpotential. Recovery from the inactivated state will be faster for more negative potentials, and will make channels available for recruitment to the open state in response to a maintained or repeated stimulus. Later we will describe how the resting R→I equilibrium and the kinetics of I→R recovery are altered by local anesthetics (Section C: also see Chapter 2).

Gating currents arise from the asymmetric displacement of charge within the membrane in response to membrane potential changes. The gating currents in excitable cells that correspond to the movement of sodium channels appear to account for the majority of the asymmetric displacement current but, because of their small size, are usually studied under conditions of zero ionic current and with the use of signal averagers. A transient outward "on gating" current seems to correlate closely with the $R \rightarrow O$ transitions of Na channels, both with respect to time and potential dependence. Upon membrane repolarization an inward "off gating" current appears. For brief depolarizations the charge moved during "off gating" equals that moved during "on gating," but for longer depolarizations the relative "off gating" charge declines. The absent charge is referred to as "immobilized," and will also be manifested in the next measure of "on gating" current, itself now reduced by charge immobilization. Charge immobilization shares many features with sodium channel inactivation and it is taken as an independent measure of channel inactivation. However, not all charge can be immobilized by depolarization; about 20% remains mobile implying that some electrically active steps occur even in inactivated channels.

d) Relationship of Sodium Permeability to the Nerve Impulse

The nerve impulse does not fall in proportion to the decrease in sodium permeability. It is quite resistant to the blockade of Na^+ channels. Drugs that block 80%–90% of the Na^+ channels only reduce the amplitude of the neuronal compound action potential by 50% (HAHIN and STRICHARTZ 1981). The reason for this is that only a fraction of the channels have time to open during the impulses normally rapid rising phase, but when some channels are blocked by drugs the rising phase is slowed and a larger fraction of the unblocked channels can open (COHEN et al. 1981). One ramification of this behavior is that any treatment that reduces the number of conducting Na^+ channels will increase the apparent potency of local anesthetics for impulse blockade. A second is that agents that block the K^+ channels, which have actions antagonistic to those of Na^+ channels, appear to decrease the impulse blocking potency of local anesthetics. This seems to be true of tetraethyl ammonium ions (FLATMAN 1968) and of several types of local anesthetics themselves (STRICHARTZ 1985). And a third is that action potentials, particularly those in fastconducting axons with a relatively high surface density of Na^+ channels, are not very sensitive indicators of Na^+ channel blockade by drugs (COHEN IS et al. 1981; COHEN CJ et al. 1984). The threshold value for firing an action potential is a more susceptible parameter of channel blockade (RAYMOND 1979), although it is also contaminanted by affects on K^+ channels. Measurements of Na^+ currents under voltage clamp is the best direct physiological determinant of the primary action of local anesthetics.

e) Pharmacological Assays

In addition to electrophysiological measurements, other assays of Na^+ channel activity are responsive to local anesthetics. Channels maintained in an open state by the addition of various "activator" drugs (CATTERALL 1975) directly catalyze the diffusive uptake of radiolabelled Na^+, a process that can be inhibited by local anesthetics (HUANG et al. 1978). In addition, the specific binding of activator molecules to excitable membranes is antagonized by local anesthetics with potencies that are comparable to those measured electrophysiologically (POSTMA and CATTERALL 1984; WILLOW and CATTERALL 1982). While neither of these assays provides the temporal resolution demanded for an analysis of Na^+ channel gating, they are useful as tools to measure steady-state dispositions of anesthetic-bound and free channels, and as a measure of anesthetic activator interactions.

A final word of caution regarding measured potencies, regardless of the assay, is appropriate here. The nature of the buffer will influence the impulse blocking and channel blocking activity of local anesthetic. Obviously, zwitterionic buffers that are restricted to the extracellular milieu will adequately control the pH and thus establish the ratio of charged to neutral anesthetic species only if present in excess well beyond the added anesthetic. Changes of extracellular pH modulate the rate and extent of resting impulse and Na^+ channel inhibition measured by infrequent stimulation (RUD 1961; RITCHIE 1975; HILLE 1977a) and the use-dependent block seen during repetitive stimulation (SCHWARZ et al. 1977; BOKESCH et al. 1984). Permeant buffers, such as CO_2-HCO_3^-, can also change the intracellular pH and will have consequences markedly different than those from "extracellular buffers" (COURTNEY 1981a; BOKESCH et al. 1984). Uptake of local anesthetics by nerve is enhanced prominently by CO_2 (BIANCHI and STROBEL 1968; BROMAGE et al. 1967). Carbon dioxide itself has mild local anesthetic properties and raises the firing threshold of axons (RAYMOND and ROSCOE 1984). In heart tissue the presence of CO_2 : bicarbonate further polarizes the resting potential and shortens the action potential duration (COURTNEY 1981a). Despite its direct effect on nerve threshold, which will increase the apparent impulse-blocking potency of any agent that inhibits sodium channels, the CO_2 : bicarbonate system actually reduces the use-dependent action of local anesthetic drugs. Finally, changes in both extracellular and intracellular pH modify the kinetics of gating of Na^+ channels (see Sect. C) and thereby influence their susceptibility to resting and use-dependent block (COURTNEY 1979; NONNER et al. 1980). The same changes that are manifested as alterations of gating properties will probably modify the binding and action of activators used in the pharmacological assays. The choice of buffer and its consistent use is essential for sensible measures of the actions of local anesthetics.

B. Structure and Physico-Chemical Properties of Local Anesthetics

Many different kinds of drugs can block conduction of nerve impulses. For instance, alcohols and many antidepressant, anticonvulsant, and antiarrhythmic drugs all have local anesthetic properties (see Chap. 2). However, local anesthetics which are clinically useful are typically composed of an aromatic ring connected to an amino group by a short alkyl chain and a hydrophilic (amide, ester, ether) bond. Figure 5 illustrates typical local anesthetics of the amino-amide type and a few others having other bonds between the ring and amino group. All of these structures are amphipathic, that is, they possess both lipophilic and hydrophilic

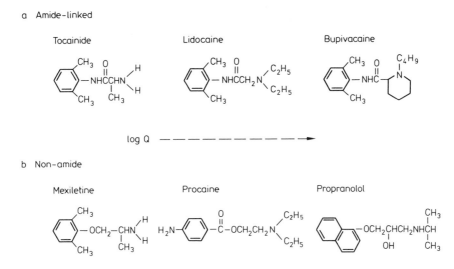

Fig. 5 a, b. Structures of typical local anesthetics. Note how some drugs have an amide link between the aromatic ring and tertiary nitrogen while others are ether- or ester-linked. Propranolol is included as an example of a beta-hydroxy ether having local anesthetic properties. Each row across increases in lipid distribution capability (octanol/water) going to the right

characteristics, generally at opposite ends of the molecule. They are also basic compounds which can add a proton to form a cation; the pKa values range from 7.5 to 10. Studies relating to the roles that each of these different portions of the molecule play in determinating the potency of local anesthetics are described below.

Before discussing the physiological actions of the various anesthetics we will review the meaning of their physico-chemical properties. Three parameters are often related to anesthetic potency and action: the molecule's mass or molecular weight, the pKa, and the hydrophobicity. In principle, these parameters can be measured directly and unambiguously, but their relevance for the interpretation of physiological potency is a less straightforward matter. Therefore, understanding the meaning of these parameters is an essential first step.

The molecular weight of a drug is known directly from its formula, although the existence of basic anesthetics as a variety of salts requires that the counterion be known for a correct determination from measured mass. The molecular weight of a compound determines how rapidly it will diffuse through free solution and, in conjunction with corresponding structural information, the size of the space within which it will fit. Because they are structured along the general design principles shown in Fig. 5, local anesthetics usually become larger by virtue of additions to the amine or the aromatic groups, located at opposite ends of the molecule.

Changes in structure around the tertiary amine group also change the pKa of the molecule, the measure of its affinity for hydrogen ions, H^+.

If BH^+ is the acid (or charged) form of an anesthetic base, B, and H_3O^+ represents all proton species in an aqueous solution, we have for the dissociation of the acid in dilute aqueous solution:

$$BH^+ + H_2O \leftrightarrow [B] + [H_3O^+] \tag{1}$$

$$K_a = \frac{[B][H_3O^+]}{[BH^+]} \qquad . \tag{2}$$

where K_a is the dissociation constant, and B, BH^+, and H_3O^+ are the activities of the species of equation (1). As we can write $pK_a = -\log K_a$ and $pH = -\log[H_3O^+]$, equation (2) can be transformed to:

$$pK_a = pH + \log\frac{[BH^+]}{B} \tag{3}$$

The activities are related to concentrations by their activity coefficients:

$$[BH^+] = f_+ \cdot (BH^+) \tag{4}$$

where f_+ is the activity coefficient for BH^+ and (BH^+) represents its concentration. For an uncharged molecule in dilute aqueous solution all of the activity coefficients approach unity and thus:

$$pK_a = pH + \log\frac{(BH^+)}{(B)} \tag{5}$$

But for an anesthetic molecule associated with a membrane the meaning of pK_a cannot be expressed so simply. At the interface of the membrane there are fixed electrostatic charges, associated with polar head groups on phospholipids, with amino acid residues of proteins, and with acidic carbohydrate substituents (e. g., sialic acid) that have basis or acidic properties and that the uptake of influence anesthetics and their apparent pK_a. About 15% of the phospholipids in nerve membranes carry at least one negative charge (STRICHARTZ 1977) and so attract protonated local anesthetics to the membrane surface. They also attract H_3O^+ and can increase the local proton concentration at the membrane surface to 10–30 times the value in bulk solution (MCLAUGHLIN et al. 1971; HILLE et al. 1975 b). Together, these two responses lead to an effective change in the pK_a of interfacially adsorbed anesthetics (MCLAUGHLIN and HARARY 1976).

In the hydrocarbon interior of the membrane, or near a protein to which an anesthetic may be bound, the effective pH will also be modified. Since both charged anesthetic and hydronium ion are at higher energies in the low dielectric medium of the membrane core than in solution, the concentration of both should be lower in this milieu. But the larger, amphipathic anesthetic suffers less of an energy increase in the membrane than does the smaller H_3O^+ resulting in the requirement for a higher (H_3O^+) in solution to produce 50% protonation of anesthetics in the membrane (WESTMAN et al. 1982). In other words, the effective pK_a of the molecule is reduced. Furthermore, the anesthetic molecule may shuttle rapidly between microscopic intramembranous regions of higher and lower dielectric, so that the apparent pK_a will represent the weighted average of this spatiotemporal distribution. Reciprocally, changes in pH that alter the degree of protonation of an anesthetic molecule will modulate the distribution ratio between regions of high and low dielectric. This interaction may produce a pH titration curve for anesthetics in membranes that is steeper than that for the equivalent protonation in a homogeneous aqueous solution.

Hydrophobicity, as it is applied to potency correlations of tertiary amine drugs, is measured by the lipid distribution coefficient, Q (or log Q). The partition coefficient, P (or log P), helps determine the distribution coefficient since the partition coefficient P measures the ratio of drug in the hydrophobic phase (often octanol) to neutral drug in the hydrophilic phase (water). Log Q, in addition, considers the fraction of the drug in the aqueous phase that is the neutral form, which, in turn, depends upon the pK_a of the drug and the prevailing pH:

$$\log Q = \log \frac{\text{neutral drug in octanol}}{\text{total drug in water}} = \log P - \log(1 + 10^{pKa - pH}) \qquad (6)$$

The log Q value is therefore smaller than log P (larger denominator) and, in addition, log Q is reduced as pH is reduced for basic substances. There is, typically, confusion in the literature as to which measurement is being provided, log P or log Q, and the reader should take care to find a precise description of just how the measurement was made.

Hydrophobicity, whether measured as P or Q values, reports the relative distributions of drugs between homogeneous aqueous and nonpolar phases. Such a distribution cannot describe the disposition of local anesthetics in real biological membranes. While octanol, or even cod liver oil (a previous "standard"), may mimic the central region of the membrane which is composed of the fatty acyl "tails" of phospholipids, the dipolar and interfacial regions of the membrane behave very differently. At the zone where the ester bonds of fatty acid-glycerol linkages in phospholipids are aligned in a plane, there is a large dipole field potential (MELNIK et al. 1977). The dipoles of the amide and ester bonds of anesthetics will be stabilized in this field, thus concentrating anesthetic molecules along this plane within the membrane. And, as noted above, the basic anesthetics will also adsorb at the surface of negatively charged membranes, although much of the adsorption is due to hydrophobic interactions (McLAUGHLIN 1975). On the basis of these facts we would not expect hydrophobicity parameters to predict the membrane uptake of anesthetics correctly, and direct measurements confirm this suspicion (UEDA et al. 1980; TRUDELL 1980). Hydrophobicity, so defined, is a parameter with limited ability to predict the true anesthetic "concentration" in a membrane.

Lastly, anesthetic molecules spend relatively brief periods in any one "phase" of the membrane. Nuclear magnetic resonance studies of phospholipid bilayer membranes show that procaine and tetracaine exchange rapidly between free solution and interfacial adsorption, and only dwell slightly longer in the deeper recesses of the membrane (BOULANGER et al. 1980, 1981). How long anesthetics remain bound to proteins remains to be reported, and the binding to sodium channels has not been measured directly, despite claims to the contrary (UEDA et al. 1980).

C. Resolution of Structural Contributions to Potency

Some aspects of the Modulated Receptor Hypothesis, which describes how local anesthetics interact with sodium channels in excitable membranes, will be reviewed at this time. This mode of drug action has important consequences for the determination of drug potencies, as will be described below. Recall that the sodium channel is triggered opened (activated) from the rest by a depolarizing stimulus and reacts further to form a different closed (inactivated) state. According to the "modulated receptor hypothesis" (HILLE 1977 b; HONDEGHEM and KATZUNG 1977), local anesthetics have very different affinitites for different states of the channel (i. e., closed or open). The development of this hypothesis and specifics of these interactions is considered in detail in Chap. 2 of this Handbook volume. The salient point which needs to be made here is that channel states associated with action potentials, the open and inactive states, are much more readily affected by anesthetic drugs. Membrane depolarization increases the fraction of channels in these states, and as a consequence, the proportion of time channels spent in both open and inactive states will be increased during periods of rapid excitation. Thus anesthetic potency appears to be greater in relatively depolarized or rapidly stimulated tissues. For this reason, it is very important, especially for in vitro assessment of anesthetic potency, to consider differences in these important operating conditions in different tissues and in different laboratory procedures.

For instance, early reports which utilize a single nerve fiber preparation held at a relatively negative membrane potential, which substantially reduces channel inactivation, reported a half-blocking concentration for sodium currents of about 1 mM for lidocaine (ARHEM and FRANKENHAEUSER 1974). Later studies, which held membrane potentials nearer to those occurring in vivo, reported a seven times greater potency for this same drug (COURTNEY et al. 1978a). Hyperpolarizing prepulses, which are normally used to condition (remove) fast sodium channel inactivation, can also reduce apparent drug potency because of their channel unblocking effects (COURTNEY 1975, 1981 b). Because of these considerations it is often difficult to develop structure/activity concepts based upon studies from several different laboratories.

Still, certain generalizations about potency dependencies on structure can be stated. Changes in structure modify certain kinetic features of drug action as well as the "tonic" blocking potency, measured at very stimulation frequencies. Some local anesthetics, particularly the larger or less lipid soluble ones, slow down the rate of "repriming" of sodium channels after they are used, the return from an inactivated to an activatable state. This kinetic characterization of drug action will be very important for determining the capability a drug has for accumulating frequency-dependent block. In general, drugs will have weaker potencies for blocking conduction at low frequencies of activity than at high frequencies of activity (COURTNEY et al. 1978 b). Sections D and E, below, will present this kinetic characterization of drug action in more detail. Chapter 2 and Sect. E describe some mechanisms involved in producing a drug action which is modulated by channel use.

I. Aromatic Groups

The aromatic group provides much of the hydrophobicity to the local anesthetic structure. In the case of the xylidine derivatives, of which lidocaine is an example, the addition of the ortho-methyl groups adds even more to the hydrophobicity of this aromatic group. In addition, these methyl groups restrict possible orientations of the carbonyl oxygen of the amide linkage to a direction perpendicular to the plane of the ring. This protrusion of the carbonyl oxygen away from the ring may provide some steric hindrance for close apposition of the ring to a lipophilic binding site, an effect which may be of importance regarding the relative potency of the amides, as described in the next section. The o-methyl groups also produce a resonance decoupling effect which makes the ring act, at the attachment site, more like an aliphatic than an aromatic group (LEO, personal communication). This effect is of importance when using the Hansch fragment technique for prediction of lipid solubility from molecular structure (HANSCH and LEO 1979).

The potency of tetracaine exceeds that of procaine by 50-fold, due largely to the addition of a butyl group at the para-amino group present on the aromatic ring of both molecules. When this *p*-amino group is derivatized and conjugated by biotin, a relatively hydrophilic moiety, the potency (for resting nerve block; i.e., "tonic potency") of tetracaine falls by a factor 50 whereas that of procaine is reduced by less than two, making the molecules almost equipotent (BUTTERWORTH et al. 1985). Although this finding illustrates the importance of aromatic hydrophobicity for apparent potency, other studies reveal that the role of these groups extends beyond unstructured hydrophobic absorption. AKERMAN has characterized a pair of anesthetic stereoisomers that contain an asymmetric carbon in the midst of two conjugated rings at the aromatic position. The isomers show weak stereospecificity, with one being 3–4 times more potent than the other, for tonic block (AKERMAN et al. 1969; HILLE et al. 1975; RANDO et al. 1985) and a larger stereospecificity (7–15) reported for use-dependent block (YEH 1980). No difference in the directly measured uptake by frog sciatic nerves or by synaptic endings was observed between the two compounds (AKERMAN 1973 a, b; ROTH et al. 1972). The results suggest that the aromatic portion of local anesthetic molecules may interact closely with a structured hydrophobic zone of the receptor, a zone which changes during stimulation.

Other experimental results are in conflict with the notion that the membrane concentration of drug, per se, determines the potency of local anesthetic molecules. Several studies on amphibian and mammalian peripheral nerve demonstrate that both the tonic and use-dependent impulse-blocking potencies of local anesthetics is enhanced by moderate cooling of the peripheral nerve (ROSENBERG and HEAVNER 1980; BRADLEY and RICHARDS 1981; BOKESCH and STRICHARTZ 1983, 1984; STRICHARTZ and ZIMMERMANN 1983). This potentiation corresponds to an increased inhibition of voltage-gated sodium channels (SCHWARZ 1979). But measurements of the anesthetic uptake by neural membranes reveal that the drug concentration in the membrane actually decreases upon cooling (BRADLEY and RICHARDS 1984). Therefore, anesthetic "concentration" probably strongly representative of hydrophobic absorption, is not the sole criterion of channel block, although changes of uptake by microscopic milieus in the membrane cannot be detected in these measurements.

II. Amide, Ester, and Ether Bonds

A relationship has been published regarding how the potency of amide-linked local anesthetics increases as the lipid distribution coefficient increases (Courtney and Etter 1983). Care was taken in these studies, which directly measured depression of sodium currents by drugs under voltage clamp, to hold the membrane at similar potential levels (to control the degree of inactivation) and to avoid rapid stimulation patterns so as to obtain the best possible measures of tonic or basal block of sodium current (see Fig. 6). These results, which are reproduced in Fig. 7, suggest that membrane-bound drug is responsible for producing the tonic block of sodium currents that is illustrated here.

What is most interesting in Fig. 7 is that the several anticonvulsant drugs, which are cyclic amides, are less potent than linear amides of equivalent lipid solubility. In addition, several non-amides, including the ethers mexiletine, alprenolol and propranolol, and the ester procaine, are much more potent than linear amides with corresponding hydrophobicity. The decreases in relative potency in going from non-amides to linear amides to cyclic amides is more clearly seen in skeletal muscle preparations than in myelinated nerve preparations (see Courtney and Etter 1983).

In a study of the potencies for equilibrium block of compound action potentials in mammalian nerves, Wildsmith et al. (1985) found similar results, with the tonic blocking potency of ester-linked compounds exceeding those of their amide-linked counterparts. It is possible that the amide bond might provide, relative to other (ether or ester) bonds, some steric hindrance for the anesthetic-receptor interaction. Recall the comments in Part I, above, regarding the "bulkiness" of the

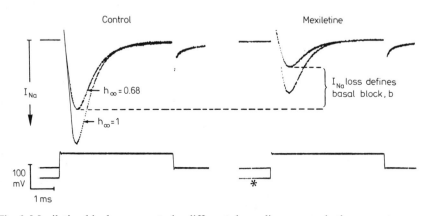

Fig. 6. Mexiletine block appears to be different depending upon whether or not one uses a conditioning hyperpolarizing prepulse. Membrane potential is stepped by 60 mV for 5 ms at an infrequent rate. Basal block is 61% if assessed using the smaller sodium current (labelled h = 0.68) where no prepulse was applied. If the larger, prepulsed (labelled h = 1) current is used, then block is estimated to be only 48% for this example (single skeletal muscle fiber). Current loss measured using a prepulse (−45 mV, 45 s long) before the channel-opening-depolarization may underestimate basal block because unblocking can occur during the prepulse for kinetically fast drugs. Such results are often interpreted as drug induced shifts in sodium inactivation. From Courtney (1981 b)

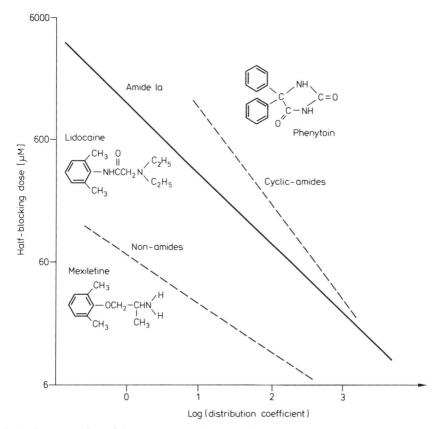

Fig. 7. Concentration of drug required to block half of sodium current at resting potential (defined by $h = 0.6–0.65$, see Fig. 9) in voltage clamped myelinated nerve preparations. Solid line represents regression fit for amide-linked local anesthetics and dashed lines the fits for nonamides (ethers and esters) and cyclic-amides (anticonvulsants). From COURTNEY and ETTER (1983)

amide bond, particularly in structures such as lidocaine which have restricting ortho methyl groups on the adjacent aromatic ring. The rigid amide-linked rings in anticonvulsant drug molecules (see Fig. 7) may present even greater steric hindrance than those in the linear amides, such as lidocaine. Their potency may, as a consequence of this hypothesized steric hindrance, be reduced compared to that of equivalent linear amides.

III. Intermediate Alkyl Chain

An amino nitrogen, typically tertiary, is attached to the aromatic portion of the ocal anesthetic via a short alkyl chain and the bonds just described. These alkyl chains are generally only 1 or 2 carbons long and, in principle, should increase lipid solubility according to their number. However, these carbons also separate two polar (hydrophilic) groups, for instance the amide-moiety and the tertiary nitrogen in the case of lidocaine. Increasing the number of intervening carbons from 1 to 2 increases the expression of the polar character of these two groups (proximity effect, see HANSCH and LEO 1979) and the resulting decrease in effective hydrophobicity can, depending on the polar groups being separated, exceed that resulting from the addition of the $-CH_2$-group in the chain. Thus, inserting a longer alkyl neck in lidocaine can actually reduce rather than increase log P. In other cases log P may increase, particularly when the groups being separated are not so polar or are already separated by more than a few carbons.

The length of the alkyl chain also may influence the ability of the terminal amine group to add a proton (pK_a), particularly for amide-linked local anesthetics. For example, when the number of carbons in the intermediate chain of lidocaine is increased from one to two, to three, the pK_a changes from 7.7, to 9.0, to 9.5, respectively (BOKESCH et al. 1983). The larger change in pK_a occurs for the initial lengthening, and is more gradual for subsequent additions. For molecular modifications of this type, the effects of reduced hydrophobicity will add to the effects of increased pK_a to lower the blocking potency of the anesthetic. This very behavior was observed in a study of series of lidocaine homologues. Lengthening the intermediate alkyl chain led to a reduction of potency, measured as the tonic blockade of compound action potentials (BOKESCH et al. 1985). Potency for use-dependent block was also reduced. When the additions were made instead on the primary alkyl groups of the tertiary amines, then the observed potency increased, even though the pK_a rose, showing that hydrophobicity, and not mass or the extent of protonation, was the dominant parameter controlling potency.

The Hansch "fragment method" for calculating partition coefficients is very useful for analyzing simple modifications of drug structure. It is also useful for estimating log P values for novel structures only slightly different from other compounds whose log P has been measured. The book that has been published on this topic (HANSCH and LEO 1979) is also valuable for its summary of 15,000 published measurements of log P values. Octanol is perhaps the most common hydrophobic solvent cited. For this reason it is used in the correlation analysis presented here, although it may not be the most appropriate solvent for depicting cell membranes (JANOFF et al. 1981).

IV. Terminal Amine

Amino groups, in amino acid side chains for example, typically have pK_a's of around 9. However, electron donating and electron withdrawing characteristics of nearby groups can substantially modify this pK_a. The amide-link in lidocaine best illustrates this effect for local anesthetics. The amide carbonyl group which is very nearby generates, via its electron withdrawing capabilities, a relatively electropositive terminal nitrogen. It is therefore much more difficult to protonate this nitrogen and this accounts for the unusually low pK_a of lidocaine and its amide-linked analogs. Increasing the intermediate alkyl chain length in lidocaine will increase its pK_a by reducing this interaction. If the amide-link is turned around, as it is in procainamide, the pK_a rises to a more typical value for amines of 9.

The pK_a of a local anesthetic will have important effects on drug distribution processes. As we elaborated in Sect. B, above, protonation will change intramembranous drug distribution and, reciprocally, distribution will alter a molecule's functional pK_a. The relatively low pK_a of the lidocaine group of drugs may account for their clinical success as local anesthetics. These drugs are more readily converted to the neutral form which is required to penetrate various hydrophobic permeability barriers in order to access the receptor sites presumed to exist within nerve membranes and inside nerves.

Once the anesthetic molecule is at a receptor site, its affinity for that site may well depend on the degree of protonation. The tonic potency of local anesthetics producing equilibrium block of sodium currents in the squid axon changed as the pH inside and outside the nerve were changed, consistent with the protonated form being at least 10 times as potent as the uncharged form, and acting from the axoplasmic side (NARAHASHI et al. 1970). When applied externally to frog nerves, tertiary amine anesthetics block more slowly and are less potent at neutral or slightly acidic extracellular pH than at alkaline pH (HILLE 1977 a). In experiments on frog muscle, the potency of extracellular lidocaine for producing use-dependent block was increased at lower extracellular pH (6 compared to 8) but almost independent of intracellular pH (SCHWARZ et al. 1977). Tonic blocking potency was also modulated by extracellular pH, with more alkaline pH conditions favoring a larger block, quite similar to the situation in frog nerve (HILLE 1977 a). In theory, changes in pH may modify the anesthetic receptor site as well as the states of the channel (COURTNEY 1979; NONNER et al. 1980), but the actions of permanently charged quaternary lidocaine and permanently neutral benzocaine are affected little by changes in external pH (SCHWARZ et al. 1977).

The effects of alkyl substitutions on the pK_a of the terminal 3°-amino group can be separated from their direct effects on size and hydrophobicity by considering the separate actions attributable to the protonated and neutral forms alone. This analysis was performed by theoretically assigning all blocking activity to either one or the other species, and then considering the changes in potency that occurred with structure, thus corrected for the changes in species ratio due to changes in pK_a (BOKESCH et al. 1985). By this approach, a strong correlation between tonic blocking potency and hydrophobicity was demonstrated for variations in the alkyl substituents on the tertiary amine. When integrated with the pH-dependent block results from squid axons and frog nerve and muscle (see above), these data imply that the 3°-amine local anesthetics act at a receptor having a hydrophobic region near their amine moiety, but that their potency is greatest when this amino group is protonated. The requirements are not contradictory if we permit the anesthetic to bind at an interfacial receptor that alternately presents both hydrophobic and hydrophilic milieus to the drug's amino region. Lipophilic interactions favor association with the former environment, and protonation stabilizes the anesthetic molecule bound in the latter disposition. Protonation reactions may be much faster than the actual drug binding reactions, and so may serve to regulate the rate of drug dissociation, a process noted by HILLE (1977 b). Consideration of such a general model is useful as an explanation for both tonic and use-dependent block, as we shall describe in Sect. E, below.

V. Stereoisomers

A weak stereospecificity has been detected for some but not all racemic pairs of local anesthetics. The stereochemistry of lidocaine derivatives containing an asymmetric carbon in their "aromatic" moiety was mentioned in a preceding passage (C.I). The tertiary amine compounds of these stereoisomers (called RAC109 I and II (see Fig. 8), when applied externally, produced about the same degree of stereo-selective block of Na^+ currents as that which resulted from the internal diffusion of their respective quaternary derivatives (HILLE et al. 1975), a result consistent with the hypothesis that both forms bind to similar sites. Direct internal and external application of the tertiary amine compounds to an infrequently stimulated squid axon produced similar differences; potencies for impulse inhibition varied by a factor of 2–3 (NARAHASHI T reported in AKERMAN 1973 b). In a more elaborate voltage clamp study, YEH (1980) showed that the measured stereospecificity (θ) for these enantiomers in squid was weakest when the axon was unstimulated during their application (initial block: $\theta = 1.04$), but increased after a train of depolarization had been applied (resting block: $\theta = 1.52$), and was strongest during a train of large depolarizations (conditioned block: $\theta = 5.64$,

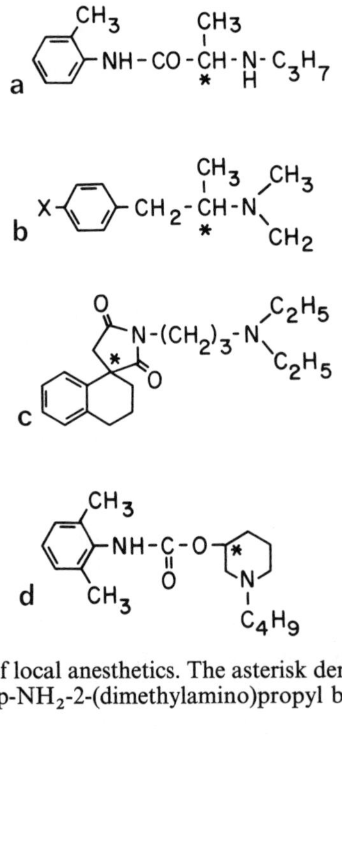

Fig. 8 a–d. Stereo-isomers of local anesthetics. The asterisk denotes the asymmetric center. a prilocaine; b p-NO_2- or p-NH_2-2-(dimethylamino)propyl benzene (see MAUTNER et al. (1980); c RAC109; d HS38

$E_m = 0$ mV; $\theta = 14.4$, $E_m = +80$ mV). The RAC109 I enentiomer was more potent during repetitive depolarizations, primarily because it bound more tightly to and dissociated more slowly from a potentiated channel state than did its stereo-isomer. The fact that this difference increased for conditioning depolarizations beyond 0 mV implies that the stereoselective attributes of the receptor functions continue to be increasingly revealed at potentials well beyond those required to open all sodium channels, or to inactivate them (HODGKIN and HUXLEY 1952). A different dependence on membrane potential was observed for the conditioned block by the quaternary derivatives of RAC109; for these compounds the stereoselectivity was the same ($\theta = 10$) for conditioning pulses of 0 mV and $+80$ mV (YEH 1980), but still greater than the initial block or resting block stereoselectivities for these compounds ($\theta = 1.2$–1.4). It thus appears that the tertiary amine drugs can discriminate differences in the local anesthetic binding site which are not detected by their quaternary analogues. Perhaps these are differences in the accessibility of protons to bound anesthetics since the asymmetric carbons are located on the drug far removed from the protonatable amine and both stereoisomers have the same pK_a ($=9.4$) in solution (AKERMAN 1973b). In fact, in an earlier set of experiments, NARAHASHI (reported in AKERMAN 1973) found a pH dependence to the stereoselective resting block of impulses by the RAC 109 compounds; $\theta = 2.0$ for external application at pH 8.0, but $\theta = 4.2$ for internal perfusion at pH 7.3. Hydrogen ion activities, however, may affect the receptor as well as the drug, and identical studies using different pH values with the permanently charged quaternary stereoisomers have not been conducted.

Other actions of the RAC 109 stereoisomers also show conformational discrimination. The class of lipophilic activator drugs, exemplified by batrachotoxin (BTX) and veratridine (VTD), bind to sodium channels and stabilize them in a conducting state (see CATTERALL 1980). The actions of both drugs are antagonized stereoselectively by the RAC 109 compounds. The binding to Na^+ channels of a BTX analogue is more rapidly reversible in the presence than in the absence of these local anesthetics, as if antagonism occurred via an allosteric inhibition, with anesthetic-bound channels having a lower affinity than free channels for BTX (POSTMA and CATTERALL 1984). The ratio of calculated affinities for the anesthetic stereoisomers was 7.2.

The veratridine-induced depolarization of frog nerves also is inhibited by the RAC 109 drugs, as well as by other local anesthetics. This inhibition is competitive in that it can be overcome by increased VTD concentrations; direct competition as well as mutual allosteric antagonism can account for this result. The stereospecificity for inhibition of the VTD response, measured at VTD concentrations that gave a half-maximal depolarization in the absence of local anesthetic, was about 3.5 (RANDO et al. 1986). Impulse inhibition in these resting nerves is somewhat less stereoselective, having values of 2.8–3.0 (AKERMAN 1973b; RANDO et al. 1986). Thus, interactions between local anesthetics and drugs that selectively stabilize open conformations of sodium channels show stereoselectivity ratios like those of weakly conditioned voltage-dependent blocks. The activator drugs, like depolarization, appear to induce changes in the channel that emphasize features which discriminate between these local anesthetic stereoisomers.

When asymmetric carbons are located elsewhere in the molecule, the stereospecificity is different. For asymmetric carbons in a branched intermediate alkyl linkage (e. g. prilocaine, propranolol) there is no difference in block (AKERMAN 1973 a, b; MAUTNER et al. 1980; COURTNEY unpublished observation in nerve and cardiac muscle), but one arises when the intermediate linkage becomes part of a hererocycle that includes the tertiary amine (AKERMAN 1973 a). The block of action potentials in infrequently stimulated frog sciatic nerves has a stereoselectivity of about 2.4 for mepivacaine isomers, a value that grows to 3.8 for the homologous bupivacaine isomers, which contain a butyl rather than a methyl substituent on the ring (see Fig. 5). When the linking bond in these molecules is changed from an amide (bupivacaine) to an amido-ester bond (HS38 isomers; see Fig. 8) the stereoselectivity increases even further to a value of 5.0. Paralleling this increase in stereoselectivity is an increase in pK_a, from 7.8 for mepivacaine to 8.1 for bupivacaine and 8.3 for HS38. An analysis of these compounds similar to the one conducted by YEH (1980) on the RAC 109 series would provide much useful information about the conformational changes at the regions of sodium channels that bind to the tertiary amine moieties of local anesthetics.

VI. Onset and Duration of Action

Several of the manipulations of drug structure discussed above will have important consequences for the onset and duration of action of local anesthetics. Drugs having higher lipid solubility and lower pK_a values appear to demonstrate more rapid onset of conduction block (COVINO and VASSALLO 1976). These results suggest that the neutral, lipid soluble form of the anesthetic is required to gain access to the receptor site most readily. Experiments on single nerve and muscle fiber preparations have confirmed this concept since many local anesthetics appear to have a faster onset of action at alkaline pH conditions, when more of the drug is in the neutral form (reviewed in STRICHARTZ 1976; RITCHIE and RITCHIE 1968; HILLE 1977a).

The duration of action of local anesthetics is also influenced by lipid solubility with the more lipophilic drugs showing the greatest duration of action (COVINO and VASSALLO 1976). Thus etidocaine, bupivacaine, and tetracaine are commonly used for regional anesthesia procedures such as obstetric anesthesia, where a block of long duration is desired. The long duration blocks by lipophilic local anesthetics probably result from their exceedingly strong partitioning into membrane structures that are associated with neurons, such as the myelin sheath. Equilibration of anesthetics between the myelin sheath and the contiguous axolemma provides a means to buffer the local membrane concentration of anesthetics. Since the myelin sheath often consists of 100-times the membrane thickness of the ensheathed axolemma, and extends over internode lengths that are 1000 times that of a single node of Ranvier (PETERS and VAUGHAN 1970), far less than 0.1% of the total anesthetic molecules partitioned into the sheath at EC50 would be sufficient to affect impulse condition if they were localized at the node. Therefore, almost all anesthetic molecules must be washed out of the myelin before axonal conduction is restored. This probably explains the long duration blocks from lipophilic anesthetics; the actual dissociation of the anesthetic molecules from their sodium channel receptor sites is a much faster process and seems a far less likely explanation (ULBRICHT 1981). High non-specific protein binding capabilities may also contribute to a drug's long duration of action (COVINO and VASSALLO 1976). Vasoconstrictors (e. g. epinephrine) can also be used to increase the time a regional anesthetic stays at high concentration at the site of regional injection.

Acidotic conditions can prolong and potentiate the action of local anesthetics once they are distributed among nerve fibers. This apparently occurs because the highly potent cationic form of the drug prevails at low pH and it will be trapped inside fibers in this form. When the pH of an anesthetic solution bathing a partially blocked nerve is changed rapidly from an alkaline to a neutral value, the block at first increases, but eventually falls to a lower level (RITCHIE et al. 1965a; STRICHARTZ, unpublished observation). This transient response is explained by a rapid protonation of anesthetics at their site of action followed by a slower redistribution of drug molecules across the nerve membrane. Additional specific effects of acidotic pH conditions will be considered in Part E, below. Acidotic potentiation of the action of local anesthetics can be significant in some clinical settings. Local anesthetics are reported to produce a faster and more profound blockade clinically when they are injected in a solution containing bicarbonate and CO_2. Local anesthetics which inadvertantly gain access to the heart during regional anesthesia procedures may be significantly more toxic during acidosis, particularly after the occurrence of anesthetic-induced seizures occur which will reduce plasma pH (CLARKSON et al. 1984).

D. Comparisons of Nerve Blocking Actions with Antiarrhythmic Actions of Local Anesthetics

Much smaller concentrations of local anesthetic are utilized in antiarrhythmic drug applications compared to those used in many nerve studies. For instance, lidocaine at 15–30 μM has significant effects on sodium channels in cardiac membranes (HONDEGHEM and KATZUNG 1977; GRANT et al. 1980; BEAN et al. 1983). Voltage clamp studies on myelinated nerve, on the other hand, use 100–250 μM lidocaine to study the depression of sodium channel function (HILLE 1977a). Why are nerve preparations and cardiac preparations so different in their sensitivity to this class of drugs?

The depressant effect that local anesthetics have on nervous excitability is modulated by the rate of use of the nerve. Ion flow through the sodium channel is more greatly depressed when the channel macromolecule is in states associated with excitation (e. g., open or inactivated states, see Fig. 9). To compare the action of local anesthetics in nerve versus heart tissues it is essential to consider differences in the operation of sodium channels in these different tissues, as well as the intrinsically different anesthetic sensitivities among the different tissues.

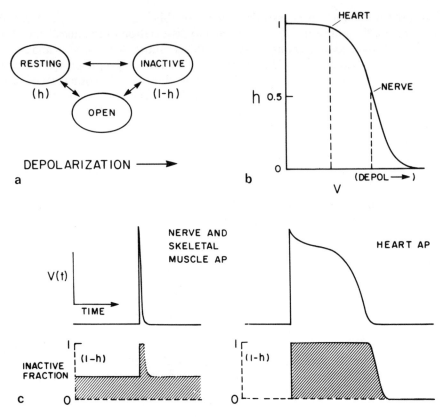

Fig. 9. a A simplified kinetic scheme uses only three states of the sodium channel: resting, open and inactive (compare to Fig. 4). Both resting and inactive states are closed or non-conducting and both may exist at the "resting" potential. Depolarization shifts the equilibria between channel states to the right, thereby causing a transient appearance of open or conducting channels and a final disposition into inactive forms. **b** Closed channels are often partitioned between resting (*h*) and inactive (1-h) fractions. The relationship between membrane potential and this h parameter is depicted here. Note that most myocardial preparations are, at their prevailing resting potentials, on a different part of this "h curve" compared to nerve (*dashed lines*). **c** Different inactivating (h-gating) behavior in nerve and cardiac tissues. In the case of nerve there is substantial inactivation (*shaded area*) at the resting potential and brief increments in inactivation occur with each action potential. In heart muscle, almost all inactivation develops with each long duration action potential

I. Sensitivity of Nerve Versus Muscle

A number of local anesthetics have been studied regarding their potency for blocking peak sodium currents in both nerve and skeletal muscle (single fiber) preparations. In these voltage clamp studies (Courtney 1981 b) care was taken to hold these preparations at similar levels of channel inactivation between test depolarizations so that drug potencies for different channel states could be more precisely compared (see below). In addition, low frequencies of depolarizing test potentials were used to avoid accumulation of frequency-dependent block of the channels. When this was done skeletal muscle fibers still appeared to be 3–5 times more sensitive than nerve to several local anesthetics. It may well be that muscle preparations are intrinsically more sensitive to the channel blocking actions of local anesthetics.

II. Different Inactivation Gating in Nerve and Heart

A substantial fraction of the sodium channels are in the inactive state at the normal resting potentials of many nerve and skeletal muscle preparations. For instance, at a typical resting potential of -80 mV in myelinated nerve about 30%–40% of the sodium channels are in the inactivated state (see Fig. 9 B). Tonic block of sodium channels by many local anesthetics, a partial block that is present in the absence of high-frequency activation, appears to be caused by a selective action of the drug on a nonactivatable form of closed channels (COURTNEY 1975). Early studies equated this nonactivatable form with the normal inactive state of sodium channels (COURTNEY 1975; HILLE 1977b). But removal of the normal inactivation reaction by either proteolytic digestion of a cytoplasmic portion of the channel (CAHALAN 1978; YEH 1978) or by reaction with chemical agents that do not cleave peptides left tonic block almost unchanged (SHEPLEY et al. 1983; STRICHARTZ and WANG 1985). Therefore, a form of the channel that exists independent of the normal inactivation reaction must account for the tonic action of local anesthetics. Recent studies on myelinated nerve suggest that this form may correspond to intermediate states that are transposed between resting, closed channels and their open forms (WANG and STRICHARTZ 1984; STRICHARTZ and WANG 1985; see Chap. 2, this volume). Additional studies which have attempted to measure the selective affinities that anesthetic drugs have for each of the different closed channel states (resting, intermediate or inactive) show that the inactive or intermediate channel states have affinities for anesthetics leading to block that are 15–30 times that associated with the resting channel state (KHODOROV et al. 1976; BEAN et al. 1983). Therefore, preparations which show some degree of either inactivation or partial activation at their resting potentials will be blocked tonically by local anesthetics in proportion to the fractional population of these states.

Differences among species as well as between sodium channels in nerve and heart are important factors in the comparative pharmacology of local anesthetics and antiarrhythmics. The peripheral nerves of mammals have impulses that are more sensitive than those of amphibians to local anesthetics. For example, the peak of the compound action potential which corresponds to impulses in large myelinated fibers is reduced by 40% tonically in rabbit vagus (in vitro) by 0.8 mM GEA968 (FALK and STRICHARTZ unpublished observation), whereas 1 mM of the same drug produces only a 15% inhibition in frog sciatic nerve (COURTNEY 1974; STRICHARTZ 1980). Use-dependent block by lidocaine (0.2 mM) in mammalian heart is potentiated maximally by one long depolarizing conditioning pulse of 100 ms duration (BEAN et al. 1983) whereas the maximum depression by 0.25 mM lidocaine in frog nerve requires many repetitive pulses of much shorter duration, (10 ms) and is affected far less by a single long depolarization (WANG and STRICHARTZ 1984). Among different drugs, for comparison, the use-dependent effects of the polar lidocaine homologue, GEA968, are optimized by trains of very brief depolarizations, as short as 0.1 ms, showing that this drug reacts rapidly and selectively with channel states that are populated early during a depolarizing pulse (STRICHARTZ and WANG 1985) whereas lidocaine selectively reacts with states that occur much later in nerve, and later still in heart. These examples show how both resting and dynamic interactions between anesthetics and channels can differ between species and, perhaps, particular organs. Keeping such variations in mind, we will continue our comparison of drug actions.

Myocardial preparations, unlike mammalian nerve, have negligible amounts of inactivation at normal resting potentials (Fig. 9 B; CHIU et al. 1979). At rest, or at potentials near maximum diastolic polarization, most channels will be in the R state, as diagrammed in Fig. 4. This holds for most healthy atrial and ventricular tissues (HAUSWIRTH and SINGH 1979), excepting specialized fibers in the SA and AV nodal regions. As a consequence, one may not observe "resting" block of myocardial sodium channels, often monitored as slowing of myocardial conduction, at slow drive rates. This is the case for lidocaine, for example, and for many other local anesthetics if care is taken to correct for the accumulation of frequency-dependent block, as will be described in Part III below.

The schematic in Fig. 9 C illustrates how very different the levels of channel inactivation are for impulses in nerve versus cardiac preparations. In the case of nerve preparations there is significant inactivation at the resting potential and only a brief increment in the level of inactivation during each brief nerve action potential. In cardiac tissues, on the other hand, almost all inactivation is attained during each cardiac action potential, an action potential that is often a hundred times longer than that in nerve.

This very different operation of the inactivation gating machinery in nerve versus cardiac preparations complicates the comparison of drug blocking potencies in these different preparations. In heart one sees little, if any, tonic block of sodium channels, and most blocking occurs during each cardiac action potential. By contrast, in nerve one sees mostly tonic block which occurs via the drug's selective action on the intermediate or inactive forms of closed channels. Action potentials in nerve can enhance the block to above the basal level of block via the drug's particularly strong affinity for intermediate, open or inactive channels (see Part V below), although the time spent in the inactive state is clearly shorter in nerve than in cardiac tissue, especially ventricular muscle. Thus, blocking of inactive channels may be functionally much more important in normally beating heart muscle than in nerve because of the long durations of cardiac action potentials. In addition, factors intrinsic to the selective affinity of local anesthetics for he various channel states may differ between nerve and cardiac muscle, as described above.

III. Factors Determining Potency in Heart

Sodium channels are responsible for the initiation of normal cardiac action potentials. If sodium channel function is depressed then cardiac conduction is slowed and, if the depression is severe enough, conduction is stopped. In order to properly assess the depressant effects of local anesthetics on cardiac conduction it is necessary to examine, in sequence, the actions these drugs have, first, at infrequent rates of myocardial excitation, then at normal heart rates, and finally at high (fibrillatory) heart rates.

Maximum rates of rise (upstroke velocities) of myocardial action potentials have been used to assess the changes in sodium channel availability which occur during exposure to local anesthetics (HONDEGHEM and KATZUNG 1977; COURT-NEY 1980a; SADA and BAN 1981; CAMPBELL 1983). [Upstroke velocities are proportional to the total ionic current crossing the membrane during nonpropagating action potentials and not to the number of available sodium channels (g_{Na}) (COHEN and STRICHARTZ 1977; STRICHARTZ and COHEN 1978) but the relationship between g_{Na} and the maximum upstroke velocity is usually a simple, monotonic function; e.g. $(dv/dt_{max})^2 \propto g_{Na}$ (COHEN I et al. 1981; COHEN CJ et al. 1984).] Normally, sodium channel availability (hence excitability) recovers within tens of milliseconds after each cardiac action potential. However, this recovery changes dramatically during exposure to drugs of the local anesthetic class. Since drug block of sodium channels is modulated by the state of the channel, block is greater after an action potential than before. Recovery from these use-induced increases in channel block occurs with widely varying time constants, ranging from a tenth of a second to tens of seconds depending upon the drug being studied. Recent results have shown that these recovery time constants are predictably dependent on drug structure; drug size (primarily) and lipid solubility (secondarily) can be used to predict where within this spectrum of block "memory" a given drug will be found (COURTNEY 1980a, b). Larger drug structures, or those having very low lipid distribution coefficients, display slower recovery kinetics. Figure 10 illustrates a test of this size/solubility hypothesis for a number of antiarrhythmics and local anesthetics. In addition, Table 1 specifies which commonly used local anesthetics should have fast or slow recovery kinetics along with specific half-time measurements for the recovery in guinea pig papillary muscle preparations.

It was clear from the original results that drugs of very low lipid solubility, such as procainamide, showed slower recovery half-times than predicted from consideration of their size alone. More recent results with bupivacaine and etidocaine suggest that only low lipid solubility modulates this otherwise size-dependent process. Etidocaine and bupivacaine display recovery kinetics (1–2 s halftimes) which are as slow, possibly even slower, than those predicted solely on the basis of molecular weight (COURTNEY 1983a). HANSCH and CLAYTON (1973) have proposed schemes to explain why exceptionally high lipophilicity actually reduces the activity of a drug; their "parabolic best-fit" concept may apply in this context. The exceptionally large lipid solubility of these two clinically important anesthetics will affect their intrinsic potency for blocking channels during myocardial action potentials, as described in the next section, even though it does not appear to facilitate their recovery kinetics.

Block of sodium channels develops during each cardiac action potential when the channel macromolecule is in states that are selectively sensitive to the drug. There is recovery from this use-induced increment in channel block during the diastolic time interval between action potentials, when the normal channel is in a low affinity state(s). If the drug is kinetically fast, as is the case for lidocaine in healthy myocardium, then there will be time for complete recovery between beats

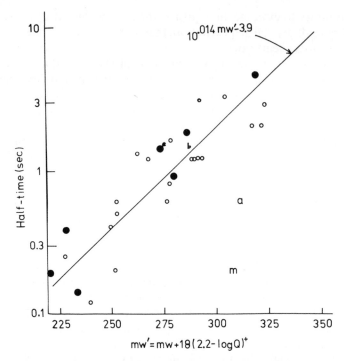

Fig. 10. The size/solubility hypothesis governing drug unblocking kinetics. A linear combination of drug size (*mw*) and lipid distribution coefficient [*mw'*=mw + 18 (2.2–log Q)] is used to predict recovery kinetics with results on 7 drugs (*filled circles*) establishing the regression line (from COURTNEY 1980a); recent studies suggest that mw' = mw if log Q greater than 2.2. Over 20 drugs with molecular weights under 340 have had their recovery half-times successfully predicted using this hypothesis; exceptions include metoprolol (*m*, SADA and BAN 1981) and aprindine derivative A777 (*a*, EHRING et al. 1982)

Table 1. Recovery half-times for local anesthetics in myocardium

	Drug	mw	mw'	HTprd	HTobs
slower/faster	Prilocaine	220	240	0.3 s	0.1 s
	Lidocaine	235	235	0.25	0.14
	Mexiletine	179	228	0.2	0.25
	Tocainide	192	229	0.2	0.38
	Mepivacaine	246	259	0.5	?
	Procaine	236	277	1.0	0.6
	Etidocaine	276	276[a]	0.9	1.3
	Bupivacaine	288	288[a]	1.35	1.4
	Procainamide	235	287	1.3	1.8

HTprd = predicted half-times from Fig. 10
HTobs = observed half-times for guinea pig papillary muscle; studies from the laboratory of K. COURTNEY.
mw' = mw + 18 (2.2 − log Q)
[a] No adjustment if log Q greater than 2.2.

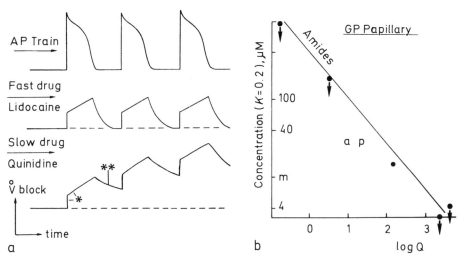

Fig. 11 a, b. Drug blocking during action potentials and AP trains. **a** Simulation shows that a train of APs evoked after a period of rest will accumulate channel block if recovery kinetics (******) are slow enough. Blocking may occur during APs via both open and inactive channel interactions (*). **b** An analysis using finite difference equations (COURTNEY 1983 b) was utilized to estimate blocking per AP for several amide-linked (*filled circles*) and ether-linked drugs (letter symbols — mexiletine, alprenolol and propranolol, left to right). Drug levels required to produce a fixed blocking effect ($K = 0.2$) are plotted against each drug's lipid distribution coefficient log Q. Significance of arrows is discussed in text

at normal rates. However, channel block can accumulate, under these same conditions, when using a drug with slower kinetics (see Fig. 11 a). A drug's "potency" for blocking myocardial excitability is then determined both by its intrinsic potency for blocking channels during individual action potentials and by its unblocking kinetics between action potentials. Myocardial drive rate will, as a consequence, be a very important determinant of the overall drug effect. Rapidly reversible drugs such as lidocaine, are selectively antiarrhythmic because their binding and dissociation to and from activated channel states occur quickly in comparison to the duration of cardiac impulses and the interpulse interval, respectively.

Structure-activity relations (SAR) regarding drug unblocking between action potentials, when the channels tend to a low affinity state, were reviewed just above. The size/solubility concept described in Fig. 10 involves unblocking rates which are usually not dose-dependent (COURTNEY 1980 a). Substantially different, dose-dependent, SAR govern the rates of blocking during the period of excitation when high affinity states occur. In order to complete these SAR inquiries, a mathematical analysis was developed that calculated an effective rate of block during each action potential in a train while block accumulated (COURTNEY 1983 b). Amide-linked drugs showed a systematic potency, inversely related to log Q, and ether-linked drugs were relatively more potent than amide-linked drugs of equivalent solubility (Fig. 11 b). These results resemble those previously described for this class of drugs regarding tonic blocking actions in nerve (Part C).

The combined effects of increased block of excitability during action potentials and unblocking between action potentials can now be considered. The arrows in Fig. 11 B designate four amide-linked local anesthetics showing slow recovery kinetics (left to rigth–procainamide, GEA 968, bupivacaine and etidocaine). These "slow" anesthetics will accumulate additional decrements of excitability at physiological heart rates. Thus, by virtue of their slower recovery halftimes, they will accumulate depression of cardiac excitability at much slower frequencies than will lidocaine and, in particular, they will accumulate block of sodium channels at normal heart rates whereas lidocaine should not. The kinetically slower drugs are, in effect, more potent at normal heart rates than is indicated by their respective positions in Fig. 11 B.

IV. Relevance to Cardiotoxicity

All local anesthetics may show a frequency-dependent modulation of their block of sodium channel function. However, only the fast-memory drugs, those having recovery half-times of a few tenths of a second, are capable of selectively blocking only high-frequency arrhythmias with little effect on myocardial conduction at normal heart rates. This kinetic feature of drug action has important consequences, as well, for the cardiotoxicity of local anesthetics (CLARKSON et al. 1984). If a kinetically slow anesthetic such as bupivacaine gains inadvertant access to the general circulation during regional anesthesia it should depress cardiac conduction at normal heart rates. This may explain why this drug has been reported to be more cardiotoxic (ALBRIGHT 1979) than the kinetically faster lidocaine. In addition, the highly lipid soluble local anesthetics such as etidocaine and bupivacaine have extremely potent depressant effects on cardiac contractility (FELDMAN et al. 1982; COURTNEY 1984 a). For example, bupivacaine is used at 0.25 the concentration of lidocaine in regional anesthesia yet has 16 times lidocaine's potency for depressing cardiac contractility (COURTNEY 1984 a). Much of the inhibition of contractility may result from interference by these drugs with voltage-dependent calcium channels in myocardial sarcolemma (LYNCH 1985; also see Chap. 7, this volume). The resulting depression of cardiac pumping can make management of patients exposed to toxic levels of these anesthetics much more difficult.

V. Importance of Intermediate, Open and Inactive Channel Blocking

The issue of whether or not sodium channels are blocked primarily in their intermediate and open states or their inactive state has important implications for both antiarrhythmic drug therapy and cardiotoxicity of these drugs. Blocking of channels occurs during action potentials, with different drugs showing different amounts of open versus inactive channel blocking. This is discerned by using voltage clamp techniques to modulate the amount of time sodium channels spent in the inactive state. When this is done, in myocardial preparations one finds that certain drugs, such as lidocaine, produce channel blocking which is steeply dependent on the time spent in the inactive state while others, such as procainamide, produce channel blocking which is not (i. e., mostly open channel block). (These results are similar to those comparing GEA 968 and lidocaine in nerve, mentioned above.) A tabulation of available results in myocardium regarding the predominant form of state-selective block by several drugs appears below:

Open channel blockers:

quinidine (COLATSKY 1982)

procainamide (COURTNEY 1983c)

Inactive channel blockers:

lidocaine (BEAN et al. 1983),

tocainide (COURTNEY 1983c)

amiodarone (MASON et al. 1983)

There is, as yet, no structure-activity clue as to which drugs preferentially block which channel state during myocardial action potentials. However, such SARs will be important for the design of drugs having specified actions. For instance, action potential durations are much shorter in atria than in ventricle and drugs which emphasize open channel blocking may thereby be relatively more efficacious in atria. Inactive channel blockers, on the other hand, may be more effective in blocking rapid repetitive firing in ventricle or damaged (depolarized) myocardium. The brief list above indicates that this may, indeed, be the case. However, the list needs to be extended to other antiarrhythmics and SAR need to be more rigorously established.

The observation that the inactive state of closed channels is more readily blocked by many drugs may have important consequences for arrhythmia therapy. Damaged or infarcted tissue will be, as a consequence, more readily affected by therapeutic drugs than healthy tissue (HONDEGHEM and KATZUNG 1977, 1980; OSHITA et al. 1980). Myocardial regions which are depolarized by tissue damage and local hyperkalemia will be more likely to show tonic block which may be completely absent in healthier tissues.

In addition, the rate of recovery from block between action potentials is markedly dependent on membrane potential. Slight depolarizations can substantially slow recovery time constants (HONDEGHEM and KATZUNG 1977; OSHITA et al. 1980) thus allowing for greater accumulation of use-dependent block at both normal and arrhythmic heart rates. Acidosis will also produce substantial slowing of recovery kinetics (GRANT et al. 1980, 1982; NATTEL et al. 1981). Both hyperkalemic and acidotic conditions should prevail in infarcted myocardium (antiarrhythmic context) and during seizure states associated with local anesthetic overdose (cardiotoxic context).

Voltage-dependent and frequency-dependent actions of local anesthetics can combine to produce both basal and cumulative blocking of myocardial excitability. This provides an exciting new structure/activity framework for development of "smart" drugs–drugs which preferentially act both where and when they are needed. Design criteria for therapeutic drugs which act selectively in damaged and arrhythmic tissues while leaving normal cardiac conduction intact are now being developed.

E. Models for Local Anesthetic Receptors

The interaction of local anesthetics with sodium channels can be visualized in different ways. An important class of such models involves identification of the different states of the sodium channel, including those new state(s) induced by drug treatment, and then specification of the kinetics of transitions between these various states. These constitute the "kinetic" models of local anesthetic action as, for example, in HILLE (1977b), HONDGEHEM and KATZUNG (1977), and KHODOROV et al. (1976). Other models involve a more physico-chemical approach in that they either implicate general membrane perturbations as responsible for local anesthesia (SEEMAN 1972, 1975; ROTH 1979; SKOU 1954) or describe the specific attributes of a binding site for local anesthetics (WATSON 1980). The kinetic class of models involves, implicitly, some specificity to the drug-receptor interaction since the sodium channel is a very specific protein with well-documented pharmacology and newly revealed biochemistry (NODA et al. 1984). HILLE (1980) and FRANKS and LIEB (1982) have provided recent, provocative critiques regarding these very different points of view.

I. Kinetic Models of Local Anesthetic Action

1. The Original Modulated Receptor Hypothesis

As mentioned above, these models of anesthetic action involve very specific interactions with the sodium channel. Not only is the membrane-bound protein defined as the receptor, but the interaction of drug with the channel is now thought to be specifically dependent upon the conformation of the channel protein. For example, open channel interactions are often characterized by higher drug affinities than are resting channel interactions. The evolution of this Modulated Receptor Hypothesis will be briefly reviewed below. Chapter 2 contains a more detailed evaluation of this hypothesis and its many ramifications in light of more current experiments.

A paper published in 1966 described the common mode of action of lidocaine and tetrodotoxin (TTX) on sodium currents in myelinated nerve preparations under voltage clamp (HILLE 1966). The effects of these two agents appeared to be selective for sodium currents over potassium currents at the drug concentrations utilized, implying that very specific membrane proteins were being affected by a drug. These two drugs are now thought to have quite different modes of action on sodium channels, with studies from Hille's laboratory over the next ten years providing much of the evidence. TTX acts from the extracellular side of the membrane to stop sodium ion flow without modifying gating properties (i. e., opening and closing rates) of the channel, at least in nerve preparations. In contrast, lidocaine and other local anesthetics interact with the channel from within the membrane phase and/or from the axoplasmic surface (NARAHASHI et al. 1970; FRAZIER et al. 1970; STRICHARTZ 1973; HILLE 1977b). These drugs do have significant effects on channel gating and channel gating, in turn, has significant effects on the drug-channel interaction. The reciprocal requirements of this drug-channel interaction are hallmarks of any modulated receptor hypothesis.

According to the original Modulated Receptor Hypothesis (MRH) the inactivated channel state had the highest affinity for local anesthetics. Open states had lower affinities and resting states the least affinity. The antagonism of tonic block by membrane hyperpolarization was evidence that reduction of the inactivated state (by voltage) removed a high affinity form of the channel (COURTNEY 1975; HILLE 1977 b). The phasic and tonic effects of 3°-amine anesthetics were successfully modelled by SCHWARZ et al. (1977) using such a kinetic scheme, but the kinetic parameters they used are not unique for this solution and other possibilities remain. A major problem encountered in such modelling is that only the resting closed and final inactivated states ever reach steady-state levels of population. The open state(s) and those intermediate between rest and open are populated only transiently and, since it appears that these are important reactive states, the phasic blocks that are achieved never correspond to true equilibrium reactions but, at best, to a dynamic steady-state when block induced by a pulse is just reversed by unblocking reactions between pulses.

2. Evolved Modulated Receptor Hypothesis

Inhibition of the formation of the inactivated channel state can be achieved in different ways, with different consequences for local anesthetic action. Proteolytic degradation of channels from the axoplasmic surface produces a selective inhibition of inactivation and a loss of use-dependent block for many, but not all, local anesthetics (CAHALAN 1978; YEH 1978). In contrast, if inactivation is inhibited by specific toxins or nondegrading reagents, use-dependent block is unaffected (SHEPLEY et al. 1983; STRICHARTZ and WANG 1985; ZABOROVSKAYA and KHODOROV 1984). Therefore, the ability of the channel to inactivate is not essential for use-dependent block. Still, some state of the channel that is modified by depolarization must selectively bind anesthetic molecules in a reaction that leads to a long-lasting non-conducting state.

3. New Schemes

Two new ways of viewing use-dependent (or, as it is often called, "phasic") block have emerged recently. In one, the additional block develops exclusively because the access to a high affinity anesthetic receptor is increased greatly by depolarization. This receptor exists in a resting channel, but is kinetically masked and thus nonreactive (STARMER et al. 1984). Depolarization changes the channel's conformation, revealing the anesthetic binding, albeit transiently, and permitting binding of the drug to some sites. Dissociation can occur between pulses. Such a model describes phasic block adequately, although it must become more explicitly detailed before it can be tested experimentally.

The second view of phasic block hypothesizes that anesthetic binding reaches equilibrium at rest and does not increase during one depolarization, but that following that depolarization, drug-bound channels only return very slowly to their resting state (STRICHARTZ and WANG 1985). Drug dissociation from such depolarization-induced states is also slow, and therefore, the fraction of drug-bound, inhibited channels accumulates during a train of sufficiently frequent depolarizations. This explanation differs slightly from the original MRH in that additional binding occurs not during the conditioning pulses, but because relaxations between pulses are too slow to permit recovery to the prestimulus conditions.

II. Physico-Chemical Models

1. Sites Outside the Pore

Theories of general anesthesia often involve postulation of some membrane disordering action of the anesthetic agents. Certain aspects of these "general membrane perturbation" theories are thought to apply to local anesthesia as well. Although many specific actions involving direct interactions with nerve sodium channels are known (and described in preceding sections of this chapter and Chap. 2) it would be worthwhile to review, at this point, some of the possible general membrane actions of local anesthetics.

Anesthetic molecules can, by dissolving in biological membranes, alter membrane function in several hypothetical ways. The appearance of Meyer-Overton type correlations (see above), which show how drug potency increases with increasing lipid solubility, suggest that membrane lipid might be the site of action. For instance the drug molecules may expand the membrane as they dissolve in it. This "critical volume hypothesis" receives much support from the phenomenon of pressure-reversal of anesthesia since pressure should only act by reducing volume. It should also be noted that high pressures can reverse conduction block by some local anesthetics (KENDIG and COHEN 1977; see MILLER 1975).

Anesthetics might also act by increasing the "fluidity" of lipid bilayers in which they are dissolved. The function of membrane proteins which are essential for nerve conduction might then be altered. Evidence has been provided showing that local anesthetics may modify bilayer fluidity (H. WANG et al. 1983; HSIA and BOGGS 1973). However, different integral proteins whose function can be measured, for instance sodium and potassium channels, are differentially sensitive to local anesthetics. Such a theory for drug action would have to be "tuned" so that each type of membrane protein might then have its own, unique microenvironment in order for this theory to explain such microscopically localized sensitivities.

To account for anesthesia, additional theories have been proposed which include phase transitions in lipid bilayers, changes in membrane thickness, and permeability changes in the bilayers. These theories and those described above are critically reviewed by FRANKS and LIEB (1982) as they apply to general anesthesia. They conclude that a protein site of action is more likely involved than a lipid site of action. The binding site is probably amphiphilic in nature since potencies correlate better with octanol than with hydrocarbon partition coefficients. Other studies show that general anesthetic agents have both general membrane perturbing and specific receptor types of action (DODSON and MILLER 1985).

The stereospecific actions of some local anesthetics would be difficult to explain using the general membrane theories of action (see C. V, above). For instance, YEH (1980) showed that the isomers of RAC 109 showed different capabilities for producing frequency-dependent blocking of sodium channels in squid giant axons. However, these stereoisomers were not that different in their tonic blocking capabilities. Perhaps the tonic block of channels is attributable to general membrane effect of the drug and the use-dependent action is caused by a different, potentially stereospecific, interaction with the drug.

III. Anesthetic Action and Channel Structure

Underlying every kinetic scheme for local anesthetic action is an attempt to relate anesthetic binding to different states and, eventually, to defined structures of the sodium channel. Early descriptions of specific receptor models reported a close correlation between drug-induced blocking reactions due to quaternary derivatives and the open conformation(s) of sodium channels (STRICHARTZ 1973). Subsequent studies showed that reversal of block by quaternary drugs during channel openings was faster when more permeant ions were outside the membrane and slower when less permeant ions were present (SHAPIRO 1977). It appeared that these drugs were occupying space along the ion pore/pathway of the channel. However, a strong antagonism between local anesthetics and the very lipophilic activators suggested that the anesthetic binding site was more hydrophobic than the ion pathway was expected to be (HUANG et al. 1978; CREVELING et al. 1983), and additional experiments indicated that the antagonism was due to an allosteric inhibition of activator (batrachotoxin) binding (POSTMA and CATTERALL 1984) and, furthermore, that there were different binding sites for neutral and charged local anesthetics producing this effect (HUANG and EHRENSTEIN 1981). Nevertheless, for inhibition of both electrically-driven and pharmacologically-activated sodium channels there is a strong correlation between hydrophobicity and potency (see Sect. C, above).

The apparent contradiction between evidence placing the anesthetic binding site in the channel and results showing a hydrophobic binding region was resolved by HILLE (1977 b) through the introduction of dual pathways to a common receptor. The 3°-amine anesthetic molecule that inhibited the channel had its protonable nitrogen in the pore, or adjacent to it, while the aromatic group nestled in a nearly hydrophobic pocket. Disposition of drugs at the site was "loose"; protonated, charged anesthetics (and quaternary derivatives) protruded into the pore, whereas unprotonated forms (and neutral drugs, like benzocaine) were more withdrawn into the membrane. (Of course, protonation of amines is a rapidly reversible process, with proton binding and unbinding probably occurring in microseconds at neutral pH, so the charge on the anesthetic molecules is perceived as an average value by slower reactions, such as channel activation or drug dissociation.) But the conclusion to HILLE's model, and its subsequent elaboration by SCHWARZ et al. (1977), is that local anesthetics are in the pore and in the membrane at the same time, on average, and that they can escape from this site either by way of the pore, to the axoplasmic compartment, or into the membrane interior, depending on their average charge.

This model is consistent with much experimental data, in the most general sense. Quaternary drugs do appear to selectively combine and leave only open channels. But attempts to correlate the binding of anesthetics to specific channel states are less successful. Sometimes channels are increasingly blocked during a pulse even before or during channel opening, showing that intermediate channel states as well as open ones can bind the drug (Strichartz and Wang 1985). Where is the binding site for this action? And is there truly only one binding site or locus on the channel that accounts for phasic block, or might different sites be revealed as the channel undergoes a sequence of conformational chanes? Although we cannot answer these specific questions now, the existing correlations between molecular features and phasic block do suggest certain attributes of the voltage-conditioned anesthetic binding site, described in the following section.

IV. Molecular Substrate for the Block Recovery Process

Block of sodium channels by local anesthetics is often enhanced by prolonged depolarization or trains of short depolarizations. After such conditioning, block then relaxes back to the tonic level with time constants which can vary by more than two orders of magnitude. Drug size appears to be the most important determinant of this kinetic process, whatever it is, which governs the repriming of sodium channel availability (Courtney 1980a; Courtney and Etter 1983). If T is the time constant of this recovery process and B is the tonic level of block then one can calculate an apparent rate of channel unblocking by $1 = (1-B)/T$. This apparent unblocking rate could represent, among other things, the rate of drug egress from the channel. This process is exquisitely size-dependent. The unblocking rate is inversely proportional to the 6th or 7th power of molecular weight, whereas free aqueous diffusion shows only a 0.3–0.5 power dependence. The dra-

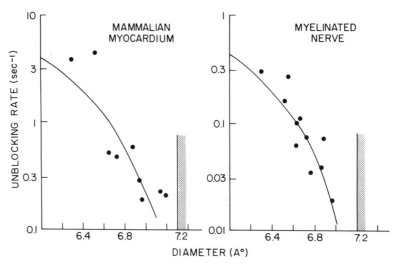

Fig. 12. Unblocking rates are fit to a cylindrical pore model using the excluded area principle $c(r-x)^2$ where r is radius of pore and x is radius of drug. Pore radius of 3.6 Å fits both myocardial observations and myelinated nerve measurements. Absolute rates of recovery from block are about 8 times faster in the warmer (35 versus 10 °C) myocardial preparations. Drugs are treated as equivalent spheres here, although they are generally more complex in shape, so that molecular weight of 300 corresponds to a molecular volume of about 180 cubic Å and equivalent spherical radius of 3.5 Å. From Courtney (1984b)

matic fall-off in repriming rates that is observed as molecular weight approaches 300 can be explained using a restrictive diffusion scheme such as a cylindrical pore model (COURTNEY 1984 b). Analysis using such a pore model gives similar pore radii for both mammalian myocardial and myelinated nerve preparations (see Fig. 12). The differences in the absolute rates of recovery might be attributable to substantial differences in temperature (35 versus 10 °C) as well as real differences in sodium channels and their microenvironments in these two very different tissues. However, other possibilities, more intimately associated with channel protein, should not be ruled out (see COURTNEY 1984 b). The "cylindrical pore" could also represent lattice spaces between the hydrocarbon chains that compose membrane.

Acknowledgements. During the writing of this review the authors received partial support from the USPHS National Institutes of Health in the form of research grants HL 24156 (to KRC) and NS/NIGMS 35647 and GM 15904 (to GRS). GS also thanks the Brigham and Women's Anesthesia Foundation for continued support.

References

Akerman B (1973 a) Uptake and retention of the enantiomers of a local anaesthetic in isolated nerve in relation to different degrees of blocking nervous conduction. Acta Pharmacol Toxicol 32:225–236

Akerman B (1973 b) Studies on the relative pharmacological effects of enantiomers of local anaesthetics with special regard to block of nervous excitation. Astra Uppsala (Research reports)

Akerman B, Camougis G, Sandberg RV (1969) Stereoisomerism and differential activity in excitation block by local anesthetics. Eur J Pharmacol 8:337–347

Albright GA (1979) Cardiac arrest following regional anesthesia with etidocaine or bupivacaine. Anesthesiology 51:285–287

Aldrich RW, Corey DP, Stevens CF (1983) A reinterpretation of mammalian sodium channel gating based on single channel recording. Nature 306:436–441

Arhem P, Frankenhaeuser B (1974) Local anesthetics: effects on permeability properties of nodal membrane in myelinated nerve fibres from Xenopus. Potential clamp experiments. Acta Physiol Scand 91:11–21

Armstrong CM, Bezanilla F (1977) Inactivation of the sodium channel: II. Gating current experiments. J Gen Physiol 70:567–590

Armstrong CM, Croop RS (1982) Simulation of Na channel inactivation by thiazin dyes. J Gen Physiol 80:641–662

Bean BP, Cohen CJ, Tsien RW (1983) Lidocaine block of cardiac sodium channels. J Gen Physiol 81:613–642

Bianchi CP, Strobel GE (1968) Modes of action of local anesthetics in nerve and muscle in relation to their uptake and distribution. Trans NY Acad Sci Ser II 30:1082–1092

Bokesch PM, Strichartz GR (1983) Temperature modulation of use-dependent local anaesthetic block. Reg Anaesth 8:49

Bokesch PM, Strichartz GR (1984) Temperature modulation of local anesthetic block in mammalian nerve. Reg Anaesth 9:46

Bokesch PM, Raymond SA, Strichartz GR (1984) Frequency-dependent block at varying pH. Reg Anaesth 9:32

Bokesch PM, Post C, Strichartz GR (1986) Structure-activity relationship of lidocaine homologues on tonic and frequency-dependent impulse blockade in nerve. J Pharmacol Exp Ther 237:773–781

Boulanger Y, Schreier S, Leitch LC, Smith ICP (1980) Multiple binding sites for local anaesthetics in membrane: characterization of the sites and their equilibria by deuterium NMR of specifically deuterated procaine and tetracaine. Can J Biochem 58:986–995

Boulanger Y, Schreier S, Smith ICP (1981) Molecular details of anesthetic-lipid interaction as seen by deuterium and phosphorous-31 nuclear magnetic resonance. Biochemistry 20:6824–6830

Bradley DJ, Richards CD (1981) Cooling potentiates the action of local anaesthetics on frog sciatic nerve. J Physiol (Lond) 312:38–39

Bradley DJ, Richards CD (1984) Temperature-dependence of the action of nerve blocking agents and its relationship to membrane-buffer partition coefficients: thermodynamic implications for the site of action of local anaesthetics. Br J Pharmacol 81:161–167

Bromage RR, Barfoot MF, Crowell DE, Truant MAP (1967) Quality of epidural blockade. III. Carbonated local anaesthetic solutions. Br J Anaesth 39:197

Butterworth JF, Moran J, Strichartz G, Whitesides G (1985) Block of neuronal sodium channels by "leashed" local anesthetics. Biophys J 47:437a

Cahalan M (1978) Local anesthetic block of sodium channels in normal and pronase-treated squid giant axons. Biophys J 23:285–311

Cahalan M, Almers W (1979) Block of sodium conductance and gating current in squid giant axons poisoned with quaternary strychnine. Biophys J 27:57–74

Campbell TJ (1983) Importance of physico-chemical properties in determining the kinetics of the effects of Class I antiarrhythmic drugs on maximum rate of depolarization in guinea-pig ventricle. Br J Pharmacol 80:33–40

Catchlove RFH (1972) The influence of CO_2 and pH on local anesthetic action. J Pharmacol Exp Ther 181:298–309

Catterall WA (1975) Co-operative activation of action potential Na^+ ionophore by neurotoxins. Proc Natl Acad Sci USA 72:1782–1786

Catterall WA (1980) Neurotoxins that act on voltage-sensitive sodium channels in excitable membranes. Annu Rev Pharmacol Toxicol 20:15–43

Chiu SY, Ritchie JM, Rogart RB, Stagg D (1979) A quantitative description of membrane currents in rabbit myelinated nerve. J Physiol (Lond) 292:149–166

Clarkson CW, Hondeghem LM, Matsubara T, Levinson G (1984) Possible mechanisms of bupivacaine toxicity: fast inactivation block with slow diastolic recovery. Anaesth Analg 63:199a

Cohen CJ, Bean BP, Tsien RW (1984) Maximal upstroke velocity as an index of available sodium conductance. Circ Res 54:636–651

Cohen IS, Strichartz GR (1977) On the voltage-dependent action of tetrodotoxin. Biophys J 17:275–279

Cohen IS, Atwell D, Strichartz G (1981) The dependence of the maximum rate of rise of the action potential upstroke on membrane properties. Proc R Soc Lond (Biol) 214:85–98

Colatsky TJ (1982) Quinidine block of cardiac sodium channels is rate- and voltage-dependent. Biophys J 37:343a

Courtney KR (1974) Frequency-dependent inhibition of sodium currents in frog myelinated nerve by GEA 968, a new lidocaine derivative. PhD thesis, Department of Physiology and Biophysics, University of Washington, Seattle, Washington

Courtney KR (1975) Mechanism of frequency-dependent inhibition of sodium currents in frog myelinated nerve by GEA-968, a new lidocaine derivative. J Pharmacol Exp Ther 195:225–236

Courtney KR (1979) Extracellular pH selectively modulates recovery from sodium inactivation in frog myelinated nerve. Biophys J 28:363–368

Courtney KR (1980a) Interval-dependent effects of small antiarrhythmic drugs on excitability of guinea-pig myocardium. J Mol Cell Cardiol 12:1273–1286

Courtney KR (1980b) Structure-activity relations for frequency-dependent block in nerve by local anesthetics. J Pharmacol Exp Ther 213:114–119

Courtney KR (1981a) Significance of bicarbonate for antiarrhythmic drug action. J Mol Cell Cardiol 13:1031–1034

Courtney KR (1981b) Comparative actions of mexiletine in nerve, skeletal and cardiac muscle. Eur J Pharmacol 74:9–18

Courtney KR (1983a) Tests of the size/solubility hypothesis. Circulation 68:296a

Courtney KR (1983b) Quantifying antiarrhythmic drug blocking during action potentials in guinea-pig papillary muscle. J Mol Cell Cardiol 15:749–757

Courtney KR (1983c) Inactive versus open channel blocking of cardiac sodium channels Biophys J 41:76a

Courtney KR (1984a) Relationship between excitability block and negative inotropic actions of antiarrhythmic drugs. Proc West Pharmacol Soc 27:181–184

Courtney KR (1984b) Size-dependent kinetics associated with drug block of sodium current. Biophys J 45:42–44

Courtney KR, Etter EF (1983) Modulated anticonvulsant block of sodium channels in nerve and muscle. Eur J Pharmacol 88:1–9

Courtney KR, Kendig JJ, Cohen EN (1978a) Frequency-dependent conduction block: the role of nerve impulse pattern in local anesthetic potency. Anaesthesiology 48:111–117

Courtney KR, Kendig JJ, Cohen EN (1978b) The rates of interaction of local anesthetics with sodium channels in nerve. J Pharmacol Exp Ther 207:594–604

Covino BG, Vassallo H (1976) Local anesthetics: mechanisms of action and clinical use. Grune and Stratton, New York

Creveling CR, McNeal ET, Daly JW, Brown GB (1983) Batrachotoxin-induced depolarization and ^{3}H-batrachotoxin-A 20α-benzoate binding in a vesicular preparation from guinea pig cerebral cortex. Mol Pharmacol 23:350–358

Dodson BA, Miller KW (1985) Evidence for a dual mechanism in the anesthetic action of an opioid peptide. Anaesthesiology 62:615–620

Ehring GR, Moyer JW, Hondeghem LM (1982) Implications from electrophysiological differences resulting from small structural changes in antiarrhythmic drugs. Proc West Pharmacol Soc 25:65–67

Feldman HS, Covino BM, Sage DJ (1982) Direct chronotropic and inotropic effects of local anesthetic agents in isolated guinea pig atria. Reg Anaesth 7:149–156

Flatman JA (1968) The action of local anesthetic agents on nerve fibres. PhD thesis, University of London

Franks NP, Lieb WR (1982) Molecular mechanisms of general anaesthesia. Nature 300:487–493

Frazier DT, Narahashi T, Yamada M (1970) The site of action and active form of local anesthetics: II. Expüeriments with quaternary compounds. J Pharmacol Exp Ther 171:45–51

Grant AO, Strauss LJ, Wallace AG, Strauss HC (1980) The influence of pH on the electrophysiological effects of lidocaine in guinea pig ventricular myocardium. Circ Res 47:542–550

Grant AO, Trantham JL, Brown KK, Strauss HC (1982) pH-dependent effects of quinidine on the kinetics of dV/dt_{max} in guinea pig ventricular myocardium. Circ Res 50:210–217

Hahin R, Goldman L (1978) Initial conditions and the kinetics of the sodium conductance in *Myxicola* giant axons: I. Effects on the time-course of the sodium conductance. J Gen Physiol 72:863–877

Hahin R, Strichartz GR (1981) Effects of deuterium oxide on the rate and dissociation constants for saxitoxin and tetrodotoxin action. J Gen Physiol 78:113–139

Hansch C, Clayton JM (1973) Lipophilic character and biological activity of drugs: II. The parabolic case. J Pharm Sci 62:1–21

Hansch C, Leo A (1979) Substituent analysis for correlation analysis in chemistry and biology. Wiley Interscience, New York

Hauswirth O, Singh BN (1979) Ionic mechanisms in heart muscle relation to the genesis and the pharmacological control of cardiac arrhythmias. Pharmacol Rev 30:5–63

Hille B (1966) The common mode of action of three agents that decrease the transient change in sodium permeability in nerves. Nature 210:1220–1222

Hille B (1977a) The pH-dependent rate of action of local anesthetics on the node of Ranvier. J Gen Physiol 69:475–496

Hille B (1977b) Local anesthetics: hydrophilic and hydrophobic pathways for the drug-receptor reaction. J Gen Physiol 69:475–496

Hille B (1980) Theories of anesthesia: general perturbations versus specific receptors. Prog Anaesthesiol 2:1–5

Hille B, Courtney K, Dum R (1975a) Rate and site of action of local anesthetics in myelinated nerve fibers. Prog Anesthesiol 1:13–20

Hille B, Woodhull AM, Shapiro B (1975b) Negative surface charge near sodium channels of nerve: divalent ions, monovalent ions, and pH. Philos Trans R Soc Lond (Biol) 270:310–318

Hodgkin AL, Huxley AF (1952) The dual effect of membrane potential on sodium conductance in the gian axon of *Loligo*. J Physiol 116:497–506

Hodgkin AL, Huxley AF, Katz B (1952) Measurement of current-voltage relations in the membrane of the gian axon of *Loligo*. J Physiol (Lond) 116:424–448

Hondeghem LM, Katzung BG (1977) Time- and voltage-dependent interactions of antiarrhythmic drugs with cardiac sodium channels. Biochim Biophys Acta 472:373–398

Hondeghem L, Katzung BG (1980) Test of a model of antiarrhythmic drug action: effects of quinidine and lidocaine on myocardial conduction. Circulation 61:1217–1226

Hsia JC, Boggs JM (1973) Pressure effect on the membrane action of a nerve-blocking spin label. Proc Nat Acad Sci USA 70:3179–3183

Huang L-YM, Ehrenstein G (1981) Local anesthetics QX572 and benzocaine act at separate sites on the batrachotoxin-activated sodium channel. J Gen Physiol 77:137–153

Huang L-YM, Ehrenstein G, Catterall W (1978) Interaction between batrachotoxin and yohimbine. Biophys J 23:219–232

Jack JJB, Noble D, Tsien RW (1975) Electric current flow in excitable cells. Oxford University Press, London, pp 261–276

Janoff AS, Pringle MJ, Miller KW (1981) Correlation of general anesthetic potency with solubility in membranes. Biochim Biophys Acta 649:125–128

Julian FJ, Moore JW, Goldman DE (1962) Current-voltage relations of the lobster giant axon membrane under voltage clamp conditions. J Gen Physiol 45:1217–1238

Kendig JJ, Cohen EN (1977) Pressure antagonism to nerve conduction block by anesthetics agents. Anesthesiology 47:6–10

Khodorov BL, Shishkova L, Peganov F, Revenko S (1976) Inhibition of sodium currents in frog Ranvier node treated with local anesthetics: role of slow sodium inactivation. Biochim Biophys Acta 433:409–435

Lynch C (1985) Local anesthetic effects upon myocardial excitation-contraction (E–C) coupling. Reg Anaesth 10:38–39

Mason JM, Hondeghem LM, Katzung BG (1983) Amiodarone blocks inactive cardiac sodium channels. Pflugers Arch 396:79–81

Mautner HG, Lorenc C, Quain P, Marquis JK, Tasaki I (1980) Synthesis and study of conformationally defined enantiomers of local anesthetics and conformationally defined enantiomers of fluorescent dyes designed to label electrically excitable membranes. J Med Chem 23:282–285

McLaughlin S (1975) Local anesthetics and the electrical properties of phospholipid bilayer membranes. In: Fink BR (ed) Molecular mechanisms of anesthesia. Raven, New York, pp 193–220

McLaughlin S, Harary H (1976) The hydrophobic adsorption of charged molecules to bilayer membranes: a test of the applicability of the Stern equation. Biochem J 15:1941–1948

McLaughlin SGA, Szabo G, Eisenman G (1971) Divalent ions and the surface potential of charged phospholipid membranes. J Gen Physiol 58:667–687

Melnik E, Latorre R, Hall JE, Tosteson DC (1977) Phloretin-induced changes in ion-transport across lipid bilayer membranes. J Gen Physiol 69:243–257

Miller KW (1975) The pressure reversal of anesthesia and the critical volume hypothesis. Prog Anaesthesiol 1:341–352

Morison DH (1981) A double-blind comparison of carbonated lidocaine and lidocaine hydrochloride in epidural anaesthesia. Can Anaesth Soc J 28:387–389

Narahashi T, Frazier D, Yamada M (1970) The site of action and active form of local anesthetics. I. Theory and pH experiments with tertiary compounds. J Pharmacol Exp Ther 171:32–44

Nattel S, Elharrar V, Zipes DP, Bailey JC (1981) pH-dependent electrophysiological effects of quinidine and lidocaine on canine cardiac Purkinje fibers. Circ Res 48:55–61

Noda M, Shimizu S, Tanabe T, Takai T, Kayano T, Ikeda T, Takahashi H, Nakayama H, Kanaoka Y, Minamino N, Kangawa K, Matsuo H, Raftery MA, Hirose T, Inayama S, Hayashida H, Miyata T, Numa S (1984) Primary structure of *Electrophorus electricus* sodium channel deduced from cDNA sequence. Nature 312:121–127

Nonner W, Spalding BC, Hille B (1980) Low intracellular pH and chemical agents slow inactivation gating in sodium channels of muscle. Nature 284:360–363

Oshita GS, Sada H, Kojima M, Ban T (1980) Effects of tocainide and lidocaine on the transmembrane action potentials as related to external potassium and calcium concentrations in guinea-pig papillary muscles. NS Arch Pharmacol 314:67–82

Peters A, Vaughn JE (1970) Morphology and development of the Myelin sheath. In: Davison AN and Peters A (eds) Myelination. Charles C Thomas, Springfield, Ill p 3–79

Pooler JP, Valenzeno DP (1983) Re-examination of the double sucrose gap technique for the study of lobster giant axons. Theory and experiments. Biophys J 44:261–269

Postma SW, Catterall WA (1984) Inhibition of binding of ^{3}H-Batrachotoxin A 20α-Benzoate to sodium channels by local anesthetics. Mol Pharmacol 25:219–227

Rando TA, Wang GK, Strichartz GR (1985) The interaction between the alkaloid neurotoxins batrachotixin and veratridine and the gating processes of neuronal sodium channels. Mol Pharmacol, vol 29 (in press)

Raymond SA (1979) Effects of nerve impulses on threshold of frog sciatic nerve fibres. J Physiol (Lond) 290:273–303

Raymond SA, Roscoe RF (1984 RF (1984) CO$_2$ as a local anesthetic. Reg Anaesth 9:43

Ritchie JM (1975) Mechanism of action of local anesthetic agents and biotoxins. Br J Anaesthesiol 47:191–198

Ritchie JM, Greengard P (1966) On the mode of action of local anesthetics. Annu Rev Pharmacol 6:405–429

Ritchie JM, Ritchie BR (1968) Local anaesthetics: effect of pH on activity. Science 162:1394–1395

Ritchie JM, Ritchie B, Greengard P (1965a) The active structure of local anaesthetics. J Pharmacol Exp Ther 150:152–159

Ritchie JM, Ritchie B, Greengard P (1965b) The effect of the nerve sheath on the action of local anesthetics. J Pharmacol Exp Ther 150:160–164

Rosenberg PH, Heavner JE (1980) Temperature-dependent nerve blocking action of lidocaine and halothane. Acta Anaesth Scand 24:314–320

Roth SH (1979) Physical mechanisms of anesthesia. Annu Rev Pharmacol Toxicol 19:159–178

Roth S, Seeman P, Akerman SBA, Chan-Wong M (1972) The action and adsorption of local anesthetic enantiomers on erythrocyte and synaptosome membranes. Biochim Biophys Acta 255:199–206

Rud J (1961) Local anesthetics. An electrophysiological investigation of local anesthesia of peripheral nerves, with special reference to Xylocaine. Acta Physiol Scand 51 (Suppl 178)

Sada H, Ban T (1981) Effects of various structurally related beta-adrenoceptor blocking agents on maximum upstroke velocity of action potential in guinea pig papillary muscles. Naunym Schmiedebergs Arch Pharmacol 317:245–251

Schwarz W (1979) Temperature experiments on nerve and muscle membranes of frogs: indications for a phase transition. Pflugers Arch 382:27–34

Schwarz W, Palade PT, Hille B (1977) Local anesthetics: Effect of pH on use-dependent block of sodium channels in frog muscle. Biophys J 20:343–368

Seeman P (1972) The membrane actions of anesthetics and tranquilizers. Pharmacol Rev 24:583–655

Seeman P (1975) The membrane expansion theory of anesthesia. Prog Anesthesiol 1:243–252

Shapiro BI (1977) Effects of strychnine on the sodium conductance of the frog node of Ranvier. J Gen Physiol 69:915–920

Shepley MP, Strichartz GR, Wang GK (1983) Local anesthetics block non-inactivating sodium channels in a use-dependent manner in amphibian myelinated axons. J Physiol (Lond) 341:62P

Sigworth FJ, Neher E (1980) Single Na$^+$ channel currents observed in cultured rat muscle cells. Nature 287:447–449

Skou JC (1954) Local anesthetics: VI. Relation between blocking potency and penetration of a monomolecular layer of lipoids from nerves. Acta Pharmacol Toxicol 10:325–337

Starmer CF, Grant AO, Strauss H (1984) Mechanisms of use-dependent block of sodium channels in excitable membranes by local anesthetics. Biophys J 46:15–28

Strichartz GR (1973) The inhibition of sodium currents in myelinated nerve by quaternary derivatives of lidocaine. J Gen Physiol 62:37–57

Strichartz GR (1976) Molecular mechanisms of nerve block by local anesthetics. Anaesthesiology 45:421–441

Strichartz G (1977) The composition and structure of excitable nerve membrane. In: Jamieson GA, Robinson DM (eds) Mammalian cell membranes, vol 3. Butterworths, London, pp 173–205

Strichartz G (1980) Use-dependent conduction block produced by volatile general anesthetic agents. Acta Anaesthesiol Scand 24:402–406

Strichartz G (1985) Interactions of local anesthetics with neuronal sodium channels. In: Covino B, Fozzard HA, Rehder K, Strichartz GR (eds) Clinical Physiology Series, American Physiological Society, Bethesda MD, p 39–52

Strichartz GR, Cohen IS (1978) V_{max} as a measure of G_{Na} in nerve and cardiac membranes. Biophys J 23:153–156

Strichartz G, Wang GK (1985) The kinetic basis for phasic local anesthetic blockade of neuronal sodium channels. In: Miller KW and Roth S (eds) Molecular and Cellular Mechanisms of Anesthetics. Plenum Publishing Corporation, New York, pp 217–226

Strichartz G, Zimmermann M (1983) Selective conduction blockade among different fiber types in mammalian nerves by lidocaine combined with low temperature. Soc for Neurosci (USA) Abstracts, p 675

Trudell JR (1980) Biophysical concepts in molecular mechanisms of anesthesia. In: Fink BR (ed) Molecular mechanisms of anesthesia, vol 2. Raven, New York, pp 261–290

Ueda I, Yasuhara H, Shieh D, Lin H-C, Lin SH, Eyring H (1980) Physical chemistry of the interaction of local anesthetics with model and natural membranes. Prog Anaesth 2:285–294

Ulbricht W (1981) Kinetics of drug action and equilibrium results at the node of Ranvier. Physiol Rev 61:785–828

Vandenberg CA, Horn R (1984) Kinetic properties of single sodium channels. Biophys J 45:11a

Wang GK, Strichartz GR (1984) Local anesthetics produce phasic block of sodium channels during activation. Biophys J 45:286a

Wang HK, Earnest J, Limbacher HP (1983) Local anesthetic-membrane interaction: A multiequilibrium model. Proc Natl Acad Sci USA 80:5297–5301

Watson PJ (1980) The mode of action of local anaesthetics. J Pharm Pharmacol 12:257

Westman J, Boulanger Y, Ehrenberg A, Smith ICP (1982) Charge and pH dependent drug binding to model membranes. A ^{2}H-NMR and light absorption study. Biochim Biophys Acta 685:315–328

Wildsmith JAW, Gissen AJ, Gregus J, Covino BG (1985) The differential nerve blocking activity of amino-ester local anaesthetics. Br J Anaesth 57:612–620

Willow M, Catterall WA (1982) Inhibition of binding of [^{3}H] batrachotoxin A 20α-benzoate to sodium channels by the anticonvulsant drugs diphenylhydantoin and carbamazepine. Mol Pharmacol 22:627–635

Yeh JZ (1980) Sodium inactivation mechanism modulates QX-314 block of sodium channels in squid axons. Biophys J 24:569–574

Yeh JZ (1980) Blockage of sodium channels by stereoisomers of local anesthetics. Progr Anaesthesiol 2:35–44

Zaborovskaya LD, Khodorov BI (1984) The role of inactivation in the cumulative blockage of voltage-dependent sodium channels by local anesthetics and antiarrhythmics. Gen Physiol Biophys (USSR) 3:517–520

CHAPTER 4

Mechanisms of Differential Nerve Block

S. A. RAYMOND and A. J. GISSEN

A. Introduction

Local anesthesia has been in active clinical use for 100 years. During the past 50 years surprisingly little change has occurred in drugs or techniques. Recently there has been a rapid increase in the demands placed on the anesthesiologist: The parturient needs pain relief but does not wish to prolong her labor by decrease in motor function. The patient with chronic pain needs relief but a clear sensorium so he may continue as an active member of society. Patients suffering from various neurological disorders with uncontrollable muscle spasms need relief without loss of sensation. These demands can be satisfied only partially with available methods of local anesthesia.

These needs have been a major motivation for investigating what has come to be called "differential nerve block", or more accurately "selective block of specific nerve fiber groups." It is logical in very sick patients to interfere with homeostatic neural mechanisms as little as possible by limiting anesthesia to only that anatomical area and those neural modalities essential to successful treatment.

The term "differential nerve block" when defined as "selective block of specific nerve fibers" implies that motor and sensory characteristics depend on activity in specific nerve fiber groups. This point of view originated in the doctrine of specific nerve energies first developed for peripheral nerves by Müller (MÜLLER 1826). There is little argument with assigning voluntary motor function to activity in large diameter, fast conducting heavily myelinated nerve fibers, and in identifying the smallest, slowest conducting nonmyelinated fibers as those associated with "slow" pain. But the correlation with size is not precise for various motor functions (such as control of intestinal tract, secretory glands, sphincters, blood vessels, and autonomic reflexes) or for other sensory modalities (such as heat, cold, proprioception, discriminatory "fast" pain, and light pressure). There is evidence that these signals can be carried simultaneously in multiple types of fibers, and that the range of fiber size involved in a particular modality overlaps substantially with fibers of other functions. It is clear that sensory modalities modulate each other centrally but such interactions are at best only qualitatively understood (ZIMMERMANN 1979; CHAPMAN 1980; WILLIS 1980; WALL 1984).

From the earliest studies of reversible "paralysis" or dissociation of motor and sensory modalities in peripheral nerves exposed to cold, pressure or local anesthetics, it has been observed that "the four customarily recognized modalities of sensation (touch, cold, warm, pain) do not become paralyzed simultaneously" (SINCLAIR and HINSHAW 1950a). During the past century the question of the order of sensory/motor loss and the underlying neural changes has been repeatedly studied, leading to what might be termed a soft consensus. Differential block is a familiar concept, but it cannot be fundamentally understood until one understands such critical issues as the role of individual peripheral fibers in sensation and what accounts for any differences in their susceptibility to drugs. The clinical objective – control of sensory and motor function – remains remote but there has been substantial progress.

In reviewing this work, we have been impressed by the extent to which critically important words such as "susceptibility", "touch", "pain", have differed in meaning and precision of use by various investigators. Thus it behooves us at the outset to attempt to clarify a few terms that we use in discussing and interpreting the findings concerning "differential block". One overriding issue is the prevailing anatomical and physiological scheme for classification of nerve fibers. This system pervades the existing work, and sharply limits the number and kind of differences among fibers that can be set forth intelligibly in a common context. To use the classification to name a group of fibers is to differentiate that group according to characteristics that are inextricably associated with contradictory or controversial findings and assumptions. How does one properly assess whether diameter or "function" is more related to drug susceptibility when fiber groups are named almost exclusively on the basis of the diameter or conduction velocities of the fibers that comprise them? Thus, we can easily speak of $A\beta$ fibers versus C fibers, but we tend to enter new territory when we consider unmyelinated visceral afferents versus unmyelinated cutaneous afferents since both groups are C-fibers. Suspecting that future investigations will deal with this problem by identifying fibers more extensively according to destination, anatomy, origin, function, and various physiological and biochemical attributes in addition to conduction velocity or diameter, we have elected to report these details wherever possible and to identify specific nerves and denote species, together with details of methods and techniques used in the studies we discuss.

Differential Rate of Block

There are two aspects of "differential block" that have been investigated since the beginnings of interest in the subject. One is 'differential rate of block' which concerns the transient case where one studies differences among fibers in some rate-limiting step during onset or recovery of block. A classical example would be diffusion barriers to local anesthetic. If one group of fibers were relatively more shielded by diffusion barriers than another, a differential block could occur during the transient phase of buildup of anesthetic even if there were no differences in susceptibility to the anesthetic at steady state. Thus, the outcome of any experiment which is concerned with the temporal order of block following the application of a blocking agent will be influenced by any and all factors governing the 'differential rate of block'.

Differential Steady-State Block

The other principal aspect that has been investigated is 'differential steady state block'. By observing the differential block to a blocking agent at steady state, one ideally hopes to infer the relative susceptibility of nerve fibers to that agent. Confusion has occurred when steady-state susceptibility is inferred from findings that specify the temporal sequence of failure following application of a blocking agent. The order of susceptibility due to a differential rate of block may be completely different from that caused by the same agent at steady state. The production of interpretable results requires care and a mature regard for the perversity of circumstance.

Phasic Block: Differential Rate vs. Differential Steady-State

The "block" referred to in either differential rate of block or differential steady state block is a "tonic block". That is, the capability of the fiber to conduct (or of the organism to sense or move) is tested in response to individual stimuli given rarely enough so that successive stimuli are independent. Tonic block is distinguished from "phasic block", which refers to an altered degree of block occurring during frequent stimulation. It is a transient change, decaying with particular kinetics after the stimulation is stopped. A differential rate of phasic block may be distinguished from a differential steady state phasic block. In both, the dependence of impulse conduction on prior impulse activity determines the level of phasic block.

Conduction Safety

Since we will be analyzing variations in the degree of "block" in terms of impulse conduction in single fibers, it is also essential to emphasize the concept of conduction safety. In essence, whether conduction block occurs is a contest between the power of the extrinsic agent and the intrinsic capacity of the nerve fiber to sustain impulse conduction – its conduction safety. The nerve impulse generates the ionic currents that sustain its propagation. Usually, more inward current is available than is needed to sustain propagation, thus defining the "margin of safety". The "safety factor" can be defined as the ratio of the current supplied by the action potential to the current required by the downstream membrane in order for active invasion of that membrane. TASAKI (1953) first measured a safety factor of 5–7 for large myelinated fibers in frog sciatic nerve by comparing the longitudinal current generated by a single isolated node stimulated electrically to the threshold current required to stimulate that node. Others have found the safety factor to be in the same range in large fibers (ICHIOKA et al. 1960; UEHARA 1958, 1960). GISSEN et al. (1982 a) cited Paintal's estimate of a safety factor of about 20 for unmyelinated fibers, but it has not been measured for small fibers.

Conduction safety may be considered to depend on 3 interrelated factors: 1) the factors influencing the "strength" of the invading action potential 2) factors governing the coupling of the action current to the uninvaded membrane and 3) factors influencing the threshold of the downstream membrane. In general it can be said that conduction will fail if the threshold rises high enough or the spike amplitude drops low enough to reduce the safety factor below 1.0 (TOMAN 1952). Thus, the safety factor can be used as a term of degree to quantify changes in the processes underlying impulse conduction in a single fiber that do not reach the point of causing (or relieving) conduction "block". As stressed by LORENTE DE NO

(1947a, p. 175) there is no margin of safety for conduction velocity. This is because even the slightest reduction of the safety factor will lessen the extent of the depolarized region ahead of the advancing impulse and/or increase the time required to raise downstream membrane to threshold. Thus we may expect changes in conduction velocity to precede conduction failure, and shifts in reaction times to precede sensory and motor "block".

B. Historical Discussion

I. Differential Tonic Block

At the turn of the century, evidence in 2 main categories pertaining to the differential action of local anesthetics began to be correlated. The first category consisted of reports concerning the order of *loss of function* with cocaine following subcutaneous injection, surface application to mucous membranes or direct application to bare nerves. The second category consisted of observations on the order of *failure of impulse conduction* in nerve fibers classified in various ways such as sensory vs. motor, or vasoconstrictor vs vasodilator (see Sinclair and Hinshaw 1950a; Sinclair 1955, for review).

No linkage was made to diameter of fibers as an important variable, nor to the possible importance of myelin. The mechanism of differential action of local anesthetics was viewed as not yet generally understood (Dixon 1905).

II. Origins of the Dominant Paradigm

The classic and influential paper by Herbert Gasser and Joseph Erlanger in 1929 added a new organizing principle, that of nerve diameter. The paper ushered in a period of more than 50 years where the prevailing view has been that differential block of *function* can be understood at the cellular level as a gradation of "susceptibility" to anesthetic: with small fibers being most susceptible and larger fibers being less so. This view was compatible with evidence that specialized functions could be linked to fibers grouped according to diameter, and that conduction velocities, which were convenient to measure, were reliably and monotonically related to diameter. Evidence for this broadly accepted idea is reviewed in Mount-castle (1980a), who concludes (p 338) that although there is considerable overlap in diameter between fibers having very different functions, the concept of parallel ordering of fiber size and fiber function is generally true. Many studies correlating diameter, conduction velocity and "modality" have been made, leading to tables (see Fig. 1) which serve to summarize the existing categorization that underlies naming and description of peripheral nerve fibers.

Gasser and Erlanger (1929) reviewed the order of failure in sensation during spinal anesthesia and peripheral nerve block. In their assessment, the evidence then available supported the notion that pain was most "susceptible" and "contact" or touch the least susceptible, with variation regarding the relative order of disappearance of cold, warmth and pain. They questioned what attribute of the fibers subserving different functions could underlie this consistency in the order of failure. They rejected the vague notions of a difference in "chemical constitution".

1. (Berthold table classifying peripheral nerve fibers)

PNS	CNS	Main morph. axon types	Main functional axon types	Functional subtypes	Effectors and receptors	Fibre diam μm	velocity m/sec	Special sub-types
		Myelinated axons	Efferent motor	α	Extratusal muscle fibres	9-20	50-120	FF FR S
				β	Extra + intrafusal muscle fibres	9-15	50-85	
				γ	Intrafusal muscle fibres	4.5-8.5 / 2-5	20-40 / 10-25	fast-γ slow-γ
		Myelinated axons	Afferent sensory	I a	Primary intrafusal ending	9-22	50-130	
				I b	Golgi tendon ending	9-22	50-130	
				II	Touch endings, Ruffini joint endings, Secondary intrafusal endings, Pacinian endings, Paciniform endings, Hairfollicle endings	5-15	25-90	
				III	Thermoreceptors, Nociceptors, Vascular wall end	1-7	6-30	
		Myelinated axons	Efferent pregangl	B	Cholinergic — Postganglionic neurons	1-3	3-15	
		Unmyelinated axons	Efferent postgangl	sC	Aminergic, Cholinergic, Purin-peptid-ergic — Smooth muscle, Heart, Glands	0.2-1.5	0.4-2	
		Unmyelinated axons	Afferent	drC	Somatic visceral — C-mechano receptors, Thermoreceptors, Polymodal-nociceptors	0.2-1.5	0.4-2	

2.

	Most Susceptible	Inter-mediate	Least Susceptible
Sensitivity to hypoxia	B	A	C
Sensitivity to pressure	A	B	C
Sensitivity to cocaine and local anesthetics	C	B	A

Table 15-1. Afferent Fiber Groups

Muscle nerve	Cutaneous nerve	Fiber diameter (μm)	Conduction velocity (m/sec)
I	Aα	13-20	80-120
II	Aβ	6-12	35-75
III	Aδ	1-5	5-30
IV*	C*	0.2-1.5	0.5-2

*Unmyelinated.

3.

TABLE 2-1. Nerve fiber types in mammalian nerve.

Fiber Type	Function	Fiber Diameter (μm)	Conduction Velocity (m/sec)	Spike Duration (msec)	Absolute Refractory Period (msec)
A α	Proprioception; somatic motor	12-20	70-120	0.4-0.5	0.4-1
β	Touch, pressure	5-12	30-70		
γ	Motor to muscle spindles	3-6	15-30		
δ	Pain, temperature	2-5	12-30		
B	Preganglionic autonomic	<3	3-15	1.2	1.2
C dorsal root	Pain, reflex responses	0.4-1.2	0.5-2	2	2
sympathetic	Postganglionic sympathetics	0.3-1.3	0.7-2.3	2	2

4.

Fig. 1. Tables classifying peripheral nerve fibers. *1.* From BERTHOLD (1978) correlating size, anatomical archetype, fiber diameter, conduction velocity, transmitter, and peripheral and organs. *2.* From GANONG (1981, p. 43) and *3.* (from MARTIN 1982, p. 163) and *4.* (GANONG 1981, p. 42) present the same categorization in more summary form with less emphasis on specialization in fibers having similar size. They show the correlation to susceptibility to blocking agents and to spike waveform and recovery processes. Note the slight differences in detail concerning conduction velocities and diameters in particular categories

Gasser and Erlanger had previously shown conduction velocity to be linearly correlated with fiber diameter in amphibian myelinated fibers (GASSER and ERLANGER 1927), and since they felt that the physicochemical processes responsible for electrical activity and impulse propagation were essentially similar in all fibers they suspected diameter might be the main parameter accounting both for differential susceptibility of function and differential action on conduction.

2

3

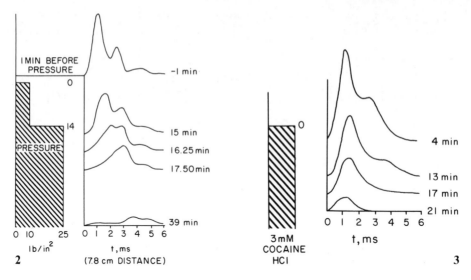

Fig. 2. Differential effect of pressure. Replotted from GASSER and ERLANGER (1929, their Figs. I, II). Sciatic nerve of bullfrog recorded in air. Seven minutes after onset of pressure at 10 lb/in^2, there was only a slight delay and rounding of the fastest elevation. Pressure was then increased to 25 lb/in^2 (1250 mmHg). Action potentials were linearized by Gasser and Erlanger to a common origin (T = 0) corresponding to arrival of the action potential in the fastest fibers in the unpressurized nerve. The elapsed time in minutes from the first increase in pressure is shown next to each trace. Note that the vertical separation between the three middle traces is expanded for clarity and is not proportional to the total duration of the experiments

Fig. 3. Differential action of cocaine. Replotted from GASSER and ERLANGER (1929, their Fig. III). The saphenous nerve of the dog was recorded in air, Aβ and Aγ elevations are shown. Action potentials were linearized by Gasser and Erlanger to a common origin (T = 0) corresponding to the arrival of the action potential in the fastest fibres in the nerve prior to addition of cocaine. The elapsed time in minutes from the addition of drug is given beside each trace

The 1929 paper consisted of 2 sorts of experiments, one with pressure and one with cocaine. Figure 2 shows the action of pressure on compound action potentials recorded from a bullfrog nerve subjected to pressure. All A wave components (α, β, and δ) of the compound AP were reduced by pressure, though it took more than 30 min for the effect to develop. The fastest (largest diameter) fibers suffered the greatest degree of delay and block; the effect does not appear to have been reversible. All components shown in the figure represent conduction velocities associated with myelinated fibers. C-fibers were not studied.

The second class of experiments were of similar design; a region of nerve between stimulating and recording electrodes was exposed to anesthetic (cocaine) in a solution confined with a 1 cm long "vulcanite" cylinder through which the nerve was threaded. With frog nerves at room temperature, the "differential action was variable, and in some nerves was insignificant or zero". For mammalian nerves recorded in air at 37 °C it was consistently observed that small fibers (i. e., slow conducting elevations in the compound action potential) tended to be blocked *before* large ones. Though in all cases a varying proportion of large fast fibers were blocked well *before* the elevations corresponding to the smaller fibers had disappeared (Fig. 3). Using reconstruction methods (review GASSER 1935 b) Gasser and Erlanger analyzed the reduction of the CAP, and concluded that temporal dispersion could not account for the drop, and that therefore there must have been an overlap in sensitivity between fibers in the $A\alpha\beta\gamma\delta$ groups. They reported that the δ group always disappeared *before* the $\alpha\beta\gamma$ complex disappeared, but not *before* the faster elevations were affected. Gasser and Erlanger also studied dilute solutions of cocaine (0.3–1.5 mM) applied over several hours, to assure homogenous diffusion of the drug within the nerve. The blocking actions were reversible. Whenever differential block was observed during onset, the reverse order was obtained during recovery. Note that their experiments tested differential *rate* of block since the traces shown in their figures were all taken as a function of delay from a dose. The incremental effects of the low concentrations with time suggest that a diffusion gradient did exist and that fibers blocked over several hours as the concentration of cocaine available to each of them became elevated.

Thus, these foundational experiments were not comprehensive in two major ways. They were essentially concerned only with differential rate of block, and they did not report the place of C-fibers in the order of blockade since the C-elevation was not discussed.

In their account, the mechanism of differential block by size was attributed to the greater "accessibility" of the protoplasm of small fibers to anesthetic than the protoplasm of large fibers on the basis of the surface to volume ratio. This explanation hinged on the assumption that local anesthetics act by "chemical combination with the protoplasm". This assumption is not compatible with evidence that local anesthetics act on the membrane, not the axoplasm (see CONDOURIS 1961 and Chap. 2, this volume), and we must look to other work to provide a mechanism for the size principle.

Gasser and Erlanger concluded that some small fibers were found to be able to conduct as long as any of the larger fibers, and that "thus, while fiber size is a determining factor in nerve susceptibility to poisons, it is not sufficiently differentiating to cause the fibers to drop out on a strictly size – basis". Gasser and Erlanger used their size principle to explain the prevailing impression that sensory fibers were more sensitive than motor fibers, by remarking that the motor fibers used in the prior studies had been larger than the often small sensory fibers in the sciatic involved in respiratory reflexes and changes in blood pressure. They also predicted that fibers signalling touch would be larger than those concerned with temperature (both cold and warmth) and that these would in turn be larger than fibers subserving pain. The paper forecast a burgeoning literature in physiology of somethesis linking function to fibers of various restricted ranges in diameter, and the predictions were successfully and convincingly supported.

Shortly after the publication of Gasser and Erlanger's paper in 1929 HEINBECKER et al. (1933) added several important findings linking the laboratory work of Gasser and Erlanger to the clinical practice of anesthesia. They reviewed the organization of the nervous system and endorsed the concept that fibers that "serve similar functional mechanisms in the body" were grouped according to size, conduction rate, elevation and wave shape of action potential and terminal connections. They concluded that "...the peripheral nervous system appears to be constructed out of specific groups of fibers, the boundaries of which do not overlap sufficiently to obscure the scheme", and proceeded to search for the fiber group mediating "painful impulses" in mixed nerves (HEINBECKER et al. 1933). Realizing that demonstrating this functional linkage would require reports on perception of pain, they performed experiments on humans and on human nerves excised from the leg of a patient with diabetic gangrene undergoing an amputation. Similar experiments were done on dogs and on excised nerves from dogs. The results were sufficient to establish a persuasive connection between activation of fibers in a specific elevation in the compound action potential having a 15–30 m/s conduction velocity and the sensation of "pricking, cutting, or abrasion".

In their subsequent report (HEINBECKER et al. 1934) they added results with nerve blocks by pressure and by procaine to the results obtained previously by differential recruitment with stimulus intensity. The experiments were performed on cat peripheral nerves (sciatic, saphenous, vagus, cervical sympathetic) exposed to anesthetic (procaine and cocaine) in a glass cylinder of 0.5 cm length. They confirmed that blocking proceeds from slower to faster conducting groups (using a blocking dose) but is never finished in one group "before" it becomes present to a significant degree in the others. They then checked the correlation between order of sensory loss in peripheral nerve blocks by procaine in 3 human volunteers and in marginal spinal anesthesia with procaine in "routine surgical patients". Essentially the same order was observed for spinal block as for peripheral nerve: increased skin temperature (signalling failure of sympathetic C-fiber vasoconstrictors due either to block of preganglionic B fibers or to direct block of the C-fibers) then loss of sensitivity to cold and warmth, then loss of "pricking pain" and pressure pain (together), then motor loss, loss of joint sense, pressure sense and the sensation of touch in that order and in close sequence with significant overlap. 9 min elapsed during the progressive loss prior to complete block in the single case selected for publication. Recovery was in rough inverse order, proceeding more slowly than onset, and beginning with return of insensitive spasmodic movement. In the peripheral nerve experiments, they reported a distinct interval between loss to cold (now associated with Aδ fibers, MACKENZIE et al. 1975; GEORGOPOULOS 1977; FRUHSTORFER and LINDBLUM 1983) which preceded the loss to warmth but they did not quantitate the thermal stimuli used ("hot metal rods", "freezing" the skin with ethyl chloride).

With these experiments the basis existed for a comprehensive synthesis concerning the design and function of the nervous system, and the approach to regional anesthesia. Subsequent contributions have mainly refined and supplemented the image of the peripheral nervous system guiding clinical practice for more than 50 years.

III. Synthesis: The Size Principle

3 main components of the synthesis were in place: 1) a schema for classifying peripheral fibers according to diameter, electrophysiology and function; 2) an ex-

perimental foundation linking human sensory experience and motor capacities to the classification, and 3) the demonstration of differential action of anesthetics on fibers so classified and on sensations so named.

Several principal lines of direct evidence had not yet been supplied, although it was widely presumed what such studies would find. Studies had not been reported on differential steady-state block, nor were there any reports concerning the unmyelinated group to test whether susceptibility to anesthetic followed the size principle in all single fibers, both myelinated and unmyelinated. How the central nervous system provided the context for interpretation of impulses in each class of fibers was recognized as an important problem (HEINBECKER et al. 1934, pp 34–35) but had not been treated experimentally.

In the next section, we trace refinements and clarifications that have contributed to this synthesis by investigators working since then. The many factors influencing differential block are highlighted in roughly the same chronological order of the investigations in which they were first discussed. Unless otherwise noted, all investigators have emphasized differential *tonic* block, though several have commented on the role of activity in Wedensky (or phasic) inhibition or in modulation of sensory or motor paralysis (HEINBECKER et al. 1934; MATTHEWS and RUSHWORTH 1957b; FRANZ and PERRY 1974; MACKENZIE et al. 1975; RUCH 1979; DEJONG 1980a; FINK and CAIRNS 1984b).

C. Confirmations, Extensions, Clarifications, and Contradictions

We use the term "size principle" to refer to the idea that differential block, of either sensory or motor *function* or of *impulse conduction* in nerve fibers, depends on the size (or conduction velocity) of the fibers. Implicit in the term is a link between size and function.

I. Confirmation and Extension of the Size Principle

1. Recruitment of Fibers and of Sensation with Stimulus Strength

The size principle accounted for differential *block* of both conduction and function, but it was also consistent with the differential *activation* of fiber groups in nerves stimulated with electrical pulses. Extracellular stimulation of axons correlates with diameter because axoplasmic resistance diminishes with cross section area. Thus, at any particular strength of stimulation, axonal segments of equal length will be more depolarized in fibers of larger diameter. This expectation is in good accord with experimental results showing a reliable order of recruitment of fibers with stimulus strength beginning with the fastest conducting and ending with the slowest conducting (GASSER 1935b; LEKSELL 1945; BURKE et al. 1975). The extent of the differential in stimulus intensity for fibers of several groups is a function of duration of stimulus pulse (BISHOP and O'LEARY 1939).

Some rare exceptions to this rule have been found. GASSER (1950) discovered a class of Aδ fibers conducting at 5–8 m/s that were activated at higher stimulus strengths than were required to fire more slowly conducting C-fibers. It has also been found that within the range of conduction velocities of C-fibers in mammalian nerves, recruitment is not orderly. A threshold stimulus excites C-fibers at both slow and fast extremes of the range (GASSER 1950; DOUGLAS and RITCHIE 1962). Nonetheless, the relation between size and recruitment is more precise than is the relation of size to drug sensitivity or the relation of size to pressure (GASSER and ERLANGER 1929; HEINBECKER et al. 1934; SINCLAIR and HINSHAW 1950 b).

Thus, there is some importance in the relation between stimulus strength and function. The early experiments correlating recruitment of elevations in compound action potential to sensation (HEINBECKER et al. 1933; GASSER 1935 b) compared sensory data from humans to neurograms obtained from excised nerves in animals. Although action potentials in one human nerve had been recorded following dissection from the amputated leg of a patient with diabetic gangrene of the foot (HEINBECKER et al. 1933), there were no examples when such recordings were made simultaneously from a stimulated nerve while the person reported the corresponding sensations.

Such a test was made more than 20 years later in an experiment performed on human patients undergoing surgical treatment for intractable pain (COLLINS et al. 1960). After lumbar laminectomy was performed, the patients were awakened from anesthesia. The sural nerve, a pure sensory nerve, had been cut in the calf, and mounted for both stimulation and monopolar recording on copper electrodes. Prior to cordotomy, the sural nerve was stimulated to provide controls so that the efficacy of the surgery in blocking pain could be assessed. At threshold intensity, $A\beta$ fibers conducting at 80–85 m/s were activated. The sensation was diversely reported as "tingling", "scraping", or "grabbing". It was not painful even for stimulating rates between 5 and 5,000 Hz. As the stimulus intensity of single shocks was increased, slower A fibers were recorded, but the same sensations were reported except that they were "stronger". Repetitions evoked a sense of urgency ("surprise", "slight anguish" or a "burning quality") but not pain. The $A\delta$ elevation appeared at a stimulus voltage 5 times higher than threshold for $A\beta$ potentials and was heralded with sensations described as "unpleasant", "stinging", and "sharp". Repeated stimulation became uncomfortable, but could be tolerated provided the patient was warned. The pain and the $A\delta$ component were reported to increase in parallel. At 20 times threshold for $A\beta$ potentials, a C-elevation appeared in response to single stimuli. These intense stimuli were also followed by multiple firings in other fibers. At this intensity patients reported a vivid increase in pain and refused to experience a second trial of repetitive stimulation. After the cordotomy, the sensations were not changed for stimuli below the intensity needed to activate $A\delta$ fibers. However, patients no longer objected to repeated stimuli at either $A\delta$ or C levels. Interestingly, given the dissociation between pain and suffering (SCHWARTZ 1950; CASSELL 1982), some patients complained of "a new unpleasantness" even in the absence of pain when given these intense stimuli.

These findings were confirmed in later less traumatic studies of human volunteers (HALLIN and TOREBJORK 1973; BURKE et al. 1975) using fascicles of median and radial nerves. In these experiments (see Fig. 4) the electrical stimulus was more localized. Percutaneous stimulating electrodes were inserted in the hand in

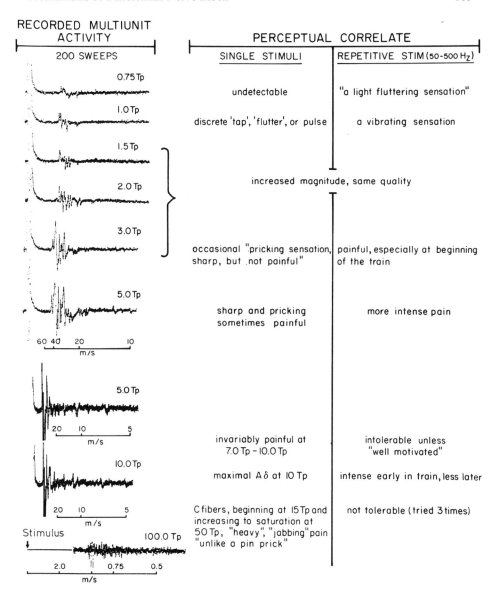

RECORDED MULTIUNIT ACTIVITY

200 SWEEPS

PERCEPTUAL CORRELATE

	SINGLE STIMULI	REPETITIVE STIM (50-500 Hz)
0.75 Tp	undetectable	"a light fluttering sensation"
1.0 Tp	discrete 'tap', 'flutter', or pulse	a vibrating sensation
1.5 Tp		
2.0 Tp	increased magnitude, same quality	
3.0 Tp	occasional "pricking sensation, sharp, but not painful"	painful, especially at beginning of the train
5.0 Tp	sharp and pricking sometimes painful	more intense pain
5.0 Tp	invariably painful at 7.0 Tp – 10.0 Tp	intolerable unless "well motivated"
10.0 Tp	maximal A δ at 10 Tp	intense early in train, less later
100.0 Tp	C fibers, beginning at 15 Tp and increasing to saturation at 50 Tp; "heavy", "jabbing" pain "unlike a pin prick"	not tolerable (tried 3 times)

60 40 20   10
m/s

20 10   5
m/s

20   10   5
m/s

Stimulus

2.0   0.75   0.5
m/s

Fig. 4. Perception during recruitment. On the left are recordings averaged over 200 sweeps of responses of median nerve fascicles to electrical stimulation in the receptive fields supplied by the median nerve. The associated descriptions as summarized from 20 experimental sessions with 6 normal subjects are given on the right. Adapted from BURKE et al. (1975)

an area of skin selected where touching evoked the most notable barrage of multi-unit action potentials in the fascicle near the wrist where intraneural tungsten recording electrodes were inserted. They were able to show a good correspondence between activation of Aδ-fibers in the neurogram and the first appearance of sharp pain in consciousness. They also described an association between activation of afferent C-fibers and the appearance of an intolerable "heavy" pain that differed in quality from pinprick.

The findings of recruitment experiments show a parallel between recruitment of fibers by size and recruitment of touch and pain. Yet it is clear that even localized electrical stimuli to the skin do not feel like natural stimuli (touch, sandpaper, pinpricks, wetness, etc.). This has been a consistent problem with electrical stimuli, and subjects have trouble describing the sensations they experience with electrical stimulation using the ordinary vocabulary derived from daily life (SINCLAIR 1955). Furthermore, such experiments are limited in design. The presence of activity in lower threshold fibers complicates the discrimination of the effects of higher threshold afferents. Differential recruitment is not a means of independently stimulating the modalities and submodalities of specialized fiber types that have been discovered. Even the traditional qualities of warm and cold, which have been linked to activity in Aδ- and C-fibers by other experiments (DYCK et al. 1972; DARIAN-SMITH et al. 1973; GEORGOPOULOS and MOUNTCASTLE 1976; MOUNTCASTLE 1980 b), were not elicited at any strength during stimulation of whole nerve (HEINBECKER et al. 1933; COLLINS et al. 1960) or even of a restricted area of skin (HALLIN and TOREBJORK 1973; TOREBJORK and HALLIN 1973, 1974, 1979; BURKE et al. 1975). This is curious considering the findings of sensory dissociation of warmth and cold during blocking procedures with anesthetics or pressure (LEWIS et al. 1931; HEINBECKER et al. 1934; SINCLAIR and HINSHAW 1950 b; VALLBO et al. 1979). Thus differential recruitment of fibers in a nerve is not well suited to test the association between fiber size and function with much precision. Recently microstimulation of single fibers in humans has been applied to the problem of associating sensation with isolated activity in fibers of particular size (TOREBJORK and OCHOA 1980; VALLBO et al. 1979) see Sect. C. 5.

Given the overlapping conduction velocities between fibers of different modalities that was stressed by GASSER (1943) which ensures that any given elevation of the compound action potential will contain several types, the difficulties in describing the muddled sensations produced by electrical stimulation are a kind of measure of the lack of precision of the link between fiber size and function. Size is a significant organizing principle in the peripheral nervous system, but it is clearly not the case that each cutaneous sensory quality is subserved by its own distinct group of fibers occupying an exclusive band in the spectrum of diameters.

2. C Fibers and Pain

a) Early Disagreements

Before 1935, the link of C-fibers to pain was controversial. It was a logical and essential extension of the size principle to establish the size of fibers subserving the sense of pain and to confirm that selective conduction block of those fibers would also selectively block the sensation of pain. The early evidence in favor of the link to C-fibers (RANSON 1931; LEWIS et al. 1931) was questioned by Heinbecker and colleagues when stimulation of vagus nerve at high C-intensity failed to evoke aversive behavior in cats, rabbits and dogs (HEINBECKER and O'LEARY 1933). In a conjoint paper testing the function of C-afferents having cell bodies in dorsal root ganglia, they expressed doubts that even cutaneous afferent C-fibers carried impulses that could be interpreted as pain (BISHOP et al. 1933). Since they could find no sensory role for afferent C-fibers, they suggested instead that such fibers were involved in reflex vasoconstriction and dilatation and concluded that all types of pain could be accounted for without invoking C-fibers.

b) Confirmation, Pressure and Anesthetic Blocks of CAP in Animals and of Sensation in Humans

Gasser's group, however, (CLARK et al. 1935) were able to correlate firing of C-fibers in cat saphenous nerve with reflexive changes in ventilation and blood pressure that would have been expected under noxious stimulation. Electrical activation of C- afferents, while A-fibers were blocked by cuff ischemia or by direct pressure on the nerve, produced reflexes similar to those caused by painful stimuli given without block. In rather deeply anesthetized cats electrical stimuli strong enough to fire $A\beta$-fibers but not $A\delta$-fibers (called B-fibers in the paper) did not generate such reflexes. Recruiting $A\delta$-fibers also had little reflex effect even when the elevation was maximal (GASSER 1935a). Only when the stimuli were strong enough to stimulate a C-wave, did respiration and heart rate change dramatically. These results in cats implicated C-fibers explicitly in reflex response to pain.

The study linked pain to activity in those C-fibers that caused withdrawal reflexes even after sympathectomy and ventral root section, i.e., afferent dorsal root C-fibers (RANSON et al. 1935). On the basis of pressure blocks, it also linked the order of sensory paralysis of delayed pain to the order of conduction block in those C-fibers, and of the faster, "sharp" pain (as well as cold) to conduction block of $A\delta$-fibers.

These experiments did not demonstrate that impulses in C-fibers produced the pain that is felt under normal conditions when larger cutaneous fibers are not blocked. They did establish that stimuli firing multiple A- and C-fibers were painful, but it was not known if activitiy in a single C-fiber could be appreciated as pain, nor whether afferent C-fibers were active tonically as were sympathetic fibers. It was not clear how the magnitude of the sensation of pain was to be correlated with the frequency of firing or firing in multiple $A\delta$- and C-fibers. The prediction that selective block of $A\delta$- and C-fibers would block pain had only been tested for acute pain from electric shock, injury, or heat; and it was not established that regional blockade of C- and $A\delta$-fibers would block all forms of pain such as chronic pain or pain from regenerating nerve (Tinel sign) as effectively as it prevented acute surgical pain.

Gasser summarized the results of the investigations of both groups by concluding that individual fibers each subserved a particular sensory quality or modality, but that in any particular elevation of the compound action potential, multiple sensory or motor functional groups would overlap in conduction velocity or diameter. Thus, not all C afferent fibers would engender pain (e. g., those in the vagus below the recurrent laryngeal branch), but some C-fibers in cutaneous nerves certainly did (GASSER 1943).

Fifteen years later SINCLAIR and HINSHAW (1950 b) compared the order of sensory loss with cuff ischemia to the order observed after injection of procaine to block ulnar and lateral popliteal nerves in humans. They showed that the order of sensory loss, particularly with procaine, depended strongly on the area of skin tested and on the intensity, size, duration and other attributes of the stimulus used to test for sensation (SINCLAIR and HINSHAW 1950 a). They questioned conclusions and prior work on the basis of the inconsistencies among stimuli and among endpoints used to test for the loss of the sensations of touch, pain, abrasion, proprioception, moptor capacity, thermal sensation, etc. Nonetheless, after controlling for such differences by using the same stimuli with the same adopted endpoint in the same population of trained subjects, they demonstrated statistically significant differences in the order of failure.

c) Differential Susceptibility of C-Fibers to Anesthetics-Empirical Contradictions

It is striking that the only evidence cited in any of the prior work corroborating the assertion that the size principle applied to C-fibers can be found in the methods section of HEINBECKER et al. (1934, p 39). The tables showed disappearance of C-waves before other elevations in a single experiment on cat saphenous nerve. Both laboratories published work concerning C-fibers (BISHOP and O'LEARY 1939; ERLANGER and GASSER 1937; ERLANGER and BLAIR 1940; ERLANGER et al. 1941; GASSER 1935 a, 1935 b, 1943 1950; GASSER et al. 1938; HEINBECKER and BISHOP 1935, HEINBECKER and BARTLEY 1940), but no account of experiments demonstrating relative susceptibility of the C-elevation to anesthetics was given, though the differential persistance of the C-wave during cuff ischemia was convincingly supported by data (GASSER 1935 b).

When new experimental studies of C-fiber susceptibility did appear, they were in conflict with the size principle. Studies using vagus, phrenic, and sciatic nerves in rabbits, guinea pigs, and frogs with 0.025% procaine (EVERETT and GOODSELL 1952) and 0.05% procaine (EVERETT and TOMAN 1954) showed overlap in the initial onset of failure in the A- and C-elevations. $A\delta$- and B-fibers failed first. In contradiction with the size principle, total block of the A-wave preceded total block of the C-elevation in vagus nerves. With sciatic nerves, total block of C usually preceded total block of A, but the rates of decline during initial onset of the block overlapped "equally". Testing differential effects with ethyl through amyl carbamates, Crescitelli found a similar order in frog sciatic nerves; first blocked were $A\delta$-fibers ("B" in the paper) then large A-fibers, then a faster C_1-component and finally the slowest conducting C_2-component (CRESCITELLI 1948, 1950). The $A\delta$- and B-group also was reported to be most susceptible to low (11 mM) sodium, blocking completely while more than 50% of the C-fibers and other A-fibers were conducting (CRESCITELLI 1952 a).

These in vitro studies indicated that susceptibility of C-fibers was not greater than the susceptibility of A-fibers as the size principle would predict on the basis of the order of disappearance of pain.

3. Differential Susceptibility Among Motor Fibers – Empirical Support for the Link Between Function, and Susceptibility to Anesthetic

In motor fibers there are two important groups with distinctly different conduction velocities: fibers from α motor neurons (100 m/s) driving contractions in skeletal muscle fibers, and γ efferent fibers (20–40 m/s) supplying intrafusal muscle fibers in spindles (LEKSELL 1945). The relative sensitivity to procaine of these two groups was tested by MATTHEWS and RUSHWORTH (1957 b). Matthews and Rushworth recorded dorsal and ventral roots in paraffin while 1.5 cm squares of filter paper soaked in 0.2% or 0.5% procaine were folded and placed over peripheral nerves containing fibers from soleus and from gastrocnemius muscles. The nerve supply was stimulated near the muscle and nerves were exposed to anesthetic in the intervening stretches between the stimulating electrodes and the recording electrodes on the roots. Figure 5 is taken from their report and shows that the γ-wave was completely blocked prior to significant reduction of the α-component in ventral root or of the elevation from spindle afferents (Group Ia) recorded in dorsal roots. The authors reported that phasic block (also called Wedenski block) was progressive following application of anesthetic. Frequency following in both α- and γ-fibers was reported to decline before low frequency compound action potentials diminished in height. The differential sensitivity of phasic block was not characterized, and there was no distinction drawn between the differential rate of block vs. block at steady state. Differences between large sensory fibers and large motor fibers in sensitivity to procaine were found not to be significant, and both were blocked at about the same rate.

The peripheral distribution of efferent fields in motoneurons is related to their size (HENNEMAN 1980), showing the pervasiveness of size as an organizing principle in motor systems as well as the sensory systems. Differential anesthesia

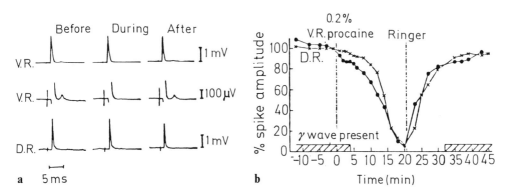

Fig. 5. a Differential block of the CAP in α vs. γ efferent fibers. Recordings from the S_1 dorsal root (*D. R.*) and ventral root (*V. R.*) recorded after stimulation of the gastrocnemius nerve exposed to 0.2% procaine. Note the failure of the γ elevations at 5 min during exposure. The recovery trace was taken 30 min after removing the procaine. **b** The relative change in the CAP of *V. R.* and *D. R.* fast A-fibers plotted from a similar experiment on the soleus motor nerve. Note the failure of the γ wave at 4 min. From MATTHEWS and RUSHWORTH (1957 b)

within the modality of voluntary motion thus would seem to be possible, but any clinical merits and hazards of this possibility do not seem to have been explored.

4. Differential Order of Functional Failure During Spinal Anesthesia

The functions most sensitive to anesthesia ought to be those subserved by the most sensitive fibers. This may be a dependable expectation for nerve blocks in the periphery where specialization of fiber type and function is well supported. However, centrally, the expectation encounters several problems. For example, although peripheral fibers have a consistent size (conduction velocity), these fibers taper to unmyelinated twigs prior to synapsis. Polysynaptic tracts and integrative systems may be fed by small or unmyelinated fibers while continuing with larger myelinated ones. Furthermore, the weakest link in function in terms of vulnerability to anesthesia may not be at the fiber level. The site of action for spinal anesthesia is not established and may differ for different functions (BROMAGE 1978). Thus, it is presently not possible to use the evidence concerning the order of block among "touch", "pain", "cold", "warm", "position sense", "voluntary and reflex motion and autonomic functions" (vasomotion and sweating) to confirm or to reject the size principle.

Nonetheless, the evidence reveals several consistencies that are relevant to the issue of mechanisms of differential block of function. Beginning in 1946, Sarnoff and Arrowood began a series of investigations with intrathecal administration of procaine hydrochloride at 0.2% via catheter so as to produce differential block (SARNOFF and ARROWOOD 1946, 1947a, b; ARROWOOD and SARNOFF 1948; ARROWOOD 1950). Using thermocouples to monitor skin temperature in 4–6 regions they found that block of sympathetic vasoconstrictors, as marked by a rise of skin temperature by 4 °C–6 °C, occurred at doses that were similar to blocking doses for loss of sensation to pinprick. The doses were well below those required to block motor flexion of toes, feet, thighs, and diaphragm. Touch, as assayed by a blunt needle, a camel's hair brush or by finger pressure, was not blocked by the doses they employed (SARNOFF and ARROWOOD 1946, 1947b). This data fit well with the size principle, but the studies did not test fiber diameter nor whether the procaine was acting on spike propagation in fibers rather than on chemically mediated transmission between cells at synapses in the dorsal horn of the spinal cord.

Subsequent authors have confirmed differential block of function with spinal anesthesia (SINCLAIR and HINSHAW 1950a, b; GREENE 1958; AHLGREN et al. 1966; WINNIE and COLLINS 1968; GHIA et al. 1979).

In differential block of function with spinal anesthesia, sympathetic outflow was most sensitive to the lowest doses of local anesthetic, blocked earliest with single doses, and block spread most rostrally. The next most sensitive modality seemed to be sharp pain, overlapping with temperature (both warm and cold), and followed by proprioception, touch, pressure, and voluntary movement. There was considerable variation from patient to patient in the order of sensitivity. The block of vasoconstriction and tonic sudomotor activity as well as pinprick and sensitivity to cold could be maintained for hours with infusion of 0.2%

procaine at levels that did not block touch, proprioception and movement. This suggested a differential steady-state susceptibility in the underlying neural systems.

Blocking of inhibitory systems in some patients who have chronic pain syndromes or who have recovered from them may release phantom limb pain or neuralgia like pains (ARROWOOD and SARNOFF 1948; AHLGREN et al. 1966; LEATH ERDALE 1957; DE JONG and CULLEN 1963). Such results reveal the importance of central integrative mechanisms in differential block of function. Stump pain in particular may develop with sympathetic block, become stronger with sensory block, worsen further with motor block and go away only as anesthesia wears off (LEATHERDALE 1957). Such unusual clinical phenomena constitute a differential "enhancement" of pain by anesthesia.

SINCLAIR and HINSHAW (1950 a) reviewed early work on differential failure of function with spinal anesthesia and stressed that the relative order of disappearance was probably affected by the stimulus used to qualify the modality and by details in methodology. GHIA et al. (1979) subsequently demonstrated that the instructions given to patients and the indicators used to test sensory or motor block affected the clinical utility of differential block for diagnosis in patients with chronic pain. Since some patients experience "block" of pain even with placebo spinals, it is clear that inferring the size of the blocked fibers from functional data is inconclusive in the absence of detailed knowledge of the central and peripheral organization of the physiological systems underlying the functions.

For example, on the basis of the size principle it was inferred that the sharp sensation of pinprick was subserved by C-fibers. Pinprick was not felt during subarachnoid infusion of 2% procaine sufficient to block tonic vasoconstriction and sweating, and the conclusion was drawn because these functions were known to be mediated peripherally by sympathetic C-fibers (ARROWOOD 1950). In fact, it appears instead that blockade of vasoconstriction and sudomotor drive reflects block of preganglionic B-fibers that have been shown in vitro to be more susceptible than C-fibers (HEAVNER and DE JONG 1974; SCURLOCK et al. 1975). Both afferent and efferent C-fibers were probably spared during the differential spinals in which aching pain was spared.

Tickle, motor capacity, touch, deep pressure, vibration sense, and position sense as determined by capacity for "appreciation of toe position" SARNOFF and ARROWOOD (1946), were not impaired or blocked in differential spinal anesthesia. This finding led to a second incorrect interpretation when it was noted that the myotatic reflex at the knee, the ankle jerk and abdominal reflexes were all blocked while position sense was unimpaired (SARNOFF and ARROWOOD 1947). It was, therefore, concluded that tendon reflexes and position sense were mediated by different fibers. On the basis of the size principle, it was further concluded that proprioception was served by large diameter myelinated fibers while the afferent arm of tendon reflexes was served by "relatively small unmyelinated fibers"; either that or the the factors of axon diameter and degree of myelinization could not be the only factors governing differential spinal block (SARNOFF and ARROWOOD 1947 b). After the discovery of the role of γ efferent fibers in contracting intrafusal spindle fibers (LEKSELL 1945), MATTHEWS and RUSHWORTH (1957 b) showed that γ-efferents were more susceptible to peripheral nerve block with procaine than were larger afferent or motor fibers. The differential inhibition of reflexes observed during differential spinal anesthesia was reinterpreted as block of γ-efferents rather than as diffeerential block of Aα afferent fibers (MATTHEWS and RUSHWORTH 1957a; NATHAN and SEARS 1961). A direct demonstration of reduced γ motor discharge during spinal anesthesia does not appear to have been done.

5. Differential Susceptibility of C-Fibers: Confirmation with Pressure and Lidocaine Blocks in Individual Units Recorded from Human Nerves

One of the consistent difficulties in the interpretation of the records of compound action potentials is that differential latency shifts among individual action potentials conducted in the fibers may act by temporal dispersion to lower the height of the compound action potential under conditions where none of the fibers are actually blocked. Thus, it is difficult to relate the number of fibers blocked to the reduction of the compound action potential. More direct evidence bearing on the dependence of conduction in individual fibers requires a shift in method. In the early 1970s, recordings of potentials in which individual A and C units could be clearly distinguished were made during blocks of peripheral nerve using lidocaine and pressure (HALLIN and TOREBJORK 1973; TOREBJORK and HALLIN 1973; MACKENZIE et al. 1975; review VALLBO et al. 1979). Individual units could also be distinguished in blocks of cat saphenous nerve under conditions where the length of the nerves exposed to anesthetic agents could be varied (FRANZ and PERRY 1974).

Vallbo and Hagbarth developed a technique for recording unit potentials from human peripheral nerve fascicles in awake, unanesthetized volunteers. This was extended to C-fibers by Torebjork and Hallin who used the technique to correlate perceptual changes during differential block of the radial nerve with lidocaine and pressure (TOREBJORK and HALLIN 1973). Their findings were confirmed in additional human studies in median and radial nerves performed by MACKENZIE et al. (1975).

a) Recruitment

At the recruitment of the first fast conducting elevation in a neural recording, the sensation is one of light touch. BURKE et al. (1975) reported that when weak electrical stimuli were given at low frequency, trained subjects felt no sensation even though discharges in a few fibers could be recorded. The subjects could not detect these discharges even when they were alerted to the stimuli. However, repetitive activation of the discharges by the same level stimuli at 200 Hz could be detected as a sense of "flutter" or vibration. As the intensities of infrequent stimuli were raised by a factor of 10 (TOREBJORK and HALLIN 1973) a sense of "pricking" was reported. Repetition with stimuli 7–10 times greater than threshold for tactile stimulation was reported as sharp and painful pricking (BURKE et al. 1975) and was correlated with the appearance of fibers conducting in the Aδ range at about 10 m/s. At 15 times the tactile threshold (Tp), a "heavy jabbing pain" appeared in the median nerve as C-fibers were recruited. This aching pain (see Fig. 4) increased in severity as the stimulus was further raised in intensity until at 50 times threshold both recruitment of C-fibers and the severity of pain felt reached a plateau (BURKE et al. 1975).

b) Lidocaine Block

Lidocaine produced a numbness and diminished perception of pain to these strong electrical stimuli, and this was correlated with failure of conduction in C-fibers (TOREBJORK and HALLIN 1973). In Fig. 6a, one sees that when lidocaine blocked some C-fibers, it blocked all of the Aδ-fibers, and many of the Aβ-fibers. MACKENZIE et al. (1975) confirmed this result and also tested sensory responses to a variety of cutaneous stimuli as well as to electrical pulses. Responses of their subjects were categorized as light touch, pinprick, pain, burning heat, warmth, cool and cold. The stimuli were delivered to an area of the finger that was associated with electrically recorded responses from the fascicle. Filaments of cotton wool were used for light touch. A manually inserted needle served for pinprick with disappearance of the sense of "sharpness" being the required endpoint. Extremes of temperature were generated by a lighted match and ice cube; more controlled thermal stimuli were produced using an irrigated copper wand. Injection of lidocaine (0.25%, 0.50%) produced transient selective block of variable depth. Figure 6b shows the diminution in C-fiber conduction that occurred 15 min after infiltration with 0.25% lidocaine at a time when the subject exhibited a hypersensitivity to cold, and an impaired warmth discrimination (tested as an inability to distinguish stimuli of 35 °C from those at 36 °C) and reduced pain perception. Mackenzie et al. reported that conduction block of individual C-fibers was generally associated with functional block of warmth and pain. Block of C-fiber potentials usually, but not always, preceded the failure of cold discrimination (distinguishing 27° from 28°). Perception of sharpness was likewise associated with Aδ unit potentials. Failure of sensitivity to touch was associated with conduction failure in fibers with conduction velocity greater than 30 m/s. In hairy skin, touch could linger after it was blocked in glabrous skin (MACKENZIE et al. 1975).

c) Pressure Block

As GASSER and ERLANGER noted in 1929, a differential block with anesthetic was a good deal less precise than it was with pressure. With pressure block, the order of failure observed by Mackenzie et al. was quite consitent with the classical view. The initial sensations following the application of pressure were dysesthesias that occurred as conduction slowed in individual fast conducting fibers. Sensation to touch began to decline in 20 to 30 minutes and failure became complete as the fast fibers failed completely. The sensations to cold failed next. This failure was preceded by an inability of the subjects to make what was otherwise an easy discrimination between 27 °C vs. 28 °C. The failure of temperature sensation was associated with block of conduction in Aδ-fibers. Then with occasional overlap as C-fibers began to block, warmth discrimination and the inability to discriminate warm temperatures 1 °C apart began to fail. Once the Aδ-fibers were blocked, ice was felt as "an odd burning". This finding is consistent with a view that the quality of cold requires conduction of impulses in some subset of Aδ-fibers in order to be perceived, and that when only C-fibers conduct, the only sensation that can

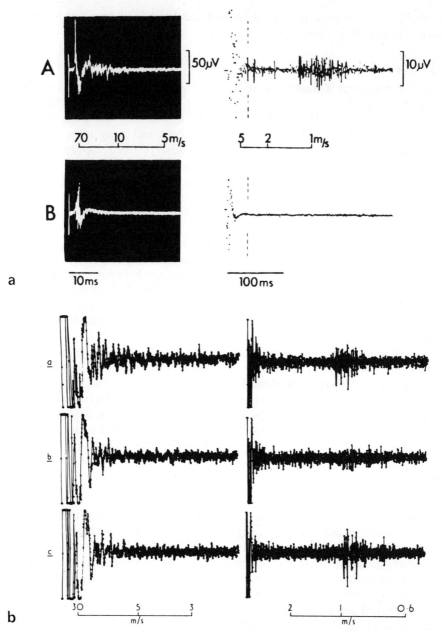

Fig. 6a, b. Monitoring of multiunit discharges in humans during differential peripheral nerve block with lidocaine. Both the left and right examples show differential block of radial nerve with lidocaine at 0.25%. Lidocaine was injected between the stimulating sites on the hand and recording electrodes in the forearm. **a** Before lidocaine, fast (5 oscilloscope traces superimposed) and slowly conducted units (50 traces averaged) appear in response to intense electrical stimuli (0.5 Hz). These were felt as a strong prolonged aching with sharp pricking (upper traces labelled *A*). At the time the lower traces were taken, weak stimuli were detected as tactile, but the intense stimuli used to produce the traces were no longer be evoked by extreme stimuli are warmth and burning pain. In experiments in vitro with cat saphenous nerve, Gasser reported that Aδ-fibers under ischemic conditions tended to fail in an order that was inconsistent with their small size. They failed with the γ elevation and failed earlier than larger A-fibers (GASSER 1935). Occasional sensory failure to cold stimuli prior to failure of the sensation of touch had been noted by LEWIS et al. (1931).

The block of the fast conducting fibers certainly reduces the tonic input from skin and muscle and reduces the number of fibers responding to touching the skin in a particular area with ice. It has been a persistent issue how the central integrating mechanisms are perturbed by such changes in the spectrum of active fibers (ZIMMERMANN 1979). The signals from C-fibers that continue to conduct when faster fibers are blocked must be interpreted against a distorted background, and it is questionable if the same sensation and perceptions would be noticed if the discharges were occurring against the normal background. Torebjork and Hallin grossly explored this question in 3 cases by anesthetizing the median nerve and ulnar nerves using 1% lidocaine. The resulting complete anesthesia of adjacent tissue did not affect the sensory dissociation in the radial nerve and produced no significant variation in the sensation experienced during preferential block of the radial nerve for pressure. Blocking neighboring afferents did not alter the tendency of subjects to select a label for their sensation from the limited range of labels that these experimenters used. Thus the perturbations caused by impulses from neighboring areas, if they exist at all, must be more refined than these experiments reveal. In later experiments, (VALLBO et al. 1979; OCHOA 1984) local microstimulation of fascicles led to unitary reactions in C-fibers. These responses were in relative isolation against the normal background. Pain followed upon repetitive activation of these individual C-fibers. At rates of 5/s the pain became severe and well localized. These experiments support a highly specific association between activity in peripheral fibers and sensation and they indicate a strong degree of independence among fibers in the sensation produced (or blocked) when they are stimulated (or when conduction is selectively blocked).

After 1 hour of nerve compression, some patients noted a dull ache that was imprecisely referred to the area served by the nerve. The ache occurred with a 10–20 min delay after the complete failure of Aδ-fiber conduction under conditions where some C-fibers were still able to conduct in response to electrical stimulation. It is not known whether discharges in afferent C-fibers were associated with this pain, which resembles tourniquet pain (COLE 1952).

These experiments with single fibers in human beings rather strikingly confirm many of the propositions of Gasser and Erlanger. They show that individual discharges in individual fibers yield highly localized perception and that the quality

---

painful. They were felt as a "blow". Pain returned with the C-fiber deflection (lower traces labelled *B* on left). From TOREBJÖRK and HALLIN (1973). **b** A less selective block. Upper traces (*a*) before lidocaine, middle traces (*b*) 15 min after the injection and lower traces (*c*) 30 min after the injection. Perception was initially normal. The middle traces were correlated with striking hypersensitivity to cold stimuli, impairment of the ability to discriminate among warm stimuli, and reduced aching in response to intense electrical stimuli. From MACKENZIE et al. (1975)

of those perceptions can be linked to the conduction velocity of the fibers being stimulated. The techniques used to produce differential block were not particularly selective. Thus, the relative susceptibility among functionally identified fibers could not be studied in detail. Tests of the steady-state susceptibility using these recording methods would seem to require a more controlled method of applying anesthetics to the nerve. The present studies are consistent with the hypothesis that susceptibility to anesthetic injected near peripheral nerves is correlated with conduction velocity. However, they do not establish the size principle, and in the next section we consider additional factors that influence differential block.

II. Contradictions of the Size Principle; Importance of Additional Factors

Studies of individual fibers in humans support specificity of function in the periphery. They also show that fibers grouped by function tend to cluster according to size, at least coarsely, with two types of overlap: 1) Different sensory fibers connected to particular receptors may overlap in peripheral connectivity, as was the case between C-unmyelinated-fibers and Aδ-myelinated fibers attached to similar mechanothermal receptors from monkey glabrous skin (GEORGOPOULOS and MOUNTCASTLE 1976, 1977; MOUNTCASTLE 1980b). 2) A group of fibers having a particular conduction velocity will include axons having several sensory and motor functions (GASSER 1943; MOUNTCASTLE 1980a).

There is no strong theoretical or molecular basis for differential failure according to fiber diameter. Fibers of various sizes intermingle in peripheral nerve, and the notion that surface to volume ratio underlies differential block by size does not follow from present understanding of the mechanism of action of local anesthetics in which "reaction with protoplasm" (GASSER and ERLANGER 1929) in the cellular interior has been replaced by interaction with molecules in the membrane of the cell surface. Surface to volume ratio may in the end be important (DE JONG 1980a), but no theory of mechanism of action of local anesthetics presently suggests why the block should be differential according to size (JACK 1975; CONDOURIS et al. 1976; DE JONG 1980b) unless there is an underlying difference in conduction safety related to size (CHIU and RITCHIE 1984). Neither is there a strong empirical basis for differential block according to the size principle.

Careful consideration of the empirical studies of differential block with local anesthetics provides ample evidence that differential block of conduction exists but the size principle does not predict the results. Table 1 summarizes many of the direct studies of tonic block with local anesthetics. The order of failure is contingent on species, type of endpoint used in the investigation, anesthetic, nerve used, and numerous other factors in addition to fiber diameter. Even by the 1950's, findings contradicting the prediction of the size principle had been made for several agents in nerves of several species. EVERETT and TOMAN (1954) following Toman's extensive review in 1952, concluded that the studies then available did "not support the older concepts of nerve block based on fiber size". Since then numerous factors in addition to fiber diameter have been invoked to account for differential block. In this section, 10 such factors are discussed.

Table 1. Anesthetic tonic block – Order of differential block of impulse conduction

Order of onset f(A, t)	Order of recovery f(A, t)	Order of steady-state f[A]	Agent A	Nerve	Preparation	End point	Conditions[a]	Approach; comments	Report
Aδ, Aγ} overlap, Aβ, Aα	Aα, Aβ} overlap, Aγ, Aδ	—	Cocaine 1:1000	Crural Saphenous Tibial Sciatic	Dog	Relative CAP	1 cm length 25° No CO_2 In vitro	Order of failure less reliable than with pressure	Gasser and Erlanger (1929)
Autonomic fibers	No comment	—	Procaine	Sciatic	Cat Frog	Relative	0.5 cm length	—	Heinbecker et al. (1934)
4–1 μ, Aδ 5–1 μ, Aγ, Aβ} overlap, Aα	Aγ, Aβ} overlap, Aα		0.5%–2%	Saphenous Vagus Cervical Sympathetic	Cat	CAP	No CO_2	—	
B(Aδ+B)	C$_2$	Aγ persists w/Aαβ blocked	Carbamates Ethyl-amyl 7–100 mM	Sciatic	38 bull frog	D$_{50}$	25 mm length No CO_2 phosphate buffer	C much more resistant than A or B	Crescitelli (1948, 1950)
Aαβ	C$_1$			Sciatic	3 R. pipiens				
Aδ, C$_1$, C$_2$ (Slower component)	Aδ, Aαβ, AδB								
A	C	—	Procaine HCl 0.025%	Vagus	Rabbit; guinea pig; cat	Relative CAP	—	"Checked" in 95% O_2/CO_2 at 37.5°C	Everett and Goodsell (1952)
C	A	—		Sciatic	Rabbit; guinea pig; cat		25° in air		
B, C} overlap, A	A, C} overlap, B	—	Procaine 0.05%–0.1%	Sciatic	Rabbit; cat; guinea pig; frog	D$_{total}$	—	Recovery slower than onset Immersed until tested	Everett and Toman (1954)
B, A, C} overlap	C, A} overlap, B	—		Vagus	Rabbit; cat; guinea pig; frog	D$_{total}$	—	"B" includes Aδ Rates of decline similar in A and C fibers	

Table 1 (continued)

Order of onset f(A, t)	Order of recovery f(A, t)	Order of steady-state f[A]	Agent A	Nerve	Preparation	End point	Conditions[a]	Approach; comments	Report
Aγ Aα	Aα Aγ } some overlap	–	Procaine 0.2%–0.5%	Sciatic	14 cats nembutal in vivo	Relative CAP	15 mm length	Slight differences in α motor + afferent Aα fibers	MATTHEWS and RUSHWORTH (1957b)
Full expression, rapid not progressive	Rapid	19–20 μ 1–2.0% 17 μ <1% 11 μ 0.25%	Urethane	Sciatic	Toad	C_{block}	2 nodes No CO_2	Block of conducted AP into isolated node, double air gap	UEHARA (1960)
Aδ (12–19 m/s) Aβ (65 m/s) Aα (80 mm/s)	Aα Aβ } same degree of overlap as during onset Aδ		Cocaine Procaine Lignocaine >1.0%	DRS$_1$[b]	13 cats	D_{total} Aδ	8 mm length 1 Hz	20% decl. of Aβ 4% decl. of Aα when Aδ was blocked	NATHAN and SEARS (1961)
–	Rapid – (2 min)	Aγδ (18–35 m/s) Aαβ (70 m/s) not blocked at all	Procaine 0.03%–0.06%	VRS$_1$[b]	Cat	C_{50} for Aδ	8 mm length	Progressive increase in dose. Stable differential block for 62 min	
Aδ (9.6–11.6 m/s) C	– –	Aδ (9.6–11.6 m/s) C	Procaine Cocaine 0.01%–0.02%	DR	Cat tail nerve	D_{total}		Isolated rootlet Aγα not blocked	
–		Phrenic (11 μ) sheath intact Sciatic (16 μ) desheathed	Alcohols Urethane Barbiturates; Tertiary amines	Phrenic Sciatic	Rat Rat or frog	C_{50}	5 mm phrenic 10 mm sciatic TRIS buffer No CO_2 22 °C		STAIMAN and SEEMAN (1974)
–		Phrenic (6 μ) sheath intact Phrenic (11 μ) Sciatic (16 μ) desheathed	Haloperidol		Rat				
–		Sciatic (16 μ) desheathed Phrenic (11 μ)	TTX						

Block characteristics	Onset / resistance	Recovery	Block values	Conditions	Block measure	Nerve	Animal/prep.	Drug / concentration	Notes	Reference
A (10 m/s) A (50–70 m/s) not blocked		of onset ½ h			block			0.25%	injured rat peripheral nerve ...	... and HALLIN (1973)
Slower myelinated Faster myelinated	Faster myelinated Slower myelinated	–		20 mm length No CO_2 4–5 Hz	D_{block}	Saphenous	4 Cats Pento-barbital	Procaine 0.5%	22 filaments, 174 unit potentials	FRANZ and PERRY (1974)
Aδ, C + slow "α" faster myelinated >70 m/s	Faster >70 m/s Aδ, C, small "α" >70 m/s			20 mm length No CO_2	D_{block}	Saphenous	Cat 20 A fibers 34 °C fibers	Procaine 0.2%	Recoveries in reverse order, unit by unit	
Required hours	A, Aδ, C together C, some resistant C units	Rapid recovery		20 mm length	C_{block}	Saphenous	Cat	Procaine 0.15% 0.02%	No differential steady-state block	
Onset over 60 min	Aδ, C, 3 Aα Aα (27 resistant units) for 60 min	–		2 mm length	C_{block}	Saphenous	Cat 30α 33δ 12C	0.2%	Variable lengths ≧2 mm exposed α = >40 m/s δ = <30 m/s Differential steady-state block	
Steady-state in ≈10 min	B (14.8 m/s) C (1.8 m/s)	Recovery to 90% in 60 min		≈25 mm length 38 °C 95% O_2, 5% CO_2	C_{50}	Cervical sympathetic trunk	Rabbit	Lidocaine 0.025–0.5 mM	Dose response curves, C_{50}-B = 0.1 mM C_{50}-C = 0.3 mM	HEAVNER and DE JONG (1974)
Steady-state ≈10 min – Prilocaine ≈20 min Amethocaine	B-C_{50} ≈ 0.15 mM C-C_{50} ≈ 0.3 mM B-C_{50} ≈ 0.005 mM C-C_{50} ≈ 0.015 mM	Recovery to 80% in 60 min		≈25 mm length	C_{50}	Cervical sympathetic trunk	Rabbit 51 trunks	Prilocaine 0.25–0.5 mM Amethocaine 0.0025–0.004 mM		SCURLOCK et al. (1975)
Steady-state ≈10 min	Recovery occurs	A(10 m/s) C_{block} = 0.3 mM A(40 m/s) C_{block} = 1.0 mM A(10 m/s) C_{block} = 5.0 mM A(41 m/s) C_{block} = 20 mM		10 or 20 mm length; 22 °C 20 cm conduction length	C_{block}	Sciatic 9 fibers 10 fibers	Bullfrog A fibers	Lidocaine 0.3–1.0 mM Benzyl alcohol	Single units Desheathed Linear increase in C_{block} with conduction velocity	STAIMAN and SEEMAN (1977)

Table 1 (continued)

Order of onset $f(A, t)$	Order of recovery $f(A, t)$	Order of steady-state $f[A]$	Agent A	Nerve	Preparation	End point	Conditions[a]	Approach; comments	Report
Steady-state ≈20 min		A(10 m/s) C_{block} = 5 nM; A(45 m/s) C_{block} = 20 nM	TTX	10 fibers			Desheathed		STAIMAN and SEEMAN (continued)
Steady-state before 30 min	Recovery to 90% in 1 h. Inverse order of onset	A-C_{50} ≈ 0.085 mM, B-C_{50} ≈ 0.34 mM, C-C_{50} ≈ 0.72 mM (Lidocaine); A-C_{50} ≈ 0.009 mM, B-C_{50} ≈ 0.013 mM, C-C_{50} ≈ 0.028 mM (Tetracaine); A-C_{50} ≈ 0.042 mM, B-C_{50} ≈ 0.084 mM, C-C_{50} ≈ 0.20 mM (Etidocaine); A-C_{50} ≈ 0.05 mM, B-C_{50} ≈ 0.13 mM, C-C_{50} ≈ 0.20 mM (Bupivacaine)	Lidocaine, Tetracaine, Etidocaine, Bupivacaine	Vagus Sciatic	Rabbit	C_{50}	10 mm length Room temp. O_2 No CO_2	Amplitude of CAP at 30 min. Desheathed. Dose response curves A (30–60 m/s) B (5–15 m/s) C (<1 m/s)	GISSEN et al. (1980)
C first, (least 220 min) B second, most A third, (intermediate)	Reversible after 12 h	B-C_{50} ≈ 0.03 mM, C-C_{50} ≈ 0.08 mM (Etidocaine); B-C_{50} ≈ 1.3 mM, C-C_{50} ≈ 2.8 mM (Lidocaine); Not achieved in 220 min (TTX)	Etidocaine, Lidocaine, TTX	Vagus Sciatic	Rabbit	C_{50}; Relative CAP at onset	10 mm length Room temp. O_2 No CO_2; 10 mm length Room temp. O_2 No CO_2	Sheath intact; Desheathed, C first affected Least degree of block at 220 min in C population	GISSEN et al. (1982a)
A} overlap C}; A} overlap C}; C	C $t_{1/2}^c$ = 29 min; A; C; A	A; C	Etidocaine 8 mM; Bupivacaine 8 mM; Etidocaine 0.08– 0.3 mM; Bupivacaine 0.04– 0.3 mM	Vagus	Rabbit	Relative CAP	10 mm Room temp O_2 No CO_2	Sheath intact	GISSEN et al. (1982b)
A	A	A							GISSEN et al. (continued)

Order of block	Comments	Conduction velocity / blocking concentration	Local anesthetic (concentration)	Nerve	Species / preparation	Measure	Conditions	Comments	Reference
Steady-state in 10 min for both A+C fibers		Aδ, B (1.25–4 m/s) A (5–37.5 m/s) C (0.5–1.2 m/s)	Lidocaine 0.2–8.0 mM	Vagus	Rabbit 99 fibers	C_{block} 30 min	20 mm length 95% O_2 5% CO_2 37°C 20 mM glucose	Single units recorded in nodose ganglion sheath intact	Fink and Cairns (1983a, b)
		Aδ C Aβ	Lidocaine 0.1–1 mM	Sural Tibial	Cat	Relative CAP	8 mm length 33°C In vivo	Differential enhanced by cooling to 25° or 14°C. Sheath intact	Strichartz and Zimmermann (1983)
Aβ } broad Aδ } overlap C		Aδ (<3 m/s) 0.19 mM Aδ (>3 m/s) 0.43 mM C (>1.4 m/s) 0.63 mM	Lidocaine	Vagus	Rabbit 36 units	C_{block}	20 mm length 95% O_2 5% CO_2 37°C 20 mM Glucose	Bracket C_{block} within 0.1 mM for single units. Values for intact sheath given here	Fink and Cairns (1984a)
C Aβ } broad Aδ } overlap		— —	Lidocaine	Vagus nodose	Rabbit	D_{block}	20 mm length	Measure delay to block for just supra-maximal dose	Fink and Cairns (1984b)
Steady-state ≈7–12 min	Restore conduction if reduce dose by 0.1 mM	Broad variation 22 m/s 0.3 mM 21 m/s 1.2 mM	Lidocaine 0.01–1.5 mM	Sciatic	Frog 11 fibers	C_{block}	>6 cm length 18°C 95% O_2 5% CO_2	Measure rise in threshold and latency for each fiber Sheath intact	Raymond and Roscoe (1984)
C Aδ Aα	Inverse of onset	—	2-chloro-/ procaine 4.9–9.8 mM Lidocaine 3.7 mM Bupivacaine 0.77–1.5 mM	Saphenous	Cat Ketamine methoxy-flurane nitrous succinyl chloride	Relative CAP to C-fiber block	—	Injection near nerve Aα 70 m/s Aδ 13 m/s C 1.2 m/s Sheath intact	Ford et al. (1984)
Aδ C } overlap Aα			Etidocaine 3.2 mM	Saphenous					

Table 1 (continued)

Order of onset f(A, t)	Order of recovery f(A, t)	Order of steady-state f[A]	Agent A	Nerve	Preparation	End point	Conditions[a]	Approach; comments	Report
Steady-state usually within 30 min	To 90%	$A\text{-}C_{50} \simeq 2.9$ mM $B\text{-}C_{50} \simeq 3.22$ mM $C\text{-}C_{50} \simeq 5.00$ mM	Procainamide	Vagus	Rabbit	C_{50} 30 min	10 mm length Room temp. 95% O_2 5% CO_2	Desheathed, Dose-response curves for each drug	Wildsmith et al. (1985)
		$A\text{-}C_{50} \simeq 0.41$ mM $B\text{-}C_{50} \simeq 0.47$ mM $C\text{-}C_{50} \simeq 0.71$ mM	Procaine						
		$A\text{-}C_{50} \simeq 0.17$ mM $B\text{-}C_{50} \simeq 0.20$ mM $C\text{-}C_{50} \simeq 0.23$ mM	Chloro-procaine						
		$A\text{-}C_{50} \simeq 0.007$ mM $B\text{-}C_{50} \simeq 0.008$ mM $C\text{-}C_{50} \simeq 0.014$ mM	Amethocaine						

A: Molecular activity of agent; given as concentrations in same units used by authors in each study.

Relative CAP: The relative temporal order of decline in components of the compound action potential.

C_{50}: Concentration at which height of component of compound action potential drops to 50% control amplitude.

C_{total}: Concentration for complete disappearance of CAP.

D_{50}: Delay between application of drug and 50% reduction of CAP.

D_{total}: Delay to complete disappearance of CAP.

C_{block}: Concentration required to block conducted impulse in a single fiber.

D_{block}: Delay to block of conduction in single fiber.

[a] Under "conditions", the first entry is the length of nerve exposed to anesthetic.

[b] DRS, VRS, are first sacral dorsal and ventral roots, respectively.

[c] $t_{1/2}$ is the time elapsed before ½ of the total change has occurred.

1. Intrinsic Differences in Conduction Safety

This "factor" includes all the unique attributes of a particular fiber other than its diameter that cause it to differ in susceptibility to blocking agents. The list below (list 1) enumerates several of the more important attributes of fibers and neurons that contribute to conduction safety. Even if an anesthetic agent were to be distributed homogeneously and were to affect explicitly only one of these attributes (such as g_{Na}, the maximum local sodium conductance), dimensional arguments do not predict that the blocking concentration would differ on the basis of size (JACK 1975; CONDOURIS et al. 1976). However, it has recently been argued that small diameter myelinated fibers might be expected to have a reduced conduction safety by virtue of a limitation on the proportional shrinkage of the internode (CHIU and RITCHIE 1984). Schwann cells were observed to reach a minimum length for fibers of 4 μ diameter. Myelinated fibers smaller than this would have disproportionately long internodes and would in theory show an increased susceptibility to anesthetics by virtue of a diminished safety factor. The size corresponds to B-fibers and small Aδ-fibers in a range for which a greater susceptibility has been observed (SCURLOCK et al. 1975; FINK and CAIRNS 1983 b).

List 1. *Factors Affecting Impulse Propagation in Nerve Membranes*

1. Tonic Parameters
   membrane potential
   potassium concentration gradient
   sodium concentration gradient
   external calcium concentration
   local electrical loading (cable constants: R_i, R_0, C, $\lambda(x)$, R_m)
   density of sodium channels (voltage governed) g_{Na}
   density of leakage channels (voltage independent)
   density of potassium channels (voltage governed) g_K
   effects of drugs on all of the above (includes pH, CO_2, hormones,
      endogenous opiates, etc.)
   local temperature
   local pressure (compression)
   density of ion pumps
   activity of ion pumps (ATP, Na, K)
   local diffusion coefficients
   degree of myelination

2. Phasic Parameters
   previous impulse activity
   local currents from active neighbors
   variations in transition kinetics or conformation of voltage
      governed channels
   metabolism and axonal transport
   blood flow (ischemia)
   trauma, disease (e.g. demyelination, injury etc.)
   trophic interactions with Schwann cells and glia

a) Empirical Evidence for Intrinsic Differences in Conduction Safety not Correlated to Size

Direct evidence that fibers of equivalent conduction velocity have widely differing susceptibility to anesthetics has been compiled for unmyelinated and myelinated fibers of rabbit vagus nerves (FINK and CAIRNS 1983 a, b, 1984 a) and for frog myelinated fibers (RAYMOND and ROSCOE 1984).

Figure 7 shows the results of applying several different concentrations of lidocaine to rabbit vagus nerve while recording from a single C-fiber. The blocking concentration is bracketed by the last two groups of traces. The concentration after equilibration for 20 min with (0.41 mM) the action potential was only de-

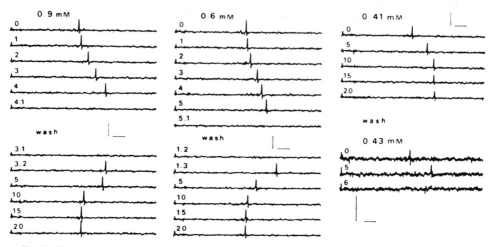

Fig. 7. Single unit response to electrical stimuli during exposure to several concentrations of lidocaine. Each group of traces shows the action potential recorded from a cell soma in the nodose ganglion activated by stimulation of a C-axon about 50 mm (FINK and CAIRNS 1984a, p 515) away from the recording electrode. Increasing latency is shown as the action potential becomes displaced to the right in sweeps taken after beginning equilibration with lidocaine. The time from lidocaine application or from the beginning of the wash is marked in minutes, to the left of each trace. The last two groups of traces bracket the blocking concentration. From FINK and CAIRNS (1984a)

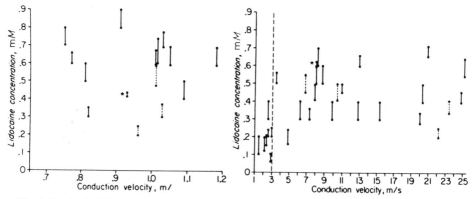

Fig. 8. Intrinsic differences among axons in susceptibility to lidocaine at steady-state. All units were recorded under matching conditions (CO_2/O_2 perfused mammalian Ringers containing glucose and bicarbonate buffer at 37 °C) from cells in rabbit nodose ganglion whose axons were stimulated about 50 mm away. The solid lines bracket the highest non-blocking concentration and the lowest blocking concentration tested in vagus nerves with sheath intact. Dashed lines bracket concentrations in desheathed preparations. The stars mark 2 desheathed preparations with lines too short to appear as dashed. From FINK and CAIRNS (1984a)

layed. After a wash, re-equilibration with 0.43 mM was sufficient to block the same unit after 6 min, indicating that the blocking concentration was less than 0.43 mM and greater than 0.41 mM (FINK and CAIRNS 1984a). Blocking concentrations were similarly bracketed for fibers of varying conduction velocity and the results are shown in Fig. 8. The bars indicate the range between the highest nonblocking concentration (lower dot) and lowest blocking concentration (upper dot) tested for each axon. These studies show quite convincingly that overlap in

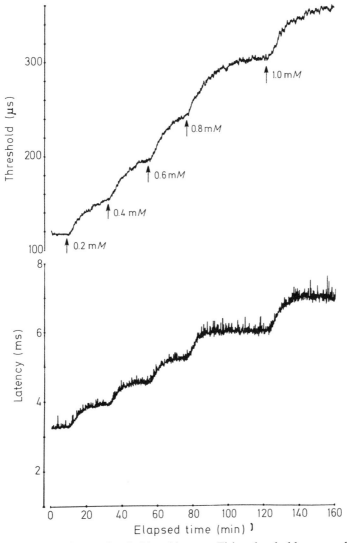

Fig. 9. Effects of lidocaine on threshold and latency. Firing threshold measured in a single myelinated axon conducting at 18.8 m/s from a frog sciatic nerve is plotted vs. elapsed time as the concentration of lidocaine was progressively increased. The lidocaine concentration is shown next to the arrows that denote the time of application. Threshold is given as duration (μs) of a current pulse having 50% probability of firing the fiber. From RAYMOND and ROSCOE (1984)

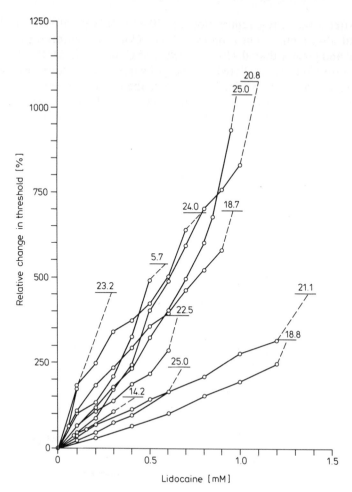

Fig. 10. Differential action of lidocaine on the threshold of A-fibers. The relative change in threshold given as the

$$\frac{(\text{present level-starting level})}{(\text{starting level})}$$

is plotted vs. successively increased concentrations of lidocaine. At each concentration the fiber was allowed to attain steady-state. The slope of each curve is related to the incremental sensitivity of each fiber to lidocaine. The blocking concentration is given by the intersection of the highest threshold reached and the degree to which a "steady state" response to the last increment in conduction had been reached by the time of block as estimated from records similar to Fig. 9. Note that the lowest incremental sensitivity did not belong to the unit that required the highest amount of lidocaine in order to be blocked. Conduction velocities for each unit in m/s are shown above the lines drawn between the last sub-blocking concentration and the concentration for which block was observed. A more slowly conducting fiber (5.7 m/s) is included for comparison with 10 fibers conducting between 18 and 25 m/s at 18 °C sensitivity to anesthetic among components of the compound action potential can be attributed, at least in part, to overlap in the steady-state sensitivity of individual fibers. The fastest conducting myelinated nerve fibers blocked in the same range of concentrations as did the unmyelinated C-fibers. The most sensitive fibers conducted at the extreme slow range for myelinated fibers. These may have been myelinated over only a portion of the length exposed to anesthetic (FINK and CAIRNS 1983a, b; 1984a).

The same conclusion is supported by evidence from frog myelinated fibers. The firing threshold for electrical stimulation and conduction latencies were measured as shown in Fig. 9 during successive increases in lidocaine concentration. As shown in Fig. 10, the sensitivity as given by the relative change in threshold per mM lidocaine differed greatly among 10 fibers that were closely matched in conduction velocity. The blocking concentrations, shown by the intersection of the highest threshold reached with a line bracketing the prior and final concentration, ranged from 0.38 mM–1.37 mM. The mechanism for the differences of susceptibility between these fibers is not apparent from these results, but it is not possible to account for them on the basis of size.

b) Empirical Evidence in Favor of the Link to Diameter

Several studies have found a positive correlation between diameter of the individual fibers and resistance to anesthetics. UEHARA (1960) measured the concentration of urethane required to block action potentials in isolated nodes from toad sciatic fibers. She tested the capabilities of the node to respond to action potentials conducting in a section of axon not exposed to anesthetic. She found that larger fibers (20 μ) took more than 3 times as much urethane (1.0%–2.0%) to block AP conduction than did small (11 μ) fibers (0.25%). The experiments were done at room temperature in excised nerves without glucose or CO_2. Differences between the experiments of Uehara and those cited in the preceeding section include the agent used, the length of nerve exposed to drug, and the method of testing conduction. In Uehara's experiments the tested node was driven by an impulse that was traveling in unexposed axon. In the experiments of Fink and Cairns and Raymond and Roscoe, at least several centimeters of the axon were exposed, and the dynamics of conduction failure reflected changes in the ability of the impulse to deliver current as well as changes in the responsiveness of the membrane receiving the current. The capability to deliver current to a load increases with the surface area occupied by the impulse, possibly accounting for the size effect seen by Uehara.

In another study (STAIMAN and SEEMAN 1977) small filaments of bull-frog sciatic fibers were recorded at 22 °C. A 1 cm length of nerve was equilibrated with blocking concentrations of lidocaine, benzyl alcohol and tetrodotoxin. The drugs were dissolved in buffered Ringer's solution without CO_2. For lidocaine, conduction velocities of 9 axons ranging from 10 m/s–45 m/s were correlated with the blocking concentration as measured by bracketing within 0.1 mM. Staiman and Seeman listed the higher concentration as that "just sufficient to prevent impulse conduction". Approximately a 3-fold change in blocking concentration so measured was correlated with a 4-fold change in conduction velocity. Using TTX,

STAIMAN SEEMAN (1977) had measured the space constant for the larger fibers at 1.89 mm. A decremental response in the region exposed to drug may have contributed to propagation of impulses in large fibers through the pool. Such an effect, if present, would act to increase the reliability of conduction across the 1 cm area, especially in large fibers having the longest space constants. Whereas with the entire conducting path exposed (RAYMOND and ROSCOE 1984), differential electrotonic spread would not be a factor (see 3, this section).

Other studies have successfully demonstrated size-related differences in steady-state susceptibility to anesthetics. In cat saphenous nerves exposed over variable lengths to 0.2% procaine, steady-state differential tonic block was found. Four Aδ (<30 m/s) units were blocked for 1 h while 4 Aα units (>40 m/s) continued to conduct (FRANZ and PERRY 1974). This "absolute differential block" (NATHAN and SEARS 1961) by size could be achieved only if less than 4 mm of nerve were exposed to anesthetic. It was not observed when 4 mm–20 mm of nerve were exposed. Clear differences in susceptibility during onset and recovery were seen as units would block in one order, and recover in the reverse order of failure, unit by unit. The susceptibility during onset was not well correlated with conduction velocity, though small myelinated fibers tended to be more sensitive than larger myelinated fibers and of approximately equal susceptibility to small C unmyelinated dorsal root fibers (FRANZ and PERRY 1974).

These studies are consistent in showing: 1) overlap in susceptibility of fibers of different diameter and 2) that individual fibers differ from each other in susceptibility according to factors other than size, although size may be important under some conditions (UEHARA et al. 1960; STAIMAN and SEEMAN 1977).

c) Unanswered Questions

To date, no one has determined in single fiber studies the differential susceptibility among nerve fibers to phasic block with anesthetics (see 8, this section). Thus it is not known whether a fiber having a high resistance to tonic block also has a high resistance to phasic block during repetitive activity.

The differences in tonic susceptibility that have been found are not well correlated with diameter. Do they correlate instead with function? This would be possible since function at best is only loosely related to diameter.

In vitro studies of single units do not make use of the normal circulation of the nerve. It is clear from diffusion studies that are mentioned in the next section that many minutes elapse for diffusion of anesthetics from the border of a nerve to fibers at its center. It is, therefore, not to be taken for granted that all fibers in excised nerves exhibit the same degree of conduction safety along their entire extent that they would show with the faster redistribution of drug expected with an intact circulation (LUNDBORG et al. 1983).

2. Diffusion

a) Delay of Block Onset

Nerve trunks vary in diameter from several mm to fine peripheral branches of 100 µ or less. Over these dimensions distribution of anesthetic will depend on bulk flow, diffusion, and vascular uptake and delivery. In the in vitro case, diffusion dominates because the nerve is usually bathed in solutions previously equilibrated with the drug. In the clinic, asymmetric delivery to one side of the trunk is common. The vasa nervorum will operate either to deliver drug (as with intravenous regional anesthesia) or to remove it (as with conventional peripheral nerve block).

BENNETT et al. (1942) used whole sciatic nerves from frogs with intact sheaths to test the relative potency of a variety of local anesthetics in blocking the conduction of the compound action potential. The nerve diameters were measured using an ocular micrometer. For 1 mm diameter nerves exposed to 10 mM procaine, it took 20 min before the height of the A-components dropped to 20% of control height. Whereas with 300 μ diameter nerves exposed to the same concentration, that level of block was achieved in about 2 min. This is definitive evidence that one component in the delay between application of the anesthetic to the outside of the nerve and the drop of the compound action potential is related to diffusion time through the nerve. Their results showed that different drugs have different "affinities" as defined by the tendency to linger during washout, but they had no evidence bearing on the issue of *differential* affinity for fibers or systems involved in different functions as had been vaguely speculated by prior authors (DIXON 1905; HEINBECKER et al. 1934). A possible differential action could be obtained if fibers of one function were located more deeply within the nerve trunk than another functional group clustered circumferentially. The differential block would apply for limited time by virtue of the transiently higher concentration at the periphery of the nerve that would result from the diffusional delay of anesthetic to the center of the nerve (LEWIS et al. 1931; DE JONG 1980 a).

The sheath (epineurium) is an important barrier to bulk flow, and depending on the agent and upon such factors as pH (CATCHLOVE 1972) it is also a factor limiting diffusion. Earlier authors had speculated regarding variations in "sheath thickness" (GASSER and ERLANGER 1929) or "efficiency of protection" (DIXON 1905) as factors accounting for susceptibility of different classes of fibers, and even in desheathed nerves, the Schwann cells, myelin and Remak bundles as well as endoneurial connective tissue and nodal gap substances permit, at least in principle, the possibility of inhomogeneous spatial distribution of diffusing anesthetic (BROMAGE 1978, pp 37–39). Nonetheless, limits on diffusion can only effect the rate at which concentration changes in the vicinity of particular fibers. They do not effect the concentrations in aqueous solutions at steady-state. Thus, to the extent that diffusion barriers are used to produce differential block, the technique is limited to differential rate of block and to a time course on the order of 10 min to several hours depending on the nature of the differential diffusion barriers, and on the affinity of anesthetics.

The nerve sheath is apparently a lipid rather than an aqueous environment, as suggested by the greater rate of access to the nerve of uncharged anesthetic molecules. The neutral form of the tertiary amine lidocaine predominates in alkaline solutions (pH 9.3) and is permeant through the sheath whereas the ratio of charged form of lidocaine to neutral form increases 100-fold at neutral pH (pH 7.3) and the time constant for anesthetic-induced reduction in the amplitude of the compound action potential following 0.3 mM lidocaine is about 5 times longer than it is in alkaline solutions (RITCHIE et al. 1965).

Once within the nerve, anesthetic molecules diffuse through a complex environment within the clefts between the axons, Schwann cells, capillaries, and fibrils of connective tissue. Nicholson and Philips have described diffusion through complex media and have derived quantiative expressions for diffusion of impermeant ions in cerebellar cortex – an electrically and structurally highly anisotropic tissue (NICHOLSON and PHILLIPS 1981). Both cations and anions were tested to determine whether long chain molecules with fixed negative charges in the extracellular space produced an asymmetric influence on the diffusion rates on the basis of the charge of the diffusing substance. No influence of the polarity of charge was found, suggesting that the polyanionic matrix hypothesized to be present around the nodes of large myelinated fibers in peripheral nerve will not retard diffusion of anionic over cationic anesthetics. However, should the matrix act as a lipid barrier to diffusion, it may well retard the diffusion of polar anesthetics of either charge to reach the node where they cross into the membrane and exert their effect.

Similarly, diffusion in peripheral nerve would be different in comparison to diffusion in extracellular fluid in 3 ways: 1) The interposition of relatively impermeant membranes of the cells in the nerve would act to squeeze the extracellular fluid into narrow clefts and thus to constrain the total volume in which molecules may distribute. This effect is quantified as the "volume fraction" (α) which expresses the fraction of the total volume occupied by ECF, and in brain it is about 20%. 2) The total path length for diffusing particle is increased as it encounters cellular obstructions in long narrow alleys, an effect called tortuosity, symbolized by lambda. The proportional increase in path length, λ, was equal to 1.55 in rat cerebellar cortex. 3) Uptake of anesthetic into cells or circulation, which will reduce the concentration gradient. The diffusion coefficient, volume fraction and tortuosity were found to be quite consistent at several depths within the cerebellar cortex even though cellular and fiber layers were quite hetereogeneous. This suggests that transport of anesthetic molecules within peripheral nerve may be well behaved when averaged over dimensions of a few microns and that it will be found to be quantitatively predictable when the diffusion equations are corrected for volume fraction, tortuosity and uptake into cellular interiors and membranes (NICHOLSON and PHILLIPS 1981).

If we take lidocaine and bupivacaine as examples, molecular weight ratios would suggest that the diffusion coefficient of bupivacaine (MW 288 g/mol) should be 90% that of lidocaine (MW 234 g/mol), and both compounds would be expected to have diffusion coefficients near 5×10^{-6} cm^2/s. Using this value we have calculated the time required for transport by diffusion alone in water to an endpoint where ½ of the initial dose of anesthetic has diffused further than certain distances $X_{1/2}$ from the source:

$X_{1/2}$	$t_{1/2}(H_2O)$
1 µ	2 ms
10 µ	200 ms
100 µ	20 s
250 µ	2 min
500 µ	8.7 min

The tortuosity of the tissue in the nerve will have the effect of increasing the path length for diffusing through a particular volume. The result would be to delay diffusion through any particular distance, which is quantitatively equivalent to dividing the diffusion coefficient by λ^2 (NICHOLSON and PHILLIPS 1982). For brain, where λ was measured in several areas to be near 1.5 (NICHOLSON and PHILLIPS 1981), this would mean that the values for $t_{1/2}$ in the above table would be multiplied by 2.4. It is likely that there is less tortuosity in peripheral nerve than in brain, but it does not yet appear to have been measured. Nonetheless for a 1 mm peripheral nerve bathed with a step increase in lidocaine, a time course on the order of 10 min was typical before attaining steady-state for blocking of the compound action potential (BENNETT et al. 1942). FINK and CAIRNS (1984a, b) have recently timed the onset of block in vagus nerve fibers and found it to be of the same order. These results suggest at least for lidocaine that diffusion is the most significant component of the delay between the shift in both concentration and the arrival of the degree of block of the compound action potential to a new steady-state level. The bulk of this delay will be accounted by the time required for anesthetic to arrive by diffusion in the fluid outside the axons.

b) Differential Access

To date there is no evidence that nerve fasicles are ensheathed with connective tissue that offers a differential diffusion barrier. However, once the anesthetic has arrived in the region of an axon, there are some possible diffusion barriers remaining that have been invoked to account for differential blockade. These are the myelin, the polyanionic gap matrix or "gap substance" (BROMAGE 1981, p 38; GISSEN et al. 1982b; FINK and CAIRNS 1984a) and the interdigitating fingers of Schwann cells (WILDSMITH et al. 1984) in A-fibers and the Schwann cell membranes collecting C-fibers into Remak bundles. The possibility that the Remak bundles constitute a diffusion barrier has been suggested as an explanation for the resistance of C-fibers to local anesthetic (TUCKER and MATHER 1980; BROMAGE 1978, pp. 41–42) but no direct evidence was offered in support. Furthermore, the existence of such a barrier would not account for the overlap and sensitivity of individual A-fibers and C-fibers at steady-state (NATHAN and SEARS 1961; FRANZ and PERRY 1974; FINK and CAIRNS 1983b, 1984a). Alternatively Gissen and collaborators have performed a series of experiments using rabbit vagus nerves at room temperature indicating the CAP for C-fibers begins to block before that of A-fibers, but that C-fibers are more resistant at steady-state (GISSEN et al. 1982b).

These investigators find that the rate of block for a variety of drugs is about the same for the C-elevation, but varies for the A-elevation. They suggested that a non-polar diffusion barrier exists at nodes in larger fibers and that it acts to retard access of charged anesthetics to the membrane in A-fibers. This simple idea is consistent with evidence that etidocaine, which was approximately 5 times more lipid soluble than bupivacaine, showed little differential action during onset. Bupivacaine was presented under similar conditions at equipotent doses and caused block in C-fibers well before it produced the same level of block in A-fibers (GISSEN et al. 1982b). The amount of block at steady-state was greater in A-fibers,

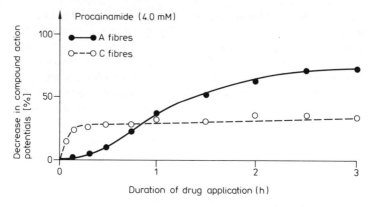

Fig. 11. Differential rate of block vs. steady-state susceptibility in large fibers and unmye-linated fibers. The per cent block of the amplitude of A and C components of the compound action potential in rabbit vagus nerves exposed to 4.0 mM procainamide for 24 °C is shown vs. elapsed time since application of the anesthetic. Steady-state blockade of the C-elevation (*dashed lines*) occurred within 15 min whereas the A-elevation (*solid lines*) became progessively blocked over 3 h, exceeding the degree of C-block only after about an hour. ●——● A-fibres; o---o C-fibres. From WILDSMITH et al. (1985)

but they did not show this sensitivity immediately. A significant interval was found where the C-elevation would transiently show a greater degree of block than the A-elevation which diminished slowly. Since these two agents have almost equal potency and are closely similar in molecular weights and diffusion coefficients, the difference in block onset was attributed to the significant difference in lipid solubility.

In a more recent study of amino ester-linked local anesthetics (WILDSMITH et al. 1985), it was also observed that the compounds having low lipid solubility were effective in producing transient differential rate of block of the C-elevation. The rate of decline of the C-elevation was consistent among the lipid soluble and the polar agents but the block of the A-elevation was progressively delayed for the less lipid soluble drugs such as procainamide. The lipid soluble agents tended to affect both groups with the same kinetics. Figure 11 shows how the larger fibers are affected slowly over the course of 3 h, and eventually reach a greater degree of block than C-fibers. C-fibers attain a steady-state condition more quickly. Without CO_2 the attainment of steady-state was dramatically slowed. Recovery from block was also quite differential. Polar drugs required hours longer in A-fibers than in C-fibers, which recovered in a few minutes. These results support Gissen's concept that A-fibers have a lipid diffusion barrier that C-fibers do not have. The idea is also consistent with clinical experience of differential rate of block in which C-fibers fail prior to A-fibers with near blocking concentrations (SARNOFF and ARROWOOD 1946; FORD et al. 1984). It has also been argued that etidocaine with its high lipid solubility, penetrates these diffusion barriers on A-fibers without the delay associated with more polar agents, and that this accounts for its rapid blockade of motor functions subserved by alpha motor neurons (WILDSMITH et al. 1985). It is well known that this block is differential with respect to epidural sensory blockade of pain which may be marginal when motor block is complete (BROMAGE 1978). FINK and CAIRNS (1984 a) cite evidence that larger myelinated fibers have deeper nodal gaps with structural differences, suggesting that a more pronounced barrier exists in the nodes of larger fibers such as α motor axons.

Taken together, this work offers the promise that polar anesthetics of low lipid solubility may be particularly useful in achieving differential block of C-fibers. A-fibers may be spared altogether if the concentration gradient of anesthetic is dissipated before diffusion to the nodal membrane is completed. Lidocaine has lower lipid solubility than either etidocaine or bupivacaine since its distribution coefficient is about 8 times less than that of bupivacaine (TUCKER and MATHER 1980). It has an intermediate pKa. It appears that the pKa of the compounds is not as closely correlated with the differential rate of block as the partition coefficient. The pKa will determine the ratio of charged to uncharged form, governing the proportion of the dose that will be more lipid soluble (see 3, this section). It would be useful to know whether lidocaine produces a comparatively greater differential rate of block of C-fibers than bupivacaine as this theory would predict. Recent evidence comparing the delay from application of anesthetic to onset of conduction failure in single fibers of rabbit vagus nerves at 37 °C with sheath intact does not support the idea that A-fibers have differential diffusion barriers to lidocaine. Fibers conducting above 15 m/s blocked with an average delay of $4.2 \min \pm 3.3$ whereas C-fibers blocked with an average delay of 7.6 ± 4.7 min (FINK and CAIRNS 1984 b). At this stage, the relative importance of the physicochemical constants of the anesthetic is not yet established, and work is needed on the micro-diffusion and distribution of agents in the area of the node and in the vicinity of unmyelinated fibers to confirm or reject the hypothesis of differential diffusion barriers.

Present studies of diffusional kinetics in isolated nodes studied in voltage clamp (ULBRICHT 1981) also do not support this concept since blocking effects of anesthetics appear with a delay of ms to seconds following application. However, microdissection of nodes is a marginal procedure yielding sucessful nodes in only a fraction of attempts, and a disruption of the structure of the nodal matrix may occur due to mechanical trauma or from the application of bathing solutions. This disruption of the matrix may not necessarily interfere with the capability of the node to manifest voltage dependent changes in conductance. Thus, a physiologically functional node may nonetheless be abnormal with respect to diffusion of substances in the nodal gap.

3. Length of Nerve Exposed

Since the work of FRANZ and PERRY (1974) it has been widely appreciated that the extent of the nerve bathed in anesthetic is an important determinant of block. Franz and Perry's explanation for why length is a factor in differential block was based on 2 propositions: 1) that internodal distances are greater in large myelinated fibers than in small diameter ones, 2) that 3 successive nodes must be "inactivated to block conduction completely" (TASAKI 1953). In steady-state block, differential action on small fibers was explained on the basis that the longitudinal extent of anesthetic was restricted by the chamber around the nerve so that small fibers might have a "critical length" of nodes poisoned where large fibers with more widely separated nodes would not. When rate of block was considered, differential action was similarly interpreted. A localized source of anesthetic would diffuse along the fibers, resulting in blockade of those having a shorter critical length before these larger fibers having a longer critical length. The dimensions involved (several mm) appear to be compatible with diffusion delays on the order of 10 min to an hour or more depending on the diffusion coefficients of the agents (FRANZ and PERRY 1974).

Many of the studies cited in Table 1 exposed a centimeter of nerve – a length which is easily manageable and which ensures that at least 3 nodes are exposed to anesthetic (TASAKI 1953; ARBUTHNOTT et al. 1980). FRANZ and PERRY (1974) found no differential block at steady-state when 4 mm or more of cat saphenous nerve was exposed. Differential block of smaller myelinated A-fibers in saphenous nerve *was* observed at steady-state (> 1 h) when only 2 mm of nerve was exposed.

However, this 1 cm limit seems likely to be insufficient to insure that length of exposure is not a factor. Exposing segments of nerve to dilute concentrations of anesthetic does not match the conditions under which Tasaki tested conduction block. In his experiments, *maximal* blocking doses of cocaine were mechanically restricted to nodes in isolated fibers. Under the more typical conditions where a nerve is exposed to a dose of anesthetic dissolved in a volume of solution, it is likely that just prior to block many nodes would remain capable of generating partial response. Such a reduced excitatory current might itself be incapable of sustaining propagation of the impulse along an indefinite length of fiber, but should greatly extend the ability of the invading impulse to depolarize the axon. Any partially responding node would not regenerate a full impulse, but the decay of the partial impulse would be prolonged in space over several successive partially responding nodes, only to fail at the last one – a process called decremental conduction (LORENTE DE NO and CONDOURIS 1959).

In a model of conduction in myelinated fibers exposed to local anesthetics, decremental conduction occurred when the maximal sodium conductance (g_{Na}) was partially reduced but not completely blocked. The action potential failed after 8–10 nodes in uniformly treated axons exposed along the entire segment (CONDOURIS et al. 1976). RUD (1961) exposed bullfrog nerve segments of 20 mm length to high concentrations of lidocaine while monitoring the action potential in a downstream region of nerve that was unanesthetized. A residual 1%–2% electronic depolarization could be detected until the region of nerve exposed to a constant concentration was increased incrementally to 31 mm. Rud did not study critical length as a function of concentration, but his work shows that depolarizing currents in large fibers may extend well beyond a 1 cm region of exposure. In an experimental study of nodes isolated in a double air gap with the rest of the fiber intact and conducting, it was observed that the node was capable of generating a response to direct electrical stimulus under narcotization that was deep enough to block response to an impulse conducted into the node along its fiber (ICHIOKA et al. 1960), indicating that the capacity to fire an impulse locally may outlast blockade of propagated impulses. Thus, if nodes generate partial responses the critical length might be extended well beyond 3 internodal lengths. The differential critical length among A-fibers and for unmyelinated fibers under conditions of decremental conduction has not been determined experimentally.

The notion that critical length for marginal blocking doses will exceed 3 internodes is supported by recent in vitro work with single fibers exposed along 2 cm or more to lidocaine. One should see no differential block among fibers if all fibers are exposed to anesthetic over a section of nerve that exceeds their critical length and if the difference in critical length completely accounts for differential block observed when lesser lengths are anesthetized (FINK, personal communication). FINK and CAIRNS (1983b, 1984a, b) have found no dependence of steady-state blocking concentration on conduction velocity in A- or C-fiber populations of rabbit vagus nerves exposed for 2 cm. No evidence of differential diffusion barriers to lidocaine was found either (FINK and CAIRNS 1984b). Among a population of single frog A-fibers exposed over 6 cm, broad differences in susceptibility to anesthetic have been found but these also were found not be be correlated with conduction velocity (RAYMOND and ROSCOE 1984). Thus, given a sufficient length of exposure, differential susceptibility according to size does not seem to occur.

In cases where anesthetic susceptibility has been closely correlated with diameter or conduction velocity, under conditions where 1 cm segments have been exposed, a component of the variation in susceptibility to anesthetic among fibers of similar conduction velocity may depend on anatomical differences among myelinated fibers. A recent review of the connection between fiber diameter, fiber circumference, axon diameter, axon circumference, and internodal distance supported the concept that internodal distance increases with all four measures of axon size. ARBUTHNOTT et al. (1980) suggested that functionally grouped classes of fibers have different functional relations between fiber size and internodal length and between fiber size and conduction velocity (see also WAXMAN 1981). Additionally, the average internodal distance may not decline in proportion to fiber diameter for fibers 4 μ in diameter and less because of a constraint imposed by the average minimum length that can be achieved by the Schwann cell (CHIU and RITCHIE 1984). These structural variations among fibers would, under the critical length hypothesis, result in variation in susceptibility of fibers. Furthermore, some fibers of the same size would have varying critical lengths.

Under in vivo conditions the distribution of anesthetic will be affected by the circulation as well as by diffusion and it might be supposed that the concentration gradient would be less well behaved. This was assessed in anesthetized cats where local anesthetics were injected subcutaneously near the saphenous nerve. The compound action potential was recorded on the peripheral side of the injection in response to supramaximal electrical stimulation given 7 cm away on the central side of the injection. 2-Chloroprocaine, lidocaine, and etidocaine at about 1/10 of the clinically used concentration were compared (FORD et al. 1984). The most lipid soluble drug, etidocaine, showed the least differential action among the Aβ-, Aδ-, and C-elevations. It also reduced the Aδ-elevation prior to the C-elevation. The least lipid soluble drug, 2-chloroprocaine, had the greatest differential action and blocked C-fibers to a greater extent than Aδ- and Aβ-elevations. The authors extended the critical length hypothesis of Franz and Perry to explain these findings, suggesting that lipid soluble drugs might be expected to pass through diffusion barriers and thus distribute evenly along the length of the nerve. Thus, etidocaine would reveal only the relative intrinsic susceptibility of fiber groups since differences in critical length would be very quickly compensated by the spread of anesthetic. On the other hand, anesthetics with low lipid solubility were hypothesized to "penetrate" the nerve irregularly with patches of high concentration and low concentration thus reducing the probability that 3 successive nodes of larger fibers would be blocked. The hypothesis of inhomogeneous distribution of less lipid soluble agents suggested by these authors seems useful, and must be considered in accounting for differences in degree of differential block among different agents.

It was observed also that the degree to which relative block among the 3 elevations was differential became reduced as the concentration of anesthetic was increased, particularly for the more lipid soluble anesthetics. This finding would fit with the explanation offered for dependence of differential block on the lipid solubility of agents, since the longitudinal dispersion of a blocking concentration would occur more quickly at higher diffusion gradients. It would also fit with Gissen's hypothesis (see 2, this section) of a lipid diffusion barrier at nopdes of larger fibers. Furthermore, it seems plausible that with highly lipid soluble drugs the myelin sheath would not act as a barrier but as a lipid solvent or medium in which anesthetics would dissolve and diffuse. This would help highly lipid soluble anesthetics to distribute along the critical length more quickly than less lipid soluble anesthetic with similar diffusion coefficient. The evidence suggests that under clinical conditions, the relation between the exposed length and the critical length is a factor determining the degree of differential block. Though, as mentioned above, we suggest that the critical length is probably greater than prior estimates based on the number of nodes needed to be *completely* blocked in order to prevent conduction in isolated fibers.

4. pH/pCO$_2$

The pCO$_2$ influences the extent of conduction block in at least three ways: 1) it modulates the pH of the extracellular solution with which it is equilibrated and this alters the ratio of charged to uncharged form of those anesthetics that are weak bases, influencing the rate of entry of anesthetic into the nerve (Catchlove 1972) as well as the potency (Hille 1968, 1977). 2) CO$_2$ is a highly permeant acid that will shift the intracellular and intra-axonal pH (Caldwell 1958) which will govern the ratio of charged to uncharged form of anesthetics in the axoplasm, and thus potency (Schwartz et al. 1979; Raymond and Bokesch 1983). 3) CO$_2$ has direct effects on membrane excitability (Lehmann 1937; Lorente de No 1947a) in the presence of anesthetics (Condouris 1961) and when present in isolation (Coraboeuf and Niedergerke 1953; Raymond and Lettvin 1978). The importance of CO$_2$ in the kinetics of block with local anesthetics has been discussed by Bromage (Bromage 1978).

Whether these complicated dynamic processes have *differential* action among nerve fibers has been little studied, although the strong influence of pCO$_2$/pH on potency of anesthetics is suggestive that differences could be large if they are present.

Recently the action of several anesthetics on the desheathed rabbit vagus nerve 23 °C–26 °C was compared at a pH of 7.4 in carbonated bicarbonate Lileys and in HEPES buffer. The rate of onset of conduction block in CO_2 solutions was dramatically faster, and the extent of block was greater than in HEPES buffered solutions (WILDSMITH et al. 1985). The blocking effect on A-fibers of more polar drugs, procaine and procainamide was much more rapid in carbonated solutions. With procainamide at 10 mM, it required 3–4 h for block of the A-elevation of the compound action potential to stabilize in carbonated solutions and required more than 8 h for block to stablize in HEPES buffered solutions. Rate modulation by pCO_2 occurred in both C-fibers and A-fibers, but the action of CO_2 appeared to be most dramatic on A-fibers. Since the pH of both solutions was 7.4, the mobility and permeability of anesthetic in the external solution should have been identical. However, the internal pH was probably lower with Co_2 buffered solutions. This would act to increase the proportion of anesthetic in the charged form in the axoplasm, thus trapping anesthetic inside the fiber, increasing the rate of onset and prolonging the duration of block. This is consistent with the observation that presence of Co_2 also slowed recovery as dramatically as it accelerated onset. The direct effect of CO_2 (CATCHLOVE 1972; RAYMOND and BOKESCH 1983) contributed to the greater degree of steady-state block seen with Co_2 (WILDSMITH et al. 1985). An acceleration of onset of anesthesia by CO_2 has been claimed during peripheral nerve and epidural block. Carbonated lidocaine showed 30% faster onset than lidocaine HCl in epidural block and saved an average of 6 min out of 14 in block of brachial plexus (review, BROMAGE 1978). Carbonation of bupivacaine caused only a slight increase in rate of onset of extradural blockade (BROWN et al. 1980), though bupivacaine – CO_2 will enhance rate of block of peripheral nerve in vitro (CATCHLOVE 1973). This speedier onset was not confirmed with carbonated lidocaine in a double blind study of epidural procedures in 20 surgical patients (MORISON 1981), but it did give significantly greater motor block than the hydrochloride.

Should a lipid diffusion barrier exist for nodes of larger A-fibers but not for Aδ- and C-fibers (GISSEN et al. 1982b; LANDON 1982; LANDON and LANGLEY 1971) one would expect to be able to modulate the differential action of local anesthetics by controlling the pH of the interstitial fluid in which they are applied. By acidifying the ECF, the dose could be rendered into the less permeant polar form, slowing access of the anesthetic to A-fibers without dramatically compromising access to the smaller myelinated fibers and unmyelinated fibers.

5. Anesthetic Species

One would hope that different compounds would differ in diffusability in the complex environment of peripheral nerve or that they would work preferentially in different ways on different classes of fibers. With regard to differential tonic block at steady-state this hope has not been sustained by facts. Most drugs studied so far lead to the same order of failure under comparable conditions (STAIMAN and SEEMAN 1974, 1977; GISSEN et al. 1980, 1982b; FORD et al. 1984; WILDSMITH et al. 1985). With regard to differential rate of block, agents with low lipid solubility seemed to produce the most, and agents with high lipid solubility the least.

The differential is greater if drugs are presented at low concentrations (FORD et al. 1984; WILDSMITH et al. 1985).

STAIMAN and SEEMAN (1974) compared a number of drugs for their effect on the compound action potential of frog sciatic nerves. They were impressed by the inconsistencies in conclusions reached in some 20 studies they reviewed concerning differential block. They claimed that none of these studies "employed techniques of equilibrium blockade", that the studies did not use a range of concentrations to establish a dose response curve and that most studies compared myelinated with unmyelinated fibers rather than fibers ranked by size within a group. In fact, UEHARA (1958, 1960) and NATHAN and SEARS (1961, 1962) had used rapidly equilibrating agents and had explicitly focused their experiments on the differential block occurring after waiting for steady-state to be established. However, Staiman and Seeman had wished to consider steady-state blocking action of drugs having a much higher membrane/buffer partition coefficient, such as dibucaine which would require more than 24 h to achieve an equilibrium distribution. Thus, they adopted an alternative to simply waiting long enough for the action potential to stabilize. Instead, using a method credited to Skou, they began by exposing the nerve to solutions well in excess of the minimum blocking concentration and then shifting to a solution of lower concentration that was adjusted to be just sufficient to prevent any recovery of the compound action potential. This method in conjunction with successive approximations was used to bracket the concentration required to achieve a reduction of a compound action potential to 50% of its control height. Staiman and Seeman compared this C_{50} for rat phrenic nerve where the mode of fiber diameter from e–m measurements was 11 μ (range 8–12 μ) to the C_{50} for rat sciatic nerve with a mode of 16 μ (no range given). In one example with haloperidol they compared the C_{50} of phrenic nerves with a mode of 6 μ from 10 day old rats. For a variety of agents (their figure 10) the action potential proved to be more sensitive for the phrenic nerve than for the sciatic. Since the length of phrenic nerve exposed to the agents was less than for the sciatic (5 mm vs. 10 mm), they attributed a difference in sensitivity to the relative diameter in the fibers of the 2 nerves.

Recognizing the likelihood of differences between sciatic and phrenic nerves even within the same species, they tested the phrenic nerves from a 10 day old rat in which nerve fibers were smaller than their adult diameter. The immature phrenic nerve also was reported to be more sensitive than adult phrenic nerves. This result was consistent with the size principle which, however, did not rule out the further possibility of other differences between phrenic nerves from adults and those from 10 day old rats.

The 18 drugs used in the study ranged from ethanol with a C_{50} of 1 M to TTX and trifluperidol at 10^{-8} M. Over the 7 decade range of relative potency, the phrenic nerve (sheath intact) was more sensitive to all but two of the agents than was the sciatic (desheathed). TTX and pentanol were the exceptions. The anomolous behavior of TTX can now be attributed to its inability to pass through the sheath. The degree of differential block was reported to be less for neutral and acidic drugs than for tertiary amines, suggesting that the level of differential block depends on the agent as well as on the intrinsic safety factor for conduction in the fiber (STAIMAN and SEEMAN 1974). Two other studies have found that various amide-linked and ester-linked tertiary amine anesthetics all showed the same degree of differential specificity for B- vs C-fibers in the cervical sympathetic trunk. These authors concluded that there was an intrinsic difference in safety factor between the B- vs C-groups, and that the evidence strongly suggested that all local anesthetics acting by blockade of Na channels would be expected to produce an equivalent relative order of blockade. These authors did not try TTX (HEAVNER and DE JONG 1974; SCURLOCK et al. 1975).

Later, STAIMAN and SEEMAN (1977) compared TTX with lidocaine and benzyl alcohol using a different paradigm where single units from bullfrog sciatic nerves were tested. The blocking concentration of TTX for 10 single units (ranging in conduction velocity from 10–45 m/s) was higher for the faster fibers and lower for the slower ones. The results with TTX were similar to those obtained with lidocaine and benzyl alcohol using a similar population of desheathed fibers.

Recently, 5 different amino-ester local anesthetics were compared for differential blocking action on A-, B-, and C-elevations of excised rabbit vagus nerves in carbonated Liley at 23 °C–26 °C and pH 7.4. All 5 agents ranging in potency from procainamide with a C_{50} of about 3 mM to tetracaine with a C_{50} of 0.007 mM, caused the same order of steady-state differential block. The A-elevation was most sensitive followed by B- and C-elevations, respectively (WILDSMITH et al. 1984).

Thus it would seem that prospects are not promising for differential steady-state block of functions subserved peripherally by C-fibers and Aδ-fibers. However, local anesthetics influence voltage-gated K^+ channels as well as Na^+ channels. And in myelinated mammalian fibers few K^+ channels seem to be at the nodes or to participate in the repolarization of the membrane during the falling phase of the action potential (CHIU et al. 1979) whereas they do in C-fibers. Blocking some K-channels in C-fibers not exposed to depolarizing agents should increase the relative conduction safety in these fibers by increasing the space constant as well as by prolonging the action potential. Often, this is the opposite of the effect desired, though it may account in part for the relative resistance of C-fibers to blockade. Some cell bodies of neurons with C-axons resist blockade for 20 min with 1 µM TTX whereas A-fiber somata block without exception in a few seconds (STANSFIELD and WALLIS 1983). Differential TTX resistance for impulse conduction in the axons of cells in the nodose ganglion exists (GISSEN et al. 1982a), but is much less dramatic. It is possible that some of the voltage-gated channels in C-fibers are TTX resistant; whether such channels, if they exist, also would be relatively more resistant to anesthetics is an intriguing possibility that remains to be established.

6. Locus of Block

The conduction safety of fibers varies along their length. One might expect that near peripheral sensory receptors where differentiation of the endings and end organs is high, opportunities would exist for differential block of function. Cutaneous polymodal nociceptors having greater sensitivity to stimuli in superficial dermis have been distinguished from those having their region of greater sensitivity in deeper dermal layers (PERL 1984). Other examples of spatial separation of receptive areas and of anatomical specialization of endings have been recently reviewed (IGGO and ANDRES 1982). The biochemistry of peripheral transduction involves peptides such as bradykinin and other pain producing substances (ZIMMERMANN 1979; ZIMMERMANN and SANDERS 1982) and it is reasonable to expect specific differential block of function to be possible in the periphery by intervention in these processes once they are better understood. With differential block of function in mind, it might be argued that "relaxants" like curare could be labeled as differential blocking agents acting preferentially on motor function. And that guanethidine, which does not block conduction (WATSON 1967), but does interfere with cross-excitation between sympathetic efferents and afferent fibers either triggering or sustaining pain in causaglia, is a differential blocking agent.

Thus it is appropriate to consider the issue of whether greater differential block might follow application of conventional agents near the entry of fibers into the CNS in spinal or epidural anesthesia (BROMAGE 1978) than by blocking a conduction path in the trunk of the peripheral nerve. Also, the broader issue of obtaining block of function by blocking synaptic conduction centrally or even by stimulation of central inhibitory systems (see factor 10) is properly an aspect of the subject of differential block. Except where differential block of sensory and motor function has been discussed, we have so far mainly considered differential block of conduction in the peripheral nerve trunk.

The issue of whether conventional anesthetics act uniformly over the surface of an axon or act preferentially at the site where it branches to form its terminal arbor and synaptic contacts has been investigated in the periphery in sympathetic ganglia. LARABEE and POSTERNAK (1952) were concerned with conduction block of axonal pathways vs conduction block of pathways having a chemical synapse in the stellate ganglia. They studied block produced by general and regional anesthetic agents on B- and C-fibers passing through the ganglia without synapsing vs. presynaptic sympathetic B-fibers synapsing onto cells having C-fibers leaving the ganglia. They found no preferential blocking action of the agents on C-fibers vs. A- and B-fibers, claiming instead, "if anything a given concentration of anesthetic blocked a smaller proportion of them (C-fibers) than of the myelinated type A- and B-fibers" (p 97). They sought to study differential block at steady-state, exposing their preparations for 30 min to sub-maximal blocking concentrations. Most of the compounds, including regional anesthetics like cocaine, acted to block conduction in the synaptic pathways rather than the axonal ones, but the difference between concentrations required to give equivalent percent reductions in compound action potentials was never greater than 10:1 and often less than 3:1. Compared to nicotine, which blocked synaptic conduction at less than 1/100 the concentration required to block axonal conduction , anesthetic agents showed a relatively low order of differential action on synapses vs. axons. The authors questioned whether anesthetic agents had their blocking action at the synaptic junction itself or by inducing failure of conduction in presynaptic terminals. Did anesthetics act preferentially on the processes of synaptic transmission in postsynaptic excitation or on the processes of axonal conduction in the small diameter presynaptic twigs of the axonal arbor?

The actions of general and regional anesthetics on postsynaptic membranes have been studied (MILLER 1975) but it is not yet established that the clinical action of general anesthetics is due to their postsynaptic actions rather than to conduction failure in fine presynaptic arbors. The differential blocking action of anesthetics at these regions appears to have been little studied though it has been occasionally discussed (BROMAGE 1978). It is known that the branch of the unipolar axon to the spinal ganglion cell is a region of relatively slowed conduction and of lower conduction safety (DUN 1955; ITO and TAKAHASHI 1960). Branch points, which abound in afferent fibers distributing in dorsal horn, are thus candidates for weak links where conduction may fail first. To what extent branching patterns in different fibers may render conduction block differential at the spinal level has not been explored.

7. Species Differences; Nerve to Nerve Differences

If the size principle alone accounted for differential susceptibility to block, it would predict that order of sensitivity would depend on diameter from nerve to nerve and across species. Small fibers in one nerve should match the sensitivity of fibers of equivalent size in another nerve and, for example, the squid giant axon should be uniquely resistant to block because of its large size. The evidence, however suggests that several issues are involved.

One issue concerns species differences. In cat cutaneous nerves, there appear to be many more C-fibers responding to light touch of the skin and to manipulation of hairs than in primates where cutaneous C-fibers fire selectively to warming or to noxious stimuli (DOUGLAS and RITCHIE 1957, 1962; MOUNTCASTLE 1980a). Whether these populations would be equivalently sensitive to blocking agents is not known. In other cases, C_1- and C_2-elevations within the C-potential have been distinguished in the compound action potential and they have been shown to be differentially susceptible to block (GASSER 1950; DOUGLAS and RITCHIE 1962). Sympathetic C-fibers which fire tonically and affect blood vessels as well as a variety of other deep organs, and drC nociceptive fibers, which are not tonically active in man (OCHOA 1984), certainly have very different physiological roles. We would expect them to show a differential phasic block because their habitual firing rates differ (see 8, this section).

We do not know of any tests of the relative susceptibility to blocking agents among sympathetic C-fibers or between somatic C-fibers and sympathetic ones. ARROWOOD and SARNOFF (1947a) reported a match in susceptibility of vasomotor and sudomotor fibers as tested in procaine spinals in human patients monitored for warming of the skin, which was the endpoint marking blocking of vasoconstrictive impulses, and for increased skin resistance, which marked the block of sudomotor drive. The result probably reflected a correspondence in sensitivity among the especially susceptible sympathetic preganglionic B-fibers (SCURLOCK et al. 1975) rather than a direct action of procaine on postganglionic C-fibers. They noted that the pain of pinprick disappeared at either slightly lower or slightly greater levels of anesthesia. Given the later work linking block of pinprick to block of Aδ-fibers (MACKENZIE et al. 1975), this fact would suggest that some of the Aδ-population was as susceptible to spinal procaine at 0.2% as were B-fibers. In other studies, (ARROWOOD and SARNOFF 1948; ARROWOOD 1950) they indicated that pain other than from pinprick persisted during differential block of pinprick sensation. At the time the authors assumed, on the basis of the size principle, that the fiber population that was spared was fast conducting and mye-linated (Aδ). Now the finding would seem more likely to indicate a relative resistance of cutaneous nociceptive C-fibers over Aδ-(and B-)fibers. However, the inference remains questionable to a degree because of uncertainties in the role of cutaneous C-fibers and the type of pain involved in these early studies. The cases seem to have been patients experiencing chronic pain such as stump pain following amputation, and the relative contributions of peripheral C-fibers and central integrative mechanisms in such chronic pain is not yet fully understood (WALL 1984).

The use of guanethidine, an adrenergic blocking agent that prevents the discharge of sensory C-fibers in response to acetylcholine (WATSON 1967) to block pain in causalgia is another likely case of differential action emerging from differences in fiber type, in this case affecting the coupling of sympathetic fibers to afferent fibers (OCHOA 1984). The agent blocks pain and thus has a differential effect on function; it does not block normal afferent conduction in sensory C-fibers including nociceptors. However, its action is not related to the size of the target fibers so much as to their biochemistry.

Another issue concerns the differences among nerves. The fiber spectrum of peripheral somatic and autonomic nerves has long been known to vary (HEIN-BECKER et al. 1934; DYCK et al. 1971). Thus, the order of relative decline in elevation of the compound action potential in one nerve may be expected to differ from that in another. Preganglionic B-fibers have been shown to be particularly sensitive to anesthetics and are more susceptible to block at steady-state than C-fibers (SCURLOCK et al. 1975). They also differ from Aδ-fibers in their afterpotentials and in resistance to anoxia and other parameters (GRUNDFEST 1939). In comparisons of cervical sympathetic trunk, where B-fibers predominate, with other nerves such as saphenous in which Aδ-fibers give rise to a similar appearing wave in the compound action potential (HEAVNER and DE JONG 1974), one might expect to see a different order of differential block of the compound action potential. Such a differential block would be associated with functional specialization of the B- and Aδ-fiber populations, not their size.

Direct evidence reveals that the relative order of block under comparable conditions does vary among nerves. With 0.05% procaine, EVERETT and TOMAN (1954), EVERETT and GOODSELL (1952) found the total block of C preceded block of A-elevations in compound action potentials from sciatic nerves of rabbits, cats, guinea pigs and frogs. On the other hand, total block of the A-elevation typically preceded total block of the C-group in vagus nerves from the same animals. Using a different endpoint, GISSEN et al. (1980) reported that C-fibers in both vagus and sciatic nerves of rabbits were more resistant to lidocaine than A-fibers. Motor fibers of the peroneal nerve in 5 of 10 cats were found to be more sensitive to cold block than sensory fibers of the same nerve matching in conduction velocity (DOUGLAS and MALCOLM 1955). Almost complete block of the compound action potential in ventral root occurred at a temperature that was insufficient to affect the dorsal root response significantly.

With respect to differential effects in different nerves in humans, (BURKE et al. 1975; MACKENZIE et al. 1975) it was found that the C-fibers of the radial nerve could be recorded regularly in response to single electrical stimuli at an intensity 5–7 times the perceptual threshold (Tp). The factor for activation of C-fibers in median nerve was usually 15–20 times Tp and never was below 10, suggesting a difference in C-fiber threshold, C-fiber population density, or in the effectiveness of the link to sensation per fiber between the two nerves.

8. Activity Dependence and Differential Phasic Block

a) Phasic Block

Nerve axons undergo oscillatory changes in their excitability and conduction velocity following impulse activity even in the absence of local anesthetics. These aftereffects of activity can be large enough to influence conduction at regions of low conduction safety, and they may last for many minutes (RAYMOND 1979; SWADLOW et al. 1980). The magnitude and time course of activity-dependent changes in excitability varies substantially among fibers (CARLEY and RAYMOND 1983) suggesting that impulse activity will elicit a differential effect on conduction safety with anesthetic drugs.

In the presence of local anesthetics, there is an incremental block of inward current measured under voltage clamp conditions following trains of depolarizing pulses. This transient increase in block and is called frequency dependent, (COURTNEY 1975), or use-dependent (STRICHARTZ 1973) block. It operates in addition to the activity dependent effects on excitability in unanesthetized membrane. Use-dependent block is implicated in the blockade of trains of conducting impulses under conditions where single impulses remain capable of conducting (COURTNEY et al. 1978). What we call phasic block is a combination of the activity-dependent changes in conduction safety that occur without anesthetic, together with those that occur when local anesthetics are present. The mechanism of phasic block produced by local anesthetics is hypothesized to involve the increased affinity of a binding site for local anesthetic that is thought to result from conformational changes occurring with depolarizations of the membrane (STRICHARTZ and WANG 1984). The mechanism of activity dependent changes in the excitability of nerve membrane that is not exposed to anesthetics has not yet been established but is thought to involve physiological processes active during recovery following nerve impulses (CONNELLY 1959; RAYMOND and LETTVIN 1978). It was long ago determined that afterpotentials in B-fibers (GRUNDFEST 1939) and C-fibers (GASSER 1950; DOUGLAS and RITCHIE 1962) differed from those in A-fibers. In particular, C-fibers show a prolonged afterhyperpolarization. The relation between the shifts in afterpotentials, which may last for a long time (CONNELLY 1959), and conduction safety has still not been elucidated.

b) Differential Phasic Block

At issue is whether phasic block can be differential. In principle, differential phasic block could occur in at least two fundamental ways, 1) because of a difference among fibers in the intrinsic sensitivity of membrane to activity with and/or without anesthetic or 2) because of a difference in the rate of impulse activity present among fibers that are equally sensitive to activity. Differences of the first type were suggested very early to explain the observation that Wedenski inhibition (the blocking of trains of impulses) was much greater during repetitive activity in autonomic (B- and C-fibers) than in somatic A- and Aδ-fibers at equivalent tonic "depression of potential amplitude" by anesthetic (Heinbecker et al. 1934, p 39). It was argued that this difference in the tendency to block trains of impulses among B-fibers and Aδ-fibers had to reflect differences in the "nature" not the size of the axons since the 1–4 μ diameter B-fibers of cervical sympathetic trunk were so similar in size to the 1–5 μ diameter Aδ-fibers of saphenous nerve. Repeated activity sped up the onset of procaine block which otherwise would require 25 min for complete block.

Matthews and Rushworth (1957b) noted that the capacity of groups of large motor and sensory myelinated fibers to generate compound action potentials for stimuli at rates between 100–500/s declined as narcosis with procaine progressed. At the time the γ-wave had been blocked for single volleys, the larger fibers could always conduct at 100 Hz, and occasionally at 300 or 500 Hz. The degree of phasic block increased monotonically with the degree of tonic block. Neither the α- or γ-fibers showed an enhanced or "supernormal" capacity for the second of a pair of pulses to pass through a region of marginal anesthetic block. Over a 1–10 ms interval following first pulse, the second compound action potential of a pair was always smaller than the first, indicating that supernormality could not offset anesthetic block, contradicting a statement made by Adrian and Lucas (Adrian 1921). Following an impulse there usually is a transient period of superexcitability or "supernormality" lasting about 1 s in frog fibers and about 200 ms in mammalian fibers. Superexcitability is enhanced by repetitive stimulation (Raymond and Lettvin 1978). Lidocaine and other local anesthetics produce a period of subexcitability that offsets the superexcitable phase. At higher doses, e. g., one-half a blocking dose and above, subexcitability is dominant and no superexcitability occurs (Raymond and Roscoe 1984). This subexcitability is associated with phasic block of conduction and is another manifestation of use-dependent block.

Repetitive activation of C-fibers tends to buildup the afterhyperpolarization (Gasser 1950; Douglas and Ritchie 1962; Rang and Ritchie 1968). In cat saphenous nerve given marginal block with 0.4 mM lidocaine, repetitive stimulation at 5 or 10 Hz on one side of the blocked region resulted in a potential at C-latency that could be recorded on the other side. Since no deflections followed single stimuli, it was argued that the recorded potential represented the activity-induced enhancement of C-fiber conduction under conditions where Aδ- and Aβ-components showed use-dependent blocks (Strichartz and Zimmermann 1983, see Fig. 12). The potential resembled the control potential recorded at C-latency prior to application of the drug. However, the C-potential has components due to the action currents and also due to the afterhyperpolarization (Gasser 1950). The observation that impulse activity promoted a C-potential but not Aβ- or Aδ-elevations indicates a differential action of activity on C-fibers and suggests that a phasic *enhancement* of conduction may exist in some fibers under conditions where anesthetics are present, and where use-dependent block may occur in other fibers.

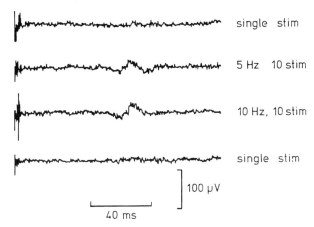

single stim

5 Hz   10 stim

10 Hz, 10 stim

single stim

100 µV

40 ms

Fig. 12. Recruitment of C-fiber conduction in 0.4 mM lidocaine by repetitive stimulation. Four traces show the electrical response recorded from cat saphenous nerve in the thigh after conduction through a 1 cm well containing lidocaine and Ringers. No response is seen following single stimuli (top and bottom traces), but a C-elevation is seen after the tenth pulse in a train at 5 Hz (second trace) and at 10 Hz (third trace) from STRICHARTZ and ZIMMERMANN (1983)

In saphenous nerve of the cat, it was observed that the maximum frequency (f_{max}) that could be conducted in individual fibers given electrical stimuli declined in parallel with the reduction in conduction velocity occurring before tonic block with procaine. The f_{max} was differentially lower in slower myelinated fibers (FRANZ and PERRY 1974). It was suggested that sensory fibers responding at high frequency would be more prone to phasic block with anesthetic than motor fibers normally functioning at frequencies "well below 30 Hz". In humans undergoing pressure block, failure to sense cold stimuli presented to the skin occurred when an Aδ-elevation could still be recorded for single electrical stimuli given at 1 Hz. However, no Aδ-elevation was detectable for a second stimulus 20 ms after the first. With pressure removed, the second stimulus became effective, and sensation for cold returned (MACKENZIE et al. 1975). This finding suggests that block of function can be expected simply by preventing repetitive firing even if occasional single stimuli can conduct in a number of fibers (MACKENZIE et al. 1975).

The earlier disappearance and higher segmental block of sympathetic vasoconstriction and sudomotor drive than block of sensation in spinal anesthesia (SARNOFF and ARROWOOD 1946) may not derive entirely from greater differential sensitivity of B-fibers to local anesthetic (SCURLOCK et al. 1975). Recently FINK and CAIRNS (1984 b) have raised the possibility that the ongoing tonic efferent activities in these fibers makes them more prone to phasic block than sensory fibers that do not fire in the absence of stimulation. They suggest that this accounts for their physiological greater sensitivity to anesthetic.

Prolonged decreases in excitability of single fibers, called "depression", follow sustained impulse activity in a normal physiological range 2–30 Hz (RAYMOND 1979). Variation among frog A-fibers in depressibility is quite pronounced (more than 500 fold) but it does not seem to be correlated with resting conduction velocity. Mammalian peripheral fibers appear to show less depression at equivalent rates of activity than do frog fibers (CARLEY 1984). Depression parallels sensory adaptation and a decline in the sensory action potential which both occur in response to repeated electrical stimuli in humans (RAYMOND and LIEF 1984). Several investigators have noted that rapid electrical stimuli at 30/s (HEINBECKER and BISHOP 1935) or more (COLLINS et al. 1960; BURKE et al. 1975) are more tolerable at the Aδ-level than repeated shocks given at sufficient intervals that the sensation does not fuse, but remains punctate. This observation has been attributed to an adaptation at the level of the central nervous system since peripheral nerve fibers fire for many hours without block at these frequencies. However, the processes responsible for depression may cause conduction failure at axonal regions of low conduction safety either in the primary afferent fibers or in the secondary pathways fed by them. Such regions may exist in the dorsal horn of the spinal cord. Local anesthetics, even at low concentration, sharply reduce the level of depression produced by impulse activity (RAYMOND and ROSCOE 1984). Depression and superexcitability also depend strongly on the pCO_2 and temperature (RAYMOND and ROSCOE 1983). Whether the action of anesthetics in inhibiting depression is differential among fibers of equivalent depressibility is not known. Post-tetanic shifts in latency in single fibers of human sural and median nerves were measured by microneurography and found to be very roughly correlated ($r = 0.53$) with pretetanic conduction velocity over the range of 15–60 m/s (MACKENZIE et al. 1977). The posttetanic slowing was measured after 2 min of tetani at 500/s, and was found to be significantly greater in patients with hereditary forms of axonal degeneration. It was also significantly greater at a skin temperature over the nerve of 33 °C than at 28 °C. Similar slowing with repetitive activity at 180–200 Hz in intraaxonal recordings of cat radial nerve fibers (IGNELZI and NYQUIST 1979 b) and cat sciatic nerve and dorsal column (IGNELZI et al. 1981) has also been reported but was found not to be correlated with the conduction velocity at rest (interpreted as fiber size).

c) Differences Among Anesthetic Agents

Both neutral and hydrophilic agents produce phasic block. The minimum frequency at which a phasic increment in block first appears varies among anesthetic agents. Some, like TTX, show little increment in phasic block of the compound action potential in frog sciatic nerves even at 50 Hz, whereas others like bupivacaine show pronounced phasic block at activity rates below 1 Hz (COURTNEY et al. 1978). It is not yet known whether these differences among agents in degree and time course of phasic block are differential among fibers classified either by size or by function.

In summary, it is presently established that phasic block depends on the pharmacological interactions underlying use-dependence convolved with the physiological processes underlying the dependence of excitability on activity. These physiological processes are themselves affected by anesthetics. Thus, the degree of *phasic* block will be a function of at least 4 variables: pCO_2, anesthetic type and concentration, activity rate, and temperature. Existing observations indicate that this function differs among fibers, but a systematic study of differential phasic block incorporating all 4 variables has yet to be done.

9. Type of Blocking Procedure and Order of Differential Block

In this paper we have primarily emphasized differential block with local anesthetics. The order of failure with other blocking agents is not always the same.

a) Block with Other Agents than Local Anesthetics

Pressure blocks conduction in two dissimilar ways: 1) a long-lasting block resulting from structural demyelination at higher pressure gradients and 2) a reversible block at lower pressures producing ischemia without notable structural pathology. Both high pressure blocks (DENNY-BROWN and BRENNER 1944; RYDEVIK 1979; review GILLIAT 1980) and lower pressure blocks affected the largest fibers preferentially. Conduction in C-fibers continues for several hours following a tourniquet (LEWIS et al. 1931; GASSER 1935b; TOREBJORK and HALLIN 1973; MACKENZIE et al. 1975; BROWN et al. 1980), though after 4 h of ischemia, endoneurial pressure within the sheath becomes an additional factor affecting conduction (LUNDBORG 1980). Aδ-fibers may be the most sensitive (GASSER 1935; MANFREDI 1970). Axoplasmic transport is affected by anoxia, though it is not known whether the extent of the effect varies among axons (LEONE and OCHS 1978; IGNELZI and NYQUIST 1979a).

Anodal polarizing currents blocked conduction in fast conducting fibers at lower currents than were required for conduction block in smaller myelinated fibers (FUKUSHIMA et al. 1975). In cat nerves, Aβ-, Aδ-, and C-elevations could be obtained in relative isolation by combining anodal polarization with ischemic pressure block (MANFREDI 1970). Both depolarizing and hyperpolarizing currents have been used to achieve differential block (ZIMMERMANN 1968; review MANFREDI 1970).

Ion pump inhibitors block conduction slowly. The block was essentially irreversible except at very low concentrations, and the C-elevation failed first in rabbit vagus nerve (FINK and CAIRNS 1983c). However, the C-elevation of the compound action potential derives from summation of afterpotentials as well as from summation of spikes in individual fibers (DOUGLAS and RITCHIE 1962) and its disappearance after ouabain may actually precede conduction block of the C-impulses. Individual frog A-fibers exposed to a similar concentration of ouabain lost their activity dependent shifts in excitability an hour or more before impulse conduction was blocked (RAYMOND and LETTVIN 1978).

Deprivation of glucose in rabbit vagus nerve affected the A-elevation much more dramatically than the C. Both elevations resisted glucose lack better without the sheath, possibly because of accumulation within the sheath of potassium leaking from the axon after ion pumps failed due to the absence of an energy source (FINK and CAIRNS 1982). Unrecoverable conduction block is produced in anoxic whole sciatic nerve preparations in the presence of glucose. Other nonmetabolized sugars do not cause the block or the nerve damage, but it is not known if these effects are differential among axons (LORENTE DE NO 1947b).

Deprivation of sodium in solutions bathing excised nerves in vitro affects C- and Aδ-fibers preferentially. Individual Aα- and Aβ-fibers overlapped C-fibers in sensitivity to low sodium (NATHAN and SEARS 1962). The order of differential block with low sodium has been found to be similar to that for local anesthetics in cases where the comparisons were made using the same techniques, same end-points and same desheathed preparations to test low sodium as to test anesthetics (CRESCITELLI 1952a; CONDOURIS 1961; NATHAN and SEARS 1962; GISSEN et al. 1982a). With the sheath intact, 3 h of exposure to 26% normal sodium reduced the A-elevation more than the C-elevation, and completely blocked the B/Aδ-elevation (SCHIMEK et al. 1984). The differential action of low sodium among nerve fibers has been explained on the basis of intrinsic differences in conduction safety rather than fiber size. The size principle does not explain the differences in susceptibility at steady-state (NATHAN and SEARS 1962) or in the differential rate of block between Aδ- and Aβ-fibers or among the C_1- and C_2-fiber groups (CRESCITELLI 1952b) or between the C-fibers and the faster A-fibers (GISSEN et al. 1982a).

Heating to 46 °C blocked conduction in rat sciatic nerves (ROSENBERG and HEAVNER 1980) and in human peroneal or median nerves following high body temperature (DHOPESH and BURNS 1976). In cat tibial nerves, heat caused differential block with 25%–100% of the C-fibers continuing to conduct while the A-elevation was blocked (ZIMMERMANN and SAUNDERS 1982). Regional cooling also produced a differential block, which was particularly effective for trains of impulses (PAINTAL 1965b; FRANZ and IGGO 1968). Greater cooling was required to block the C-elevation, especially where the length of the cooled region exceeded 2 mm (DOUGLAS and MALCOLM 1955). Among myelinated fibers no relationship was found between the diameter of the fiber and susceptibility to cold block (PAINTAL 1965a; FRANZ and IGGO 1968). Combining cooling with local application of lidocaine enhanced differential selectivity of the block for C-fibers and blocked the activity-induced increase of the C-elevation that was observed with lidocaine alone (STRICHARTZ and ZIMMERMANN 1983).

A variety of long lasting chemical agents have been used to block nerve conduction and have been found to produce differential effects. Phenol produces a reversible blocking effect at low concentrations (less than 0.1%) that is greater for the A-elevation than for the C (DODT et al. 1983; AMAGASA et al. 1984). At higher concentrations (0.75%–1.0%) an irreversible block of C-fibers was produced while conduction was preserved in a significant fraction of A-fibers (DODT et al. 1983). Above 2% the neurolytic effects of phenol are considered non-selective (WOOD 1978). Ammonium salts have also been claimed to block C-fibers while sparing touch or motor function (review KATZ and JOSEPH 1980). The local application of hyposmotic solutions in peripheral nerves produced block by a combination of pressure, dilution of ionic gradients, and possibly neurolytic damage (KATZ and JOSEPH 1980; SCHIMEK et al. 1984). Acute application of Capsaicin acts by still unknown mechanisms to block development of C-fibers in neonatal mice (JANCSO et al. 1977) and to cause C-axons to discharge in mature animals. The discharge depletes substance P and somatostatin. Capsaicin blocks active transport and inhibits conduction in C-afferents from hours to days (review NAGY 1982). The compound is an important model for a possible class of agents that will interfere with impulse conduction selectively. It also alters functional connectivity of peripheral fibers within the CNS (WALL 1982; WALL et al. 1982).

b) The Basis of Differential Block

The several studies cited in this section indicate that the order of conduction failure in differential block appears to be contingent on the blocking agent. This is best explained by noting that the mechanisms of differential block are multiple, reflecting the numerous ways to interfere with the process of conduction. In the preceding section, specific procedures that acted to limit sodium influx during action potentials such as TTX and lowering of extracellular sodium tended to have a differential blocking action similar to that shown by local anesthetics, which also lower sodium influx. Other procedures such as cooling, pressure or poisoning ion pumps had very different effects, and have very different actions on the nerve. In principle, a unified approach to differential block would best be achieved by considering in detail the processes involved in impulse propagation in fibers of various function. Any process that is required to support conduction may be controlled, and numerous procedures can be devised to target them. To maximize the differential aspect of conduction block, processes should be selected that differ among fibers. These run the gamut from K-channel density to recovery mechanisms (see COHEN and DEWEER 1977). We discuss this approach somewhat further in section D, where the value of understanding molecular mechanisms of conduction block is considered in light of the limitations on our capacity to predict effects of agents or conduction in different fibers. In our opinion, these limits derive from a lack of knowledge concerning the differential physiology of fibers having different functions.

10. Central Integration and Differential Block of Function

The outcome of differential block of axons in the periphery is contingent on the functional effects of the block at the level of the CNS. To some extent differential effects on function can be obtained by localized blocking within the CNS (TASKER et al. 1980; YOUNG et al. 1984). Electrical stimulation of peripheral fibers may be analgesic, differentially "blocking" central systems involved in sensing pain. This has been demonstrated for a variety of noxious stimuli and chronic pain conditions including causalgia (MEYER and FIELDS 1972) and acute pain from electrical stimulation of tooth pulp (BAKLAND 1973).

Similarly, stimulation of powerful descending pathways originating in rostroventral medulla (see FIELDS and BASBAUM 1978, 1979; FIELDS 1984 for reviews) produces profound analgesia sufficient for surgery in rats (REYNOLDS 1967). Various analgesic systems exist that can be distinguished anatomically (FIELDS et al. 1983) and pharmacologically (LEWIS et al. 1984). They are already exploited clinically in the placebo effect but the development of optimal therapeutic techniques awaits further knowledge of how to activate them and of what specific effects can be reliably produced.

Together with other clinical observations concerning the role of culture, expectation, training, and concurrent electrical or natural stimulation (WALL 1971; DAWSON 1971; CHAPMAN 1980; CASSELL 1982; PRICE 1984)) on perception of pain, work on descending systems confirms the importance of central integrative processes in governing what will be felt and how intensely it will be perceived (MELZACK and WALL 1965; WALL 1980). Thus differential block of specific functions may be approached not only by conduction block but by activation of existing systems whose role is to modulate sensory inputs and to suppress motor or autonomic activity.

With regard to the ultimate goal of selective control of autonomic functions, difficulties extend beyond the lack of a suitable technique for differential blockade for particular groups of sympathetic and parasympathetic fibers. Much is known about neural controls involved in thirst, hunger, vasomotion, and organ function in liver, pancreas (GERICK et al. 1976). and in kidney but not yet at the level of specific roles for individual fibers (JANIG 1982). The role of visceral afferents in pain and dysfunction in bone, muscle and other deep organs is not well established, especially in cancer, infectious disease or in chronic conditions following surgery or trauma. This lack of knowledge concerning functional and physiological differentiation among unmyelinated fibers will be a significant obstacle to achieving control of autonomic systems.

D. Summary and Conclusion

In the preceding discussion of selected studies of differential block drawn from the literature of the last 50 years, several important notions have emerged. Differential blockade of sensation, motor function, autonomic regulation and impulse conduction, groups of fibers and in individual fibers certainly occurs. It is usually a differential rate of block, especially in the clinical environment, and seems to be influenced by attributes of the agent that govern its differential access by diffusion to large and small fibers such as its pKa or lipid solubility (GISSEN et al. 1982b). The order of sensitivity or order of sequence of block varies according to the blocking agent and the particular experimental conditions and endpoint adopted. Some familiar notions are supported by the evidence; for example, blocks with pressure or ischemia tend to produce an inverse order of sensitivity among fibers and among sensations than do blocks with anesthetics (HALLIN and TOREBJORK 1973; MACKENZIE et al. 1975). However, the results often contradict the size principle as a solitary explanation of relative susceptibility to anesthetic (e. g., EVERETT and TOMAN 1954; SCURLOCK et al. 1975; GISSEN et al. 1982a, b; FINK and CAIRNS 1984a). Other factors found to modulate the order of failure and the degree of anesthetic block included temperature, pH, nerve activity, nerve type, duration of drug exposure, CO_2 tension, shifts in central integrative processing, etc.

At present we believe that the evidence bearing on differential block cannot be easily organized within the existing categorization to yield a consensus that is very useful as a guide to clinical practice. In vitro experiments do yield consistent results, but often these results are contingent upon attributes of highly nonclinical conditions such as a constant concentration of anesthetic in the solution bathing a desheathed nerve having no circulation of blood. Experiments designed to mimic clinical situations also yield consistents results (e. g., TOREBJORK and HALLIN 1973; FORD et al. 1984) but do so where conditions are too uncontrolled to permit much analysis of mechanism. Nonetheless we see trends in the emphasis of recent studies that together with implications of other work suggest a framework for research with the promise of providing the clinician with significantly increased capabilities and the neuroscientist with an improved understanding of how the peripheral nervous system communicates with the central nervous system.

I. The Notion of Functional Specificity

Even though our understanding of the operations underlying information handling in the CNS is too limited for full appreciation of the significance of the detailed functional specificity of peripheral fibers, the existing knowledge certainly suggests that if techniques for producing selective blockade of impulse conduction in peripheral fibers categorized by function were available, selective blockade of those same selected functions would follow upon blockade of those fibers, at least in patients without nerve injury. After nerve injury or deafferentation, functional specificity may remain in the periphery but activation of sensory systems may produce unusual results, such as triggering chronic pain with light touch (TASKER et al. 1980). Furthermore, available evidence does not exclude the possibility that differential sensory block among modalities would occur perceptually even if peripheral fibers were to fail isotropically with anesthetic regardless of diameter or functional specificity. Somesthetically, broad dimming of all inputs such that the probability of conduction block increased equally among fibers could nonetheless be *perceived* as an ordered failure of sensory (and motor) function. The quantitative rules used by CNS to interpret inputs and organize outputs are not yet proven to be constrained to follow the common assumption that differential block of function proves differential block of conduction in the peripheral network of functionally specialized fibers.

At present, work on the susceptibility to anesthetics of individual conducting fibers is just beginning. Recent in vitro studies of single rabbit vagus A- and C-fibers (FINK and CAIRNS 1984a b) and frog sciatic A-fibers (RAYMOND and ROSCOE 1984) showed considerable variation among individual fibers in susceptibility to steady-state tonic block with lidocaine. It is not known, however, whether the differences in susceptibility are related to function, since none of the population of axons studied has been characterized other than on the basis of conduction velocity, which was not at all well correlated with susceptibility.

II. A Distributed Model of Conduction Safety

The data on susceptibility of single units to lidocaine forces the conclusion that intrinsic differences in conduction safety exist among fibers. The studies also strongly suggest that such differences do not originate solely on the basis of fiber size. The parameter of conduction safety does not characterize a fiber along its entire length. Conduction safety has long been known to be reduced at branch points and in axon teledendra (DUN 1955; ITO and TAKAHASHI 1960; KRNJEVIC and MILEDI 1959; RAYMOND and LETTVIN 1978; GROSSMAN et al. 1979; SWADLOW et al. 1980; SMITH 1980). It is also contingent temporally, varying from moment to moment with impulse activity (RAYMOND 1979), local ionic gradients (MALENKA et al. 1981) and CO_2 tension (RAYMOND and ROSCOE 1983). Thus it is real-

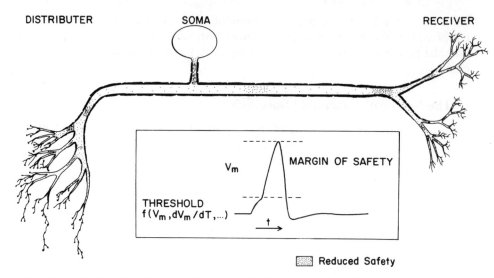

Fig. 13. A visualization of conduction safety distributed over the cellular surface. Note that threshold is represented as depending on many parameters including several in list 1. The margin of safety is pictured here with reference to the action potential though it could equally well be defined in terms of currents. The margin of safety is set by convolving the spike generating influence and the local threshold for activation of a patch of membrane. Dot density is used here to represent possible regional variations in conduction safety

istic to consider conduction safety as a distributed parameter, a variable with a domain over the entire intricate geometry of the excitable membrane. Figure 13 illustrates this point.

The utility of this image of the neuron extends beyond its correspondence with neurophysiological findings. With anesthesia, conduction will tend to fail first wherever the safety factor is reduced below unity. Other things being equal, block may therefore occur at much lower concentrations at the weak links in the chain of impulse propagation. These regions of low conduction safety exist in space, where they depend on the static geometry of the fiber and on its molecular anatomy. They also exist in time wherever prior activity or phasic properties of anesthetics have transiently lowered the safety factor.

Once conduction safety is mapped onto the entire surface of the neuron, it becomes easier to see the relevance of studies of axons in peripheral nerve to the mechanism of general anesthesia. The image is also useful because it stresses that failure of conduction depends on how anesthetics act on all the properties of the axon that influence its local capability to propagate the nerve impulse, including leakage conductance, internal resistivity, channel densities, and local metabolic systems active during recovery from impulse activity.

It is not known if a fiber having a higher conduction safety than another in the periphery maintains its relatively greater degree of conduction safety over its entire extent. However, tests of recovery of threshold for electrical stimulation following impulse trains in frog myelinated fibers show that for 10 or more nodes along a given fiber, there is great similarity in recovery processes even though fibers differ by a factor of 100 from each other. Fibers differ, but the nodes of one fiber are consistent with each other (CARLEY and RAYMOND 1983).

1. Long Lasting Differential Control

There is also a trend for research on differential block to become concerned with long lasting procedures. Differential block has figured primarily in acute blocks for surgery or for differential diagnosis in pain (AHLGREN et al. 1966; WINNIE and COLLINS 1968). However, the need to develop treatments for various chronic pain syndromes has led to procedures that produce differential block for extended times. Phenol block is differential for C-fibers and may be either persistent or reversible depending on concentration and duration of exposure (DODT et al. 1983). High temperature (55 °C) applied to a nerve selectively blocks A-fiber conduction for weeks but spares C-fibers (ZIMMERMANN 1968; ZIMMERMANN and SANDERS 1982). The capacity of capsaicin to reduce the number of C-fibers has been studied with respect to pain, and found to be associated with a long term analgesia in rats (WALL 1982; WALL et al. 1982). This work has led to a recognition that the organization of receptive fields in dorsal horn and other alar plate derivatives is dynamic, with alterations following nerve damage (WALL 1979; WALL and DEVOR 1982), C-fiber stimulation, and acute treatment of peripheral nerve with capsaicin (WALL 1984; OCHOA 1984). The basis of the phenomenon may involve shifts in conduction safety of normally blocked axon branches since the expansions of receptive fields of cord cells in the marginal layer in LII and LIII begin to occur within minutes of a skin burn – too fast to be accounted for by sprouting (WALL 1984). Reorganization also occurs in the cortex after dorsal roots are cut (FRANK 1980) and during epidural blockade (METZLER and MARKS 1979).

Differential activation of A-fibers by electrical stimulation has been effective over days or even weeks in causalgia (MEYER and FIELDS 1972; LINDBLOM and MEYERSON 1975). Differential surgical block of sympathetic outflow has long been an effective treatment for causalgia and trigeminal neuralgia (RUCH 1979). The evidence suggests the operation of as yet unclear processes. As the long term trophic and informational interactions between fibers in dorsal horn become better understood (WALL 1984), we may expect to control such processes to medical advantage.

2. Activity-Dependence of Conduction Safety and Phasic Block with Anesthetics

It is known that impulse activity causes significant changes in threshold that linger for minutes to hours (RAYMOND 1979). The relationship of this activity-dependence to function is not known, though as with anesthetic susceptibility there are significant differences in activity-dependence among fibers. The phasic block produced in the presence of anesthetics (COURTNEY et al. 1978) has been shown in large frog fibers to interact with normal dependence of excitability on previous impulse activity (RAYMOND and ROSCOE 1984). No tests of this interaction have been reported in small fibers so it is not known how differential the processes are.

At present there is no theory that successfully accounts for the dependence of excitability on impulse activity either with or without anesthetic present. The activity-dependent changes in excitability without anesthetic have not been studied using voltage clamp methods.

3. The Shape of a New Paradigm

In place of the size principle we suggest a new paradigm that does not contradict experimental or clinical findings. Fibers clearly differ in conduction safety. Likewise, regions of a given fiber may differ in conduction safety from each other. Size is but one feature of a neuron that has been found to be loosely correlated with function and with differential susceptibility to blocking agents. However, clinical utility depends more directly on understanding of differential block of function then differential block of fibers of different size.

This requires expansion of knowledge in at least two areas: 1) Increased understanding of the functional roles of individual fibers; 2) a greatly enlarged empirical base that shows the differential sensitivities and physiological properties among fibers classified by function. At present these needs would be most directly met by experimental work in which susceptibility is tested in the same fibers that are studied in detail for "function". Most investigators now classify and categorize function with short verbal descriptions. Even though these categories may not prove to be optimal, the level of detail reached by sensory and motor physiologists already highlights the gap in our knowledge regarding the relative susceptibility to block of fibers so classified. It is important to test susceptibility of fibers grouped by function and individuated by records of their firing patterns. It would be even more informative to accumulate this knowledge for several regions of each neuron.

The principle proposed to organize this new information is the image of peripheral fibers classified by coding and by the detailed microanatomy of their distribution, with a dynamic map of conduction safety as influenced by impulse activity and by blocking agents acting alone or in combination. While full attainment of this image is remote, it seems likely that clinical practice in regional anesthesia will eventually see the development of procedures for selective control of function. This seems likely to begin first with combinations of techniques such as stimulation, cooling, ischemia, and control of parameters influencing diffusion of anesthetic agents. New agents directly aimed at influencing phasic block await the further clarification of processes involved. To enhance specificity, increased advantage should be taken of the areas where fibers are themselves most highly differentiated: in their peripheral endings and receptors and in their central terminations. With an accelerated understanding of central integration of messages encoded in peripheral fibers, we may expect more selective technologies for delivering anesthetics to specific fibers selected on the basis of surface antigens or relative dependence on particular metabolic processes (DODD et al. 1984). These notions present anesthesia research in differential block with a complex challenge. At issue, it seems to us, is a fundamental expansion of nature of academic anesthesiology to become a discipline more resembling a branch of engineering in its capacity to analyze and to control sensory and motor functions.

Acknowledgements. The authors are grateful to Dr. John Butterworth, Dr. Honorio Benzon, and Dr. Thomas Rando for comments on the manuscript. The secretarial services of Ms. Rachel Abrams were superb, and we thank her for her help. We had support from USPHS GM 30160, USPHS GM 35647 and the Brigham and Women's Hospital Anesthesia Foundation.

References

Adrian ED (1921) The recovery process of excitable tissues. Part II. J Physiol (Lond) 55:193–225

Adrian ED (1932) The mechanism of nervous action. University of Pennsylvania Press, Philadelphia

Ahlgren EW, Stephen CR, Lloyd EAC, McCollum DE (1966) Diagnosis of pain with a graduated spinal block technique. JAMA 195:125–128

Amagasa S, Ando K, Sakai M, Kato Y, Ichiyanagi K (1984) Phenol exerts greater effects on larger nerve fibers. Pain (Suppl. 2):S 10

Arbuthnott R, Boyd IA, Kalu KU (1980) Ultrastructural dimensions of myelinated peripheral nerve fibers in the cat and their relation to conduction velocity. J Physiol (Lond) 308:125–157

Arrowood JG (1950) Differential spinal block with particular reference to hypertensive patients. Proc R Soc Med 43:919–928

Arrowood JG, Sarnoff SJ (1948) Differential spinal block: use in the investigation of pain following amputation. Anesthesiology 9:614–622

Bakland LK (1973) Electroanalgesia by transalveolar and transdental stimulation. Thesis, Harvard School of Dental Medicine, Boston, MA

Bennett AL, Wagner JC, McIntyre AK (1942) The determination of local anesthetic potency by observation of the nerve action potential. J Pharmacol Exp Ther 75:125–136

Berthold CH (1978) Morphology of normal peripheral axons. In: Waxman SG (ed) Physiology and pathobiology of axons. Raven, New York, pp 3–63

Bischoff A (1979) Congenital insensitivity to pain with anhidrosis: a morphometric study of sural nerve and cutaneous receptors in the human prepuce. In: Bonica JJ (ed) Advances in pain research and therapy, vol 3. Raven, New York, pp 53–65

Bishop GH, O'Leary J (1939) B and C nerve fibers. Am J Physiol 126:434

Bishop GH, Heinbecker P, O'Leary J (1933) The function of the non-myelinated fibers of the dorsal roots. Am J Physiol 106:647–669

Boyd IA, Kalu KU (1979) Scaling factor relating conduction velocity and diameter for myelinated afferent nerve fibres in cat hind limb. J Physiol (Lond) 289:277–297

Bromage PR (1978) Epidural analgesia. Saunders, Philadelphia, PA

Brown DT, Morison DH, Covino BG, Scott DB (1980) Comparison of carbonated bupivacaine and bupivacaine hydrochloride for extradural anaesthesia. Br J Anaesth 52:419–422

Burgess PR, Yu WJ, Clark FJ, Simon J (1982) Signaling of kinesthetic information by peripheral sensory receptors. Annu Rev Neurosci 5:171–187

Burke D, Mackenzie RA, Skuse NF, Lethlean AK (1975) Cutaneous afferent activity in median and radial nerve fascicles: a microelectrode study. J Neurol Neurosurg Psychiatr 38:855–864

Caldwell PC (1958) Studies on the internal pH of large muscle and nerve fibres. J Physiol (Lond) 142:22–49

Carley LR (1984) Characterizing and comparing the aftereffects of activity at successive nodes of Ranvier from frog sciatic nerve fibers. Ph D Thesis, Dept Electrical Engineering and Computer Science, MIT, Cambridge, Mass

Carley LR, Raymond SA (1983) Comparison of the aftereffects of activity between nodes of Ranvier. Soc Neurosci (Abstr) 9:1049. 24

Cassell EJ (1982) The nature of suffering and the goals of medicine. N Engl J Med 306:639–645

Catchlove RFH (1972) The influence of CO_2 and pH on local anesthetic action. J Pharmacol Exp Ther 181:298–309

Catchlove RFH (1973) Potentiation of two different local anaesthetics by carbon dioxide. Br J Anaesth. 45:471–475

Chapman CR (1980) Pain and perception: comparison of sensory decision theory and evoked potential methods. Res Pub Assoc Res Nern Ment Dis 58:111–142

Chiu SY, Ritchie JM (1984) On the physiological role of internodal potassium channels and the security of conduction in myelinated nerve fibers. Proc R Soc Lond (Biol) 220:415–422

Chiu SY, Richie JM, Rogart RB, Stagg D (1979) A quantitative description of membrane currents in rabbit myelinated nerve. J Physiol (Lond) 292:149–166

Clark D, Hughes J, Gasser HS (1935) Afferent function in the group of nerve fibers of slowest conduction velocity. Am J Physiol 114:69–76

Clifton GL, Coggleshell RE, Vance WH, Willis WD (1976) Receptive fields of unmyelinated ventral root afferent fibres in the cat. J Physiol (Lond) 256:573–600

Coggleshell RE, Applebaum ML, Fazen ML, Stubbs TB, Sykes MT (1975) Unmyelinated axons in human ventral roots: a possible explanation for the failure of dorsal rhizotomy to relieve pain. Brain 98:157–166

Cohen LB, DeWeer P (1977) Structural and metabolic processes directly related to action potential propagation. Handbook of Physiology Chap 5, American Physiological Society, Washington, pp 137–159

Cole F (1952) Tourniquet pain. Anaesth. Analg 31:63–64

Colquhoun DJ, Ritchie JM (1972) The interaction at equilibrium between TTX and mammalian non-myelinated nerve fibers. J Physiol (Lond) 221:533–553

Collins WF Jr, Nulsen FE, Randt CT (1960) Relation of peripheral nerve fiber size and sensation in man. Arch Neurol 3:381–385

Condouris GA (1961) A study on the mechanism of action of cocaine on amphibian peripheral nerve. J Pharmacol Exp Ther 131:243–249

Condouris GA, Goebel RH, Brady T (1976) Computer simulation of local anesthetic effects using a mathematical model of myelinated nerve. J Pharmacol Exp Ther 196:737–745

Connelly CM (1959) Recovery processes and metabolism of nerve. Rev Mod Phys 31:474–484

Coraboeuf E, Niedergerke R (1953) Kohlensäure- und pH-Wirkung an der markhaltigen Einzelfaser des Froschs. Pflügers Archiv 258:103–107

Courtney KR (1975) Mechanism of frequency-dependent inhibition of sodium currents in frog myelinated nerve by the lidocaine derivative GEA968. J Pharmacol Exp Ther 195:225–236

Courtney KR, Kendig JJ, Cohen EN (1978) Frequency-dependent conduction block: the role of nerve impulse pattern in local anesthetic potency. Anesthesiology 48:111–117

Crescitelli F (1948) Carbamate conduction block in frog nerve fibers. Am J Physiol 155:82–91

Crescitelli F (1950) A temperature differentiation on the dual action of amyl carbamate on frog nerve. J Cell Comp Physiol 35:261–272

Crescitelli F (1952a) Some features in responses of different nerve fiber types to a deficiency of sodium. Am J Physiol 169:1–10

Crescitelli F (1952b) Modification in responses to sodium of nerve fibers treated with drugs. Am J Physiol 169:638–648

Darian-Smith I, Johnson OK, Dykes R (1973) "Cold" fiber population innervating palmar and digital skin of monkey: responses to cooling pulses. J Neurophysiol 36:325–346

Dawson GD (1971) Brain mechanisms. In: Remond A (ed) Handbook of EEG and clinical neurophysiology Vol 9, Elsevier, Amsterdam, pp 44–56

Denny-Brown D, Brenner C (1944) Lesion in peripheral nerve resulting from compression by spring clip. Arch Neurol Psychiatr 52:1–19

Dhopesh VP, Burns RA (1976) Loss of nerve conduction in heat stroke. NEng J Med 294:557–558

Didisheim JC, Posternak JM (1959) Anesthésie différentiale du nerf sciatique de la grenouille. Helv Physiol Acta 17:242–253

Dixon WE (1905) The selective action of cocaine on nerve fibres. J Physiol (Lond) 32:87–94

Dodd J, Jahr CE, Jessel TM (1984) Neurotransmitters and neuronal markers at sensory synapses in dorsal horn. In Kruger L, Liebeskind JC (eds) Advances in pain research and therapy, vol 6. Raven, New York, pp 105–121

Dodt HU, Strichartz GR, Zimmermann M (1983) Phenol solutions differentially block conduction in cutaneous nerve fibers of the cat. Neurosci Lett 42:323–327

Douglas WW, Malcolm JL (1955) The effect of localized cooling on conduction in cat nerves. J Physiol (Lond) 130:53–71

Douglas WW, Ritchie JM (1957) Non-medullated fibers in the saphenous nerve which signal touch. J Physiol (Lond) 139:385–399

Douglas WW, Ritchie JM (1962) Mammalian non-myelinated nerve fibers. Physiol Rev 42:297–334

Douglas WW, Ritchie JM, Straub RW (1960) The role of non-myelinated fibers in signalling cooling of the skin. J Physiol (Lond) 150:266–283

Dun FT (1955) The delay and blockage of sensory impulses in the dorsal root ganglion. J Physiol (Lond) 127:252–264

Dyck PJ, Lambert EH, Nichols PC (1972) Quantitative measurements of sensation related to compound action potential and number and sizes of myelinated and unmyelinated fibers of sural nerve in health, Friedrich's ataxia, hereditary sensory neuropathy and tabes dorsalis. In: Cobb WA (ed). Handbook of EEG and clinical neurophysiology, Vol 9, Somatic sensation. Elsevier, Amsterdam pp 83–118

Erlanger J, Blair EA (1940) Facilitation and difficilitation effected by nerve impulses in peripheral fibers. J Neurophysiol 3:107–127

Erlanger J, Gasser HS (1937) Electrical signs of nervous activity. University of Pennsylvania Press, Philadelphia, pp 1–221

Erlanger J, Blair EA, Schoepfle GM (1941) A study of the spontaneous oscillations in the excitability of nerve fibers, with special reference to the action of strychnine. Am J Physiol 134:705–718

Everett GM, Goodsell JS (1952) The greater resistance to procaine of slow fiber groups in some peripheral nerves. J Pharmacol Exp Ther 106:385

Everett GM, Toman JEP (1954) Procaine block of fiber groups in various nerves. Fed Proc 13:352–353

Fields HL (1984) Brainstem mechanisms of pain modulation. In: Kruger L, Liebeskind JC (eds) Advances in pain research and therapy, vol 6. Raven, New York, pp 242–252

Fields HL, Basbaum AI (1978) Brainstem control of spinal pain-transmission neurons. Annu Rev Physiol 40:217–248

Fields HL, Basbaum AI (1979) Anatomy and physiology of a descending pain control system. In: Bonica JJ (ed) Advances in pain. Research and therapy, vol 3, pp 427–440

Fields HL, Vanegas H, Hentall ID, Zorman G (1983) Evidence that disinhibition of brain stem neurons contributes to morphine analgesia. Nature 306:684–686

Fink BR, Cairns AM (1982) A bioenergetic basis for peripheral nerve fiber dissociation. Pain 12:307–317

Fink BR, Cairns AM (1983a) Test of differential block by lidocaine in individual nerve fibers. Reg Anesth 8:36–37

Fink BR, Cairns AM (1983b) Differential peripheral axon block with lidocaine: unit studies in the cervical vagus nerve. Anesthesiology 59:182–186

Fink BR, Cairns AM (1983c) A new approach to differential peripheral nerve fiber block. Na$^+$, K$^+$-ATPase inhibition. Anesthesiology 59:127–131

Fink BR, Cairns AM (1984a) Differential slowing and block of conduction by lidocaine in individual afferent myelinated and unmyelinated axons. Anesthesiology 60:111–120; 515

Fink BR, Cairns AM (1984b) Differential block times of individual axons. Reg Anesth 9:36

Fitzgerald M (1983) Capsaicin: action on peripheral nerves. A review. Pain 15:109–130

Ford DJ, Raj PP, Pritam S, Regan KR, Ohlweiler D (1984) Differential peripheral nerve block by local anesthetics in the cat. Anesthesiology 60:28–33

Frank JI (1980) Functional reorganization of cat somatic sensory motor cortex Sml after selective dorsal root rhizotomies. Brain Res 186:458–462

Franz DN, Iggo A (1968) Conduction failure in myelinated and non-myelinated axons at low temperatures. J Physiol (Lond) 199:319–345

Franz DN, Perry RS (1974) mechanisms for differential block among single myelinated and non-myelinated axons by procaine. J Physiol (Lond) 236:193–210

Fruhstorfer H, Lindblom U (1983) Vascular participation in deep cold pain. Pain 17:235–241

Fukushima K, Yohara O, Kato M (1975) Differential blocking of motor fibers by direct current. Pflugers Arch 358:235–242

Ganong WF (1981) Review of medical physiology. Lange, Los Altos, pp 31–45

Gasser HS (1935a) Changes in nerve-potentials produced by rapidly repeated stimuli and their relation to the responsiveness of nerve to stimulation. Am J Physiol 35–50

Gasser HS (1935b) Conduction in nerves in relation to fiber types. Res Publ Assoc Res Nerve Ment Dis 23:44–62; 15:35–59

Gasser HS (1943) Pain-producing impulses in peripheral nerves. Res Publ Assoc Res Nerv Ment Dis 23:44–62

Gasser HS (1950) Unmedullated fibers originating in dorsal root ganglia. J Gen Physiol 33:651–690

Gasser HS, Erlanger J (1927) The role played by the sizes of the constituent fibers of a nerve trunk in determining the form of its action potential wave. Am J Physiol 80:522–547

Gasser HS, Erlanger J (1929) Role of fiber size in establishment of nerve block by pressure or cocaine. Am J Physiol 88:581–591

Gasser HS, Grundfest H (1939) Axon diameters in relation to the spike dimensions and the conduction velocity in mammalian A-fibers. Am J Physiol 127:393–414

Gasser HS, Richards CH, Grundfest H (1938) Properties of the nerve fibers of slowest conduction in the frog. Am J Physiol 123:299–306

Georgopoulos AP (1977) Stimulus-response relations in high-threshold mechanothermal fibers innervating primate glabrous skin. Brain Res 128:547–552

Georgopoulos AP, Mountcastle VB (1976) Functional properties of primary afferent units probably related to pain mechanisms in primate glabrous skin. J Neurophysiol 39:71–83

Gerick JE, Charles MA, Grodsky GM (1976) Regulation of pancreatic insulin and glucagon secretion. Annu Rev Physiol 38:353

Ghia JN, Toomey TC, Mao W, Duncan G, Gregg JM (1979) Towards an understanding of chronic pain mechanisms: the use of psychologic tests and a refined differential spinal block. Anesthesiology 50:20–25

Gilliatt RW (1980) Acute compression block. In: Sumner AJ (ed). The physiology of peripheral nerve disease, Chap 9. Saunders, Philadelphia, pp 287–315

Gissen AJ, Covino BG, Gregus J (1980) Differential sensitivities of mammalian nerve fibers to local anesthetic agents. Anesthesiology 53:467–474

Gissen AJ, Covino BG, Gregus J (1982a) Differential sensitivity of fast and slow fibers in mammalian nerve: II. Margin of safety for nerve transmission. Anesth Analg 61:561–569

Gissen AJ, Covino BG, Gregus J (1982b) Differential sensitivity of fast and slow fibers in mammalian nerve: III. Effect of etidocaine and bupivacaine on fast/slow fibers. Anesth Analg 61:570–575

Greene NM (1958) Area of differential block in spinal anesthesia with hyperbaric tetracaine. Anesthesiology 19:45–50

Grossman Y, Parnas I, Spira ME (1979) Differential conduction block in branches of a bifurcating axon. J Physiol (Lond) 295:282–305

Grundfest H (1939) Properties of mammalian B-fibers. Am J Physiol 127:252–262

Hallin RG, Torebjork HE (1973) Electrically induced A and C-fibre responses in intact human skin nerves. Exp Brain Res 16:309–320

Hallin RG, Torebjork HE (1976) Studies on cutaneous A and C-fibre afferents. Skin nerve blocks and perception. In: Zotterman Y (ed) Sensory functions of the skin in primates. Pergamon, Oxford, pp 137–149

Heavner J, de Jong RH (1974) Lidocaine blocking concentrations for B- and C-fibers. Anesthesiology 40:228–233

Heinbecker P, Bartley SH (1940) Action of ether and nembutal on the nervous system. J Neurophysiol 3:219–236

Heinbecker P, Bishop GH (1935) The mechanism of painful sensations. Res Publ Assoc Res Nerve Ment Dis 15:226–238

Heinbecker P, O'Leary J (1933) The mammalian vagus nerve – a functional and histological study. Am J Physiol 106:623–646

Heinbecker P, Bishop GH, O'Leary J (1933) Pain and touch fibers in peripheral nerves. Arch Neurol Psychiatr 29:771–789

Heinbecker P, Bishop GH, O'Leary J (1934) Analysis of sensation terms of nerve impulses. Arch Neurol Psychiatr 31:34–53

Hille B (1968) Pharmacological modifications of the sodium channels of frog nerve. J Gen Physiol 51:199–219

Hille B (1977) The pH-dependent rate of action of local anesthetics on the node of Ranvier. J Gen Physiol 69:475–496

Henneman E (1980) Organization of the spinal cord and its reflexes. In: Mountcastle VB (ed) Medical physiology. Mosby, St. Louis, pp 762–786

Hunt CC, McIntyre AK (1960a) Properties of cutaneous touch receptors in cat. J Physiol (Lond) 153:88–98

Hunt CC, McIntyre AK (1960b) An analysis of fibre diameter and receptor characteristics of myelinated cutaneous afferent fibres in cat. J Physiol (Lond) 153:99–112

Ichioka M, Uehara Y, Seikichi K (1960) On the local response of a single node of Raniver under various conditions. Jpn J Physiol 10:235–245

Iggo A (1960) Cutaneous mechanoreceptors with afferent C-fibres. J Physiol (Lond) 152:337–353

Iggo A, Andres KH (1982) Morphology of cutaneous receptors. Annu Rev Neurosci 5:1–33

Ignelzi RJ, Nyquist JK (1979a) Observations on fast axoplasmic transport in peripheral nerve following repetitive electrical stimulation. Pain 7:313–320

Ignelzi RJ, Nyquist JK (1979b) Excitability changes in peripheral nerve fibers after repetitive electrical stimulation. J Neurosurg 51:824–833

Ignelzi RJ, Nyquist JK, Tighe WJ (1981) Repetitive electrical stimulation of peripheral nerve and spinal cord activity. Neurol Res 3:195–208

Ito M, Takahashi I (1960) Impulse conduction through spinal ganglion. In: Katsuki Y (ed) Electrical activity of single cells. Ikagu Shoin, Tokyo, pp 159–179

Jack JJB (1975) Physiology of peripheral nerve fibers in relation to their size. Br J Anaesth 47:173–182

Jancso G, Kiraly E, Jancso-Gabor A (1977) Pharmacologically induced selective degeneration of chemosensitive primary sensitive neurons. Nature 270:741–743

Jänig W (1982) The autonomic nervous system. In: Human physiology. Schmidt RF, Thews G (eds) Springer, Berlin, pp 111–149

Jong, de RH (1980a) Clinical physiology of local anesthetic action. In: Neural blockade in clinical anesthesia and management of pain, Chap 2. Cousins MS, Bridenbaugh PO (eds). JP Lippincott Co., Philadelphia, pp 21–44

Jong, de RH (1980b) Editorial views: differential nerve block by local anesthetics. Anesthesiology 53:443

Jong, de RH, Cullen SC (1963) Theoretical aspects of pain: bizarre pain phenomena during low spinal anesthesia. Anesthesiology 24:628–635

Katz J, Joseph (JW (1980) Neuropathology of neurolytic and semidestructive agents. In: Cousins MJ, Bridenbaugh PO (eds) Neural Blockade. Lippincott, Philadelphia, pp 122–132

Krnjević K, Miledi R (1959) Presynaptic failure of neuromuscular propagation in rats. J Physiol (Lond) 149:1–22

LaMotte RH (1984) Cutaneous nociceptors and pain sensation in normal and hyperalgesic skin. Adv Pain Res Ther 6:69–82

Landon DN (1982) The structure of the nerve fiber. In Culp WJ, Ochoa J (eds) Abnormal nerves and muscles as impulse generators. Oxford University Press, New York, p 27–53

Landon DN, Langley OK (1971) The local chemical environment of nodes of Ranvier: a study of cation binding. J Anat 108:419–432

Larrabee MG, Posternak JM (1952) Selective action of anesthetics on synapses and axons in mammalian sympathetic ganglia. J Neurophysiol 15:91–114

Leatherdale RAL (1956) Phantom limb pain associated with spinal analgesia. Anaesthesia 11:249–251

Lehmann JF (1937) The effect of changes in pH on the action of mammalian. A nerve fibers. Am J Physiol 118:600–612

Leksell L (1945) The action potential and excitatory effects of small ventral root fibers to skeletal muscle. Acta Physiol Scand (Suppl) 31:1–84

Leone J, Ochs S (1978) Anoxic block and recovery of axoplasmic transport and electrical excitability of nerve. J Neurobiol 9:229–245

Levine JW, Terman GW, Shavit Y, Nelson LR, Liebeskind JF (1984) Neural, neurochemical, and hormonal bases of stress-induced analgesia. In: Kruger L, Liebeskind JC (eds) Advances in pain research and therapy, vol 6. Raven, New York, pp 277–288

Lewis T (1942) Pain. MacMillan, London, pp 1–192

Lewis T, Pickering GW, Rothchild P (1931) Centripetal paralysis arising out of arrested bloodflow to the limbs including notes on a form of tingling. Heart 16:1–32

Lindblom U, Meyerson BA (1975) Influence on touch, vibration and pain of dorsal column stimulation in man. Pain 1:251–270

Lorente de Nó R (1947a) Carbon dioxide and nerve function. In: Studies from the Rockefeller Institute for Medical Research, New York, vol 131, p 148–194

Lorente de Nó R (1947b) Effects of sugars and other substances upon nerve. A study of nerve physiology. Studies from the Rockefeller Institute for Medical Research, New York, vol 131, pp 195–243

Lorente de Nó R, Condouris GA (1959) Decremental conduction in peripheral nerve: integration of stimuli in the neuron. PNAS 45:592–617

Lundborg G (1980) Intraneural microcirculation and peripheral nerve barriers. Techniques for evaluation – clinical implications. In: Omer GE, Spinner M (eds) Managment of peripheral nerve problems. Saunders, Philadelphia, pp 903–916

Lundborg G, Myers R, Powell H (1983) Nerve compression injury and increased endoneurial fluid pressure. A "miniature compartment syndrome". J Neurol Neurosurg Psychiatr 46:1119–1124

Mackenzie RA, Burke D, Skuse NF, Lethlean AK (1975) Fibre function and perception during cutaneous nerve block. J Neurol Neurosurg Psychiatr 38:865–873

Mackenzie RA, Skuse NF, Lethlean AK (1977) A micro-electrode study of peripheral neuropathy in man: 2. Response to conditioning stimuli. J Neurol Sci 34:175–189

Malenka RC, Kocsis JD, Ransom BR, Waxman SG (1981) Modulation of parallel fiber excitability by postsynaptically mediated changes in extracellular potassium. Science 214:339–341

Manfredi M (1970) Differential block of conduction of larger fibers in peripheral nerve by direct current. Arch Ital Biol 108:52–71

Martin JH (1982) Somatic sensory system I: receptor physiology and submodality coding. In: Kandel ER, Schwartz JF (eds) Principles of neural science. Elsevier, New York, pp 157–169

Matthews PBC (1982) Where does Sherrington's "muscular sense" originate? Muscles, joints, corollary discharges? Annu Rev Neurosci 5:189–218

Matthews PBC, Rushworth G (1957a) The selective effect of procaine on the stretch reflex and tendon jerk of soleus muscle when applied to its nerve. J Physiol (Lond) 185:245–262

Matthews PBC, Rushworth G (1957b) The relative sensitivity of muscle nerve fibres to procaine. J Physiol (Lond) 135:263–269

Mayer DJ, Price DD, Becker DP (1975) Neurophysiological characteristics of the anterolateral spinal cord neurons contributing to pain perception in man. Pain 1:51–58

Melzack R, Wall PD (1965) Pain mechanism: a new theory. Science 150:971–979

Mendell LM, Henneman E (1979) Input to motoneuron pools and its effects. Chapt 27. In: Mountcastle VB (ed) Medical physiology, vol 1. Mosby, St. Louis, pp 742–761

Mendell LM, Wall PD (1965) Responses of single dorsal cord cells to peripheral cutaneous unmyelinated fibers. Nature 206:97–99

Metzler J, Marks PS (1979) Functional changes in cat somatic sensory-motor cortex during short-term reversible epidural blocks. Brain Res 177:379–383

Meyer GA, Fields HL (1972) Causalgia treated by selective large fibre stimulation of peripheral nerve. Brain 95:163

Miller K (1975) The pressure reversal of anesthesia and the critical volume hypothesis. In: Fink BR (ed) Molecular mechanisms of anesthesia, vol 1. Raven, New York, pp 341–351

Morison DH (1981) A double-blind compression of carbonated lidocaine and lidocaine hydrochloride in epidural anaesthesia. Can Anaesth Soc J 28:387–389

Mountcastle VB (1980a) Sensory receptors and neural encoding: Introduction to sensory processes. In: Mountcastle VB (ed) Medical physiology, vol 1. Mosby, St. Louis, pp 327–347

Mountcastle VB (1980b) Pain and temperature sensibilities. In: Mountcastle VB (ed) Medical physiology, vol 1. Mosby, St. Louis, pp 391–427

Müller J (1826) Zur vergleichenden Physiologie des Gesichtssinnes des Menschen und der Thiere nebst einem Versuch über die Bewegungen der Augen und über den menschlichen Blick. Cnoblock, Leipzig

Nagy JI (1982) Capsaicin's action on the nervous system. Trends in Neuroscience 5:362–365

Nathan PW, Sears TA (1961) Some factors concerned in differential nerve block by local anaesthetics. J Physiol (Lond) 157:565–580

Nathan PW, Sears TA (1962) Differential nerve block by sodium-free and sodium-deficient solutions. J Physiol (Lond) 164:375–394

Nicholson C, Phillips JM (1981) Ion diffusion modified by tortuosity and volume fraction in the extracellular microenvironment of the rat cerebellum. J Physiol (Lond) 321:225–257

Nicholson C, Phillips JM (1982) Diffusion in the brain cell microenvironment. Lectures on Mathematics in the Life Sciences 15:103–122

Ochoa J (1984) Peripheral unmyelinated units in man: structure, function, disorder and role in sensation. Kruger L, Liebeskind JC (eds). Advances in Pain Research Therapy, vol 6. Raven, New York, pp 53–68

Ochoa J, Torebjörk HE (1983) Sensations evoked by intraneural microstimulation of single mechanoreceptor units innervating the human hand. J Physiol (Lond) 342:633–654

Ochoa J, Torebjörk HE, Culp WJ, Schady W (1982) Abnormal spontaneous activity in single sensory nerve fibers in humans. Muscle nerve 5:574–577

Paintal AS (1965a) Block of conduction in mammalian myelinated fibers by low temperatures. J Physiol (Lond) 180:1–19

Paintal AS (1965b) Effects of temperature on conduction in single vagal and saphenous myelinated nerve fibres of the cat. J Physiol (Lond) 180:20–49

Perl ER (1980) Afferent basis of nociception and pain: evidence from the characteristics of sensory receptors and their projections to the spinal dorsal horn. Res Publ Assoc Nerv Ment Dis 58:19–45

Perl ER (1984) Characterization of nociceptors and their activation of neurons in the superficial dorsal horn: first steps for the sensation of pain. In: Kruger L, Liebeskind JC (eds) Advances in pain research and therapy, vol 6. Raven, New York, pp 23–51

Price DD (1984) Roles of psychophysics, neuroscience and experimental analysis in the study of pain. In: Kruger L, Liebeskind JC (eds), Advances in pain research and therapy, vol 6. Raven, New York, pp 341–355

Rang HP, Ritchie JM (1968) On the electrogenic sodium pump in mammalian non-myelinated nerve fibers and its activation by various external cations. J Physiol (Lond) 196:183–221

Ranson SW (1931) Cutaneous sensory fibers and sensory conduction. Arch Neurol Psychiatr 26:1122–1144

Ranson SW, Droegenmueller WH, Davenport HK, Fisher C (1935) Number, size and myelination of the sensory fibers in the cerebrospinal nerves. Res Publ Assoc Nerv Ment Dis 15:3–34

Raymond SA (1979) Effects of nerve impulses on threshold of frog sciatic nerve fibres. J Physiol (Lond) 290:273–303

Raymond SA, Bokesch PM (1983) Effects of CO_2/bicarbonate vs an organic buffer on nerve threshold and local anesthetic block at varying pH. Anesthesiology 59:A 295

Raymond SA, Lief PA (1984) Psychological assessment of adaptation to transcutaneous electrical nerve stimulation. Pain, Suppl 2:569

Raymond SA, Lettvin JY (1978) Aftereffects of activity in peripheral axons as a clue to nervous coding. In: Waxman SG (ed) Physiology and pathobiology of axons. Raven, New York, pp 203–225

Raymond SA, Roscoe RF (1984) Effects of lidocaine on threshold of nerve axons. Reg Anesth 9:51

Raymond SA, Roscoe RF (1983) Aftereffects of nerve impulses on threshold of frog sciatic fibers depends on pH (pCO_2). Soc Neurosci Abstracts 9:513

Reynolds DV (1969) Surgery in the rat during electrical analgesia induced by focal brain stimulation. Science 164:444–445

Ritchie JM (1982) Sodium channel density in excitable membranes. In: Culp WJ, Ochoa J (eds) Abnormal nerves and muscles as impulse generators. Oxford University Press, New York, pp 168–190

Ritchie JM, Ritchie B, Greengard P (1965) The effect of the nerve sheath on the action of local anesthetics. J Pharmacol Exp Ther 150:160–164

Rosenberg PH, Heavner JE (1980) Temperature-dependent nerve blocking action of lidocaine and halothane. Acta Anesth Scand 24:314–320

Ruch TC (1979) Pathophysiology of Pain. In: Ruch TC, Patton HD (eds) Physiology and biophysics. Saunders, Philadelphia, pp 272–324

Rud J (1961) Local anesthetics: an electrophysiological investigation of local anesthesia of peripheral nerves with special reference to xylocaine. Acta Physiol Scand 51 (Suppl) 178:1–171

Rydevik B (1979) Compression injury of peripheral nerve. PhD thesis, Department of Anatomy, University of Gothenburg

Sarnoff SJ, Arrowood JG (1946) Differential spinal block – a preliminary report. Surgery 20:150–159

Sarnoff SJ, Arrowood JG (1947 a) Differential spinal block: II. The reaction of sudomotor and vasomotor fibers. J Clin Invest 26:203–216

Sarnoff SJ, Arrowood JG (1947 b) Differential spinal block: III. The block of cutaneous and stretch reflexes in the presence of unimpaired position sense. J Neurophysiol 10:205:210

Sarnoff SJ, Arrowood JG, Chapman WP (1948) Differential spinal block. IV. The investigation of intestinal dyskinesia, colonic artery and visceral afferent fibers. Surg Gynecol Obstet 86:571

Schimek F, Sumi SM, Fink BR (1984) Differential effects of hyposomatic hyponatric swelling on A- and C-fibers. Anesthesiology 60:198–204

Schwartz HG (1950) Neurosurgical relief of intractable pain. Surg Clin North Am 30:1379–1389

Schwarz W, Palade PT, Mille B (1977) Local anesthetics: effect of pH on use-dependent block of sodium channels in frog muscle. Biophys J 20:343–368

Scurlock JE, Heavner JE, de Jong RG (1975) Differential B- and C-fibre block by an amide- and an ester-linked local anesthetic. Br J Anaesth 47:1135–1139

Sessle BJ (1979) Is the tooth pulp a "pure" source of noxious input? In: Bonica JJ (ed) Advances in pain research and therapy, vol 3. Raven, New York, pp 245–260

Sinclair DC (1955) Cutaneous sensation and the doctrine of specific energy. Brain 78:584–614

Sinclair DC, Hinshaw JR (1950a) Sensory changes in procaine nerve block. Brain 73:224–243

Sinclair DC, Hinshaw JR (1950 b) A comparison of the sensory dissociation produced by procaine and by limb compression. Brain 73:480–498

Sinclair DC, Hinshaw JR (1951) Sensory changes in nerve blocks induced by cooling. Brain 74:318–355

Smith DO (1980) Mechanisms of action potential propagation failure at sites of axonal branching in the crayfish. J Physiol (Lond) 301:243–259

Staiman A, Seeman P (1974) Impulse-blocking concentration of anesthetics, alcohols, anticonvulsants, barbiturates, and narcotics on phrenic and sciatic nerves. Can J Physiol Pharmacol 52:535–550

Staiman A, Seeman P (1977) Conduction-blocking concentration of anesthetics increase with nerve axon diameter: studies with alcohol, lidocaine and tetrodotoxin on single myelinated fibers. J Pharmacol Exp Therap 201:340–349

Stansfeld CE, Wallis DI (1983) Differences in tetrodotoxin (TTX) sensitivity in group A- and C-cells of the rabbit nodose ganglion. J Physiol 341:14P–15P

Strichartz GR (1973) The inhibition of sodium currents in myelinated nerve by quaternary derivatives of lidocaine. J gen Physiol 62:37–57

Strichartz GR, Wang GK (1986) The kinetic basis for phasic local anesthetic blockade of neuronal sodium channels. In: Roths, Miller K (eds) Molecular and cellular mechanics of anesthetics. Plenum, New York, pp 217–226

Strichartz GR, Zimmermann (1983) Selective conduction blockade among different fiber types in mammalian nerves by lidocaine combined with low temperature. Soc Neurosci (Abstr) 9:675

Swadlow HA, Kocsis JD, Waxman SG (1980) Modulation of impulse conduction along the axon tree. Annu Rev Biophys Bioeng 9:143–179

Tanner JA (1962) Reversible blocking of nerve conduction by alternating current excitation. Nature 195:712–713

Tasaki I (1953) Nervous transmission. Thomas, Springfield, Ill, pp 164

Tasaki I (1982) Physiology and electrochemistry of nerve fibers. Academic, New York, pp 1–348

Tasker RR, Organ LW, Hawrylyshyn P (1980) Deafferentation and Causalgia. Res Publ Assoc Res Nerv Ment Dis 58:305–334

Toman JEP (1952) Neuropharmacology of peripheral nerve. Pharmacol Rev 4:168–218

Torebjörk HE, Hallin RG (1973) Perceptual changes accompanying controlled preferential blocking of A- and C-fibre responses in intact human skin nerves. Exp Brain Res 16:321–332

Torebjörk HE, Hallin RG (1974) Responses in human A- and C-fibres to repeated electrical intradermal stimulation. J Neurol Neurosurg Psychiatr 37:653–664

Torebjörk HE, Hallin RG (1979) Microneurographic studies of peripheral pain mechanisms in man. In: Bonica JJ et al. (ed) Advances in pain research and therapy. Raven, New York, pp 121–131

Torebjörk HE, Ochoa JL (1980) Specific sensations evoked by activity in single identified sensory units in man. Acta Physiol Scand 110:445–447

Torebjörk HE, Ochoa JL, Schady W (1984a) Referred pain from intraneural stimulation of muscle fascicles in median nerve. Pain 18:145–156

Torebjörk HE, LaMotte R, Robinson CT (1984b) Peripheral neural correlates of magnitude of cutaneous pain and hyperalgesia: simultaneous recordings in humans of sensory judgements of pain and evoked responses in nociceptors with C-fibers. J Neurophysiol 51:341–355

Tucker GT, Mather LE (1980) Absorption and disposition of local anesthetics: pharmacokinetics. In: Cousins MJ, Bridenbaugh PO (eds) Neural blockade. Lippincott, Philadelphia, pp 45–85

Uehara Y (1958) Conduction of nervous impulses in NaCl deficient media. Jpn J Physiol 8:282–291

Uehara Y (1960) Narcotic and NaCl deficiency as blocking agents. Jpn J Physiol 10:267–274

Ulbricht W (1981) Kinetics of drug action and equilibrium results at the node of Ranvier. Physiol Rev 61:785–828

Urban BJ, McKain CW (1982) Onset and progression of intravenous regional anesthesia with dilute lidocaine. Anesth Analg 61:834–838
Vallbo AB, Hagbarth KE, Torebjörk HE, Hallin BG (1979) Somatosensory, proprioceptive, and sympathetic activity in human peripheral nerves. Physiol Rev 59:919–957
Wall PD (1971) Somatosensory mechanisms. In: Remond A (ed) Handbook EEG and clinical neurophysiology, vol 9. Somatic sensation. Elsevier, Amsterdam pp 1–6
Wall PD (1979) Changes in damaged nerve and their sensory consequences. In: Bonica JJ (ed) Advances in pain research and therapy, vol 3 Raven, New York, pp 39–52
Wall PD (1980) The role of substantia gelatinosa as a gate control. Res Publ Assoc Res Nerv Ment Disease 58:205–231
Wall PD (1982) The effect of peripheral nerve lesions and of neonatal capsaicin in the rat on primary afferent depolarization. J Physiol (Lond) 329:21–35
Wall PD (1984) Mechanisms of acute chronic pain. In: Kruger L, Liebeskind JC (eds) Advances in pain research and therapy, vol 6. Neural mechanisms of pain. Raven, New York, pp 95–104
Wall PD, Devor M (1982) Consequences of peripheral nerve damage in the spinal cord and in neighboring intact peripheral nerves. In: Culp WJ, Ochoa J (eds) Abnormal nerves and muscles as impulse generators. Oxford University Press, New York, pp 588–603
Wall PD, Fitzgerald M, Nussbaumer JC, Loos H van der, Devor M (1982) Somatotopic maps are disorganized in adult rodents treated with capsaicin as neonates. Nature 295:691–693
Watson PJ (1967) Interaction between acetylcholine and guanethidine on sensory C-fibers. Eur J Pharmacol 1:407–413
Waxman SG (1981) Cellular aspects of conduction in myelinated nerve fibers in relation to clinical deficit. In: Dorfman LJ, Cummins KL, Leifer LJ (eds) Conduction velocity distributions: a population approach to electrophysiology of nerve. AR Liss, New York, pp 1–15
Wildsmith JAW, Gissen AJ, Gregus J, Covino BG (1985) The differential nerve blocking activity of amino-ester local anaesthetics. Br J Anaesth 57:612–620
Willis WD (1980) Neurophysiology of nociception and pain in the spinal cord. Res Pub Assoc Res Nerve Ment Dis 58:77–92
Winnie AP, Collins VJ (1968) The Pain Clinic. I. Differential neural blockade in pain syndromes of questionable etiology. Med Clin North Am 52:123–129
Wood KM (1978) The use of phenol as a neurolytic agent: a review. Pain 5:205–229
Young RF, Feldman RA, Kroening R, Fulton W, Morris J (1984) Electrical stimulation of the brain in the treatment of chronic pain in man. In: Kruger L, Liebeskind JC (eds) Advances in pain research and therapy, vol 6. Raven, New York, pp 289–303
Zimmermann M (1968) Selective activation of C-fibers. Pfluegers Arch 301:329–333
Zimmermann M (1979) Peripheral and central nervous mechanisms of nociception, pain, and pain therapy: facts and hypotheses. In: Bonica JJ (ed), Advances in pain research and therapy, vol 3, Raven, New York, pp 3–32
Zimmermann M, Sanders K (1982) Responses of nerve axons and receptor endings to heat, ischemia, and algesic substances. Abnormal excitability of regenerating nerve endings. In: Culp WJ, Ochoa J (eds) Abnormal nerves and muscles as impulse generators. Oxford University Press, New York, pp 513–532
Zotterman Y (1939) Touch pain and tickling: an electrophysiological investigation on cutaneous sensory nerves. J Physiol (Lond) 95:1–28

CHAPTER 5

Pharmacokinetics of Local Anesthetics

G. R. ARTHUR

A. Introdcuction

Utilizing the pharmacokinetics of local anesthetic agents has different emphasis than for most other drugs, as these agents are applied directly to the site of their action rather than being transported in the blood stream to this site. Toxic reactions to local anesthetics are usually associated with the accidental intravenous injection of drug. but toxic effects can occur in normal usage. A knowledge of how the body handles these agents will help in understanding why these reactions can occur and also their different pharmacological behaviour.

B. Factors Affecting the Interpretation of Local Anesthetic Blood Concentrations

I. Units of Expression

It is necessary to state exactly in what terms both the dose of drug and its concentrations in blood are expressed. Lidocaine hydrochloride BP is prepared as the hydrated salt so: 1.00 g lidocaine hydrochloride monohydrate ≡ 0.94 g lidocaine hydrochloride ≡ 0.81 g lidocaine base (SCOTT et al. 1972). Blood concentrations of a drug are frequently expressed in terms of its base and dose of drug expressed as its salt. It is important to bear this in mind when relating these two pieces of information.

Table 1. Blood/Plasma concentration ratios and plasma protein binding of local anesthetic agents. TUCKER and MATHER (1975)

Agent	Blood/plasma concentration ratio	Plasma protein binding (%)
Prilocaine	1.00[a]	55[b]
Lidocaine	0.84	70
Mepivacaine	0.92	80
Etidocaine	0.58	95
Bupivacaine	0.73	95

[a] ARTHUR (1981).
[b] ERIKSSON (1966).

Concentrations of local anesthetics are generally determined in plasma or whole blood and it should be realized that these values are not interchangeable. TUCKER and MATHER (1975) demonstrated this in a group of volunteers receiving amide type local anaesthetic agents. Drug concentrations were determined in both arterial plasma and arterial blood and the plasma concentrations were found to be in excess of the blood concentrations. These differences are accentuated in the highly plasma protein bound local anesthetic agents (Table 1).

II. Sampling Site

Another factor determining drug concentration in blood is the sampling site. Figure 1 illustrates whole blood concentrations of prilocaine hydrochloride from three different sampling sites (femoral artery, portal vein and hepatic vein) in dogs during and after intravenous infusion of this drug (ARTHUR 1981). During the infusion, arterial concentrations are in excess of the portal venous concentrations as drug is absorbed by tissues which the arterial system supplies with blood. Prior to sampling, the only tissues which the arterial blood containing drug has perfused are the lung and heart. On terminating the infusion, the tissues begin to release the drug they have absorbed and hence the portal venous concentrations exceed arterial concentrations. Because the main site of metabolism of the amide type local anesthetics is the liver, the hepatic venous concentrations will be less than the other sampling sites. As a result of this, any post hepatic venous blood sample will contain less drug than a peripheral venous sample taken at the same time. Arterial/venous blood concentration differences were also described by TUCKER and MATHER (1975).

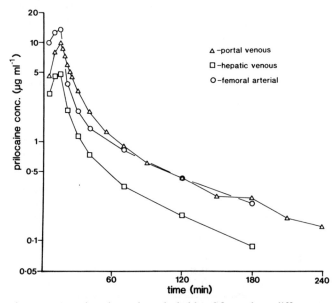

Fig. 1. Prilocaine concentrations in canine whole blood from three different sampling sites, resulting from the intravenous infusion of 10 mg kg^{-1} prilocaine over a 15 min period

III. Plasma Protein Binding

The percentage binding of the amide type local anesthetics to plasma proteins reported in Table 1 relates only to concentrations of drug around 1 μg ml^{-1}. TUCKER et al. (1970) demonstrated that as total concentration of drug in plasma increased, there was a marked decrease in the amount of drug bound. At 20 μg ml^{-1} the amount of bupivacaine bound decreased from 95%–65%, the amount of mepivacaine bound decreased from 80%–40% and the amount of lidocaine bound decreased from 70%–30%. As it is the unbound drug in blood which is most readily available for uptake by tissue and also for metabolism and excretion, it is important to know what factors will affect plasma protein binding.

1. Factors Affecting Protein Binding

The major protein complex to which these drugs bind has been identified as α_1-acid glycoprotein (PIAFSKY and KNOPPERT 1978; ROUTLEDGE et al. 1980). In a study of patients with elevated α_1-acid glycoprotein due to cancer, JACKSON et al. (1982) showed a significant decrease in the amount of unbound lidocaine when compared against normal control subjects. Other studies have shown α_1-acid glycoprotein changes to be correlated with changes of lidocaine free fractions. WOOD and WOOD (1981) studying mothers and newborns found higher free fractions of lidocaine in neonatal blood than maternal blood, and higher free fractions in pregnant then in nonpregnant women. A significant correlation between plasma α_1-acid glycoprotein concentration and amount of bound lidocaine was demonstrated. A similar relationship between mother and newborn for bupivacaine protein binding has also been reported (MATHER and THOMAS 1978). Conversely, no significant change in etidocaine binding was found between pregnant and nonpregnant women, nor was any change seen during labor (MORGAN et al. 1982). Elevated plasma concentration of α_1-acid glycoprotein in trauma cases, after myocardial infarction and during uremia have been shown to be associated with increased lidocaine binding (EDWARDS et al. 1982; ROUTLEDGE et al. 1981a; GROSSMANN et al. 1982). The effects of heparin on plasma protein binding of drugs has been of some concern. However, it was indicated by BROWN et al. (1981) that these effects were mainly artifacts caused in vitro by the action of triglyceride lipases. The use of oral contraceptives by women reduces the protein binding of lidocaine (WOOD and WOOD 1981; ROUTLEDGE et al. 1981 b) and a reduced concentration of α_1-acid glycoprotein by estrogens is thought to be the factor influencing this change. At low serum concentrations of lidocaine, it was found that smokers had a lower amount of free drug present (McNAMARA et al. 1980). Increases in the amount of α_1-acid glycoprotein in smokers was implicated as the causal factor here. At higher serum concentrations (9 μg ml^{-1}), although smokers had a slightly lower amount of free drug present than the non-smokers, the difference was not as pronounced. It was suggested that at higher concentrations, high affinity binding sites were saturated and binding to low affinity sites on albumin accounted for most of the binding.

Studies on the effect of pH on protein binding indicated an increase in the amount of free drug present when pH is lowered (BURNEY et al. 1978; McNAMARA et al. 1981). Experiments using dog plasma (COYLE and DENSON 1982) have shown the effects of lowered pH on protein binding to be much less pronounced for bupivacaine than for lidocaine. As it is mostly the unionized form of the local anaesthetic agents which is bound to plasma protein, the probable mechanism for this reduction of binding is the increase in cationic form of drug, as pH is lowered.

Changes in the amount of unbound local anaesthetic agents are unlikely to affect biotransformation rates. Within clinical concentrations, the hepatic extraction of etidocaine is approximately 75% even though it is 95% protein bound. In general, the rate limiting factor in the metabolism of these drugs is hepatic blood flow. However, alterations in plasma protein binding can change what may be regarded as a toxic blood concentration of the amide type local anesthetics.

C. Metabolism

The distinct difference in the metabolic pathways of the ester type and the amide type local anesthetic agents is that the initial metabolic step for the amides is generally dealkylation of the amine nitrogen and for the esters is hydrolysis.

I. Ester Type Local Anesthetics

Hydrolysis by plasma pseudocholinesterase accounts for a majority of the metabolism of the ester type agents. However, the liver is also involved in the extraction and metabolism of these compounds. The rate of hydrolysis is exceedingly rapid (Table 2) and the half lifes of elimination of procaine and chloroprocaine are less than 1 min (DUSOUICH and ERILL 1977; REIDENBERG et al. 1972; FOLDES et al. 1965) although an elimination half-life of 8.3 min has been reported for procaine in anesthetised patients (SEIFEN et al. 1979). The predominant metabolite resulting from the hydrolysis of procaine like compounds is para-aminobenzoic acid (Fig. 2). This metabolite has been implicated in the occurrence of allergic reactions which can occur following the administration of these ester type drugs.

A beneficial result of this rapid metabolism is that, should a toxic reaction occur, related to high blood concentrations of these drugs, then the toxic reaction would be of very short duration. The only major problem that may arise is when

Table 2. Rate of hydrolysis of ester type local anesthetic agents

	Rate of hydrolysis[a] (μM ml^{-1} h^{-1})	Half life of elimination (s)
Procaine	1.2	43[c]
Chloroprocaine	4.7	21[b]
Tetracaine	0.3	–

[a] FOLDES et al. (1965).
[b] O'BRIEN et al. (1979).
[c] DUSOUICH and ERILL (1977).

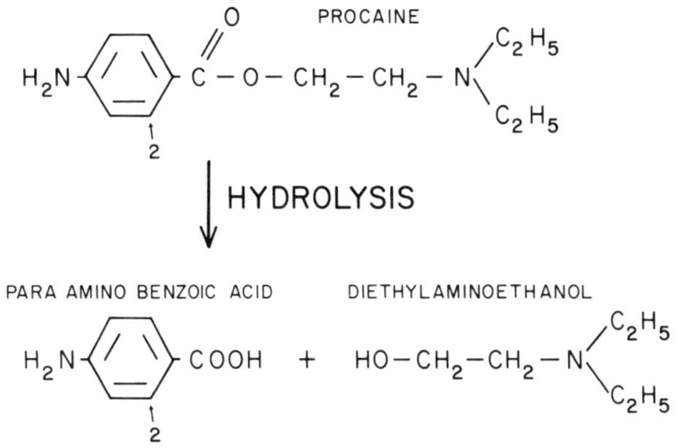

PROCAINE

H₂N—⟨benzene ring, position 2⟩—C(=O)—O—CH₂—CH₂—N(C₂H₅)(C₂H₅)

↓ HYDROLYSIS

PARA AMINO BENZOIC ACID   DIETHYLAMINOETHANOL

H₂N—⟨benzene ring, position 2⟩—COOH + HO—CH₂—CH₂—N(C₂H₅)(C₂H₅)

Fig. 2. Metabolic pathway of procaine (and chloroprocaine) by hydrolysis. (The addition of Cl at position 2 on the benzene ring gives chloroprocaine and its subsequent metabolite 2-chloro-4-amino benzoic acid)

an ester type agent is administered to patients with atypical pseudocholinesterase. These patients will be unable to metabolize ester type agents to any great extent and the possibility for a prolonged toxic reaction exists. However, in a study of patients receiving phospholine iodide, which reduced serum pseudocholinesterase activity to not less then 20% of normal values, chloroprocaine metabolism was not greatly affected (LANKS and SKLAR 1980). Bupivacaine, to a greater extent than the other amide type local anesthetics, has been reported to reduce the rate of chloroprocaine hydrolysis in human serum (LALKA et al. 1978). The clinical effects of this inhibition were not thought to affect the duration of anesthesia. A similar study (RAJ et al. 1980) implicated bupivacaine and neostigmine as agents capable of reducing chloroprocaine hydrolysis rates.

A majority of the para-aminobenzoic acid formed after procaine metabolism is excreted unchanged, or as a conjugated product in the urine (BRODIE et al. 1948). Studies on the urinary excretion of 2-chloro-4-aminobenzoic acid in man, after intravenous infusion of chloroprocaine, indicated up to 65% recovery of total dose over a 90 min period. Approximately 85% of the metabolite recovered was in the form of a conjugate (O'BRIEN et al. 1979).

II. Amide Type Local Anesthetics

It is generally accepted that the amide type local anesthetic agents are metabolized exclusively by the liver, with the exception of prilocaine. Very little of the parent drug is excreted in the urine. Values for urinary excretion have been quoted as 3% for lidocaine (KEENAGHAN and BOYES 1972), <1% for prilocaine (MATHER 1972, cited in MATHER and TUCKER 1978), 1% for mepivacaine (MEFFIN et al. 1973), <1% for etidocaine (THOMAS et al. 1976) and <1% for bupivacaine (FRIEDMAN et al. 1982). The processes involved in the hepatic metabolism of the amide type local anesthetics have been previously reviewed (HANSSON 1971; BOYES 1975; MATHER and TUCKER 1978).

1. Lidocaine

Lidocaine metabolism has been most extensively studied and a majority of an administered dose in man has been identified in terms of excreted metabolites (Boyes 1975). Initially, the lidocaine undergoes N-dealkylation to form monoethylglycinexylidide (MEGX). This can undergo further dealkylation to glycinexylidide (GX) or, in common with GX, it can be hydrolyzed to form 2,6-xylidine which in turn is hydroxylated giving 4-hydroxy-2,6-xylidine. This is the major metabolite which is excreted in the urine (Fig. 3).

Although relatively small amounts of MEGX and GX are recovered in the urine, they are of importance as they have the capability of causing toxic reactions similar to those of the parent compound. Although these two metabolites are less toxic than lidocaine, they have been implicated in the occurrence of toxic reactions during lidocaine administration (Nation et al. 1977; Halkin et al. 1975).

2. Bupivacaine

N-dealkylation of bupivacaine is the best characterized metabolic step for this drug. The resulting breakdown product, 2-pipecoloxylidine (PPX), has been measured in the urine of man, accounting for 5% of the administered dose (Reynolds

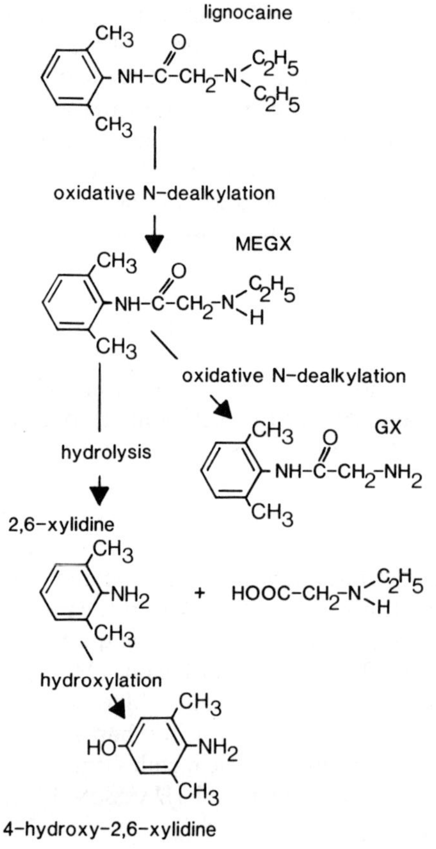

Fig. 3. Partial metabolic pathway of lidocaine

1971; FRIEDMAN et al. 1982). Although the monkey has been shown to excrete 52% of a given dose of bupivacaine as pipecolic acid, the hydrolysis product of PPX (GOEHL et al. 1973), it is not thought that this reaction is as important in man (BOYES 1975; REYNOLDS 1971). Other metabolites identified in the monkey included hydroxylation products of both the parent compound and PPX. GOEHL et al. (1973) also demonstrated a small amount of bupivacaine excretion, together with its metabolites, in the feces of monkeys (6%), this being due to biliary secretion of the drug.

3. Mepivacaine

Although very similar in structure to bupivacaine, the N-dealkylation step to form PPX accounts for only 1% of the dose excreted in the urine and a majority of the recovered metabolites appear as conjugated hydroxylated products (THOMAS and MEFFIN 1972; MEFFIN et al. 1973). Further metabolites were identified by MEFFIN and THOMAS (1973) and combined, these account for approximately half the administered dose of drug.

4. Prilocaine

Metabolic studies of prilocaine in humans are limited. In a study using liver and kidney preparations from rats (GEDDES 1965), it was suggested that the initial metabolic step was hydrolysis of the amide link to form ortho-toluidine and N-

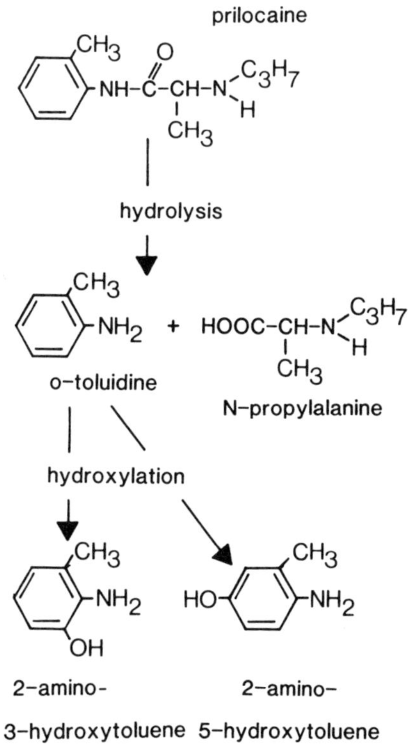

Fig. 4. Metabolic pathway of prilocaine

propylalanine. Later work (Akerman et al. 1966 b) identified 2 further metabolic products in the urine of rats and cats which were the hydroxylation products of ortho-toluidine (Fig. 4). It is thought that these hydroxylated metabolites are directly involved in the occurrence of methemoglobinemia seen occasionally after the administration of prilocaine. Enzyme activity in the liver responsible for prilocaine hydrolysis has been located in the microsome fraction (Akerman and Ross 1970) and has the same pH dependency profile as reported for the hydrolysis of MEGX (Hollunger 1960).

The lung has been suggested as a possible site of extra-hepatic prilocaine metabolism (Akerman et al. 1966a; Arthur 1981). However, these results from in vitro tissue incubation studies have not been confirmed in vivo using the dog as an experimental model (Arthur 1981).

5. Etidocaine

A large number of etidocaine metabolites have been identified (Vine et al. 1978; Thomas et al. 1976; Morgan et al. 1977). However, recovery of these metabolites in urine accounts for less than 40% of an administered dose. In common with the other amide type local anesthetics, etidocaine undergoes N-dealkylation and can also be hydroxylated on the aromatic ring. Hydrolytic metabolism appears to be of less importance than for lidocaine and prilocaine, with less than 10% of the dose appearing in the urine as both 2,6-xylidine and its hydroxylated product, as opposed to over 70% for lidocaine.

D. Pharmacokinetics in Man

The most commonly quoted data on the pharmacokinetics of the most widely used amide type local anesthetics is that of Tucker and Mather (1975, 1979). Table 3 illustrates the pharmacokinetic parameters of these agents from this work and also data from Arthur et al. (1979) for the less commonly used amide type local anesthetic, prilocaine. The data for these local anesthetics, excluding prilo-

Table 3. Pharmacokinetic parameters for the amide type local anesthetic agents in man (see text)

Parameter	Prilocaine[a]	Lidocaine	Etidocaine	Mepivacaine	Bupivacaine
$t_{1/2}$ clim.	93	96	162	114	162
V_D^b	410	212	666	150	209
V_{Dss}	261	91	133	84	73
Cl	2.84	0.95	1.11	0.78	0.58

$t_{1/2}$ elim. ($\equiv t_{1/2}\beta$) = Half-life of elimination (min).
$V_D\beta$ = Apparent volume of distribution based on the elimination phase of the drug (l).
V_{Dss} = Apparent volume of distribution at steady state (l).
Cl = Clearance (l min^{-1}).
[a] The data for prilocaine is based on a two compartment model. The values for the other drugs are based on a three compartment model.

caine, are based on arterial whole blood concentrations after a short intravenous infusion of drug. The data for prilocaine was determined from venous plasma concentrations after an intravenous infusion. However, as prilocaine has a whole blood/plasma concentration ratio of 1, there will be no difference between blood or plasma data. For the parameters quoted, there will be little difference between venous and arterial data.

As stated earlier, very small amounts of these drugs are excreted unchanged in the urine and the major site of their metabolism is the liver. Because of this, the clearance values for these drugs should be a product of hepatic blood flow and hepatic extraction of drug. Thus, clearance of these drugs is limited by hepatic blood flow and hepatic function. This was verified by TUCKER et al. (1977), using data from previous studies (TUCKER and MATHER 1975; WIKLUND 1977 a, b). The values for hepatic extraction ratios in Table 4 are quoted from this work. This data was derived from continuous intravenous infusions of these agents to human volunteers. Over a period of 150 min, cardiac output increased significantly with both lidocaine and bupivacaine but not with etidocaine. However, with all three drugs, an increase in hepatic blood flow was noted. Concomitant with this increase, there was a slight reduction in the hepatic extraction ratio for lidocaine, a more dramatic reduction for bupivacaine and virtually no effect on the extraction ratio of etidocaine. As a result of these factors hepatic clearance of lidocaine and etidocaine increased marginally over 150 min, whereas the value for bupivacaine decreased over the same time period. These effects were found to be positively correlated with blood concentrations of these drugs.

The clearance value for prilocaine of 2.84 l min^{-1} indicates that there is a high degree of extra hepatic metabolism of this drug as it is impossible for the liver to clear a greater volume of blood than that passing through it. AKERMAN et al. (1966 a) reported that in vivo lung and kidney preparations were capable of metabolizing prilocaine. As only a very low level of pulmonary extraction would be necessary to account for this extrahepatic metabolism, the lung seemed to be the most likely organ to account for this metabolism. However, it has not been possible to show this using the anesthetized dog as an experimental model (ARTHUR 1981). The possibility of human pulmonary and/or renal metabolism still exists.

The volume of distribution relates to a hypothetical volume required to account for the amount of drug in the body. Etidocaine is the most lipid soluble of these compounds and, as would be expected, has the largest volume of distribu-

Table 4. Hepatic extraction and biochemical properties of the amide type

Local anesthetics	HE	pKa[a]	Lipid[a] solubility
Lidocaine	0.72	7.7	2.9
Etidocaine	0.74	7.7	141
Bupivacaine	0.40	8.1	27.5
Mepivacaine	0.51	7.6	0.8
Prilocaine	–	7.7	1.0

[a] From COVINO and VASSALLO (1976).

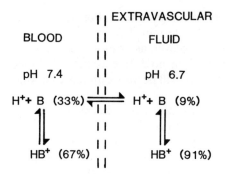

Fig. 5. Representation of a mechanism for the accumulation of a basic amine in tissue ($p_{Ka} = 7.7$). $B =$ un-ionised compound, $HB^+ =$ ionised compound

tion. Bupivacaine which is the second most lipid soluble of these drugs has an apparent volume of distribution similar to that of mepivacaine and lidocaine which are considerably less lipid soluble (see Table 4). So, lipid solubility is obviously not the only factor controlling tissue uptake of these drugs. As it is the unionized form of these local anesthetic drugs which is most readily absorbed from the blood, any differences in their pKa values would affect the amount of drug readily available for absorption. With the exception of bupivacaine, this group of drugs have very similar pKa values, hence, the ratios of ionized to unionized form will be very similar at a given pH. Plasma protein binding of the amide type local anesthetics has no apparent effect on their tissue uptake. Tissue protein binding on the other hand may play a significant role in determining the apparent volumes of drug distribution. It would appear that all these factors together with the chemical structures of these drugs make some contribution towards determining their tissue uptake.

Figure 5 represents one of the mechanisms for the accumulation of a basic amine in tissue. In this case, the tissue pH illustrated is 6.7 determined for dog lung by EFFROS and CHINARD (1969). Effects of protein binding are ignored in this model. As uncharged base is absorbed by the tissue, it equilibrates between the uncharged base and the charged cationic form of the drug. As there is a greater proportion of the cationic form of the basic amine in the tissue, a concentration gradient will be maintained, resulting in a greater concentration of drug in the tissue. This blood to tissue gradient will be greatly enhanced in the presence of intracellular binding of the drug cation, the mechanism for which has been proposed by FEINSTEIN and PAIMRE (1969).

The half-lives of elimination for this group of drugs indicate that after the redistribution phase, lidocaine and prilocaine concentrations in blood decrease more rapidly than the other amide type local anesthetics. Bupivacaine and etidocaine persist in the circulation the longest with a half-life of elimination of 2.7 h.

E. Factors Affecting Pharmacokinetics of Local Anesthetics

I. Lung Uptake of Local Anesthetics

As previously stated, the lung has been implicated as an extrahepatic site of prilocaine metabolism from in vitro studies using lung slices (AKERMAN et al. 1966a).

This has not been confirmed by studies in vivo. Nevertheless, the lung plays an important role in the distribution of amide type local anesthetics in the body.

In a study of intravenous regional anesthesia (TUCKER and BOAS 1971) it was suggested that the lung could absorb large quantities of local anesthetics after cuff release and thus reduce the high first pass concentrations of these drugs. Lung uptake of lidocaine in volunteers receiving a 0.5 mg kg^{-1} intravenous bolus injection of lidocaine was found to be 60% over a 15–20 s period (JORFELDT et al. 1979). This would represent a substantial portion of the volume of distribution of this drug if the uptake persisted. However, drug is released from the lung quite rapidly after the high initial uptake. The effect of lung uptake is reduced as the dose of drug administered is increased. A 0.5 mg kg^{-1} intravenous bolus injection of lidocaine in pigs resulted in a 40% first pass lung uptake of drug but when the dose was increased to 2.0 mg kg^{-1} this value was reduced to 28% indicating a dose-dependent uptake by the lung (BERTLER et al. 1978). As a result of this, it can be assumed that in the case of an inadvertent intravenous injection of a clinical dose of local anaesthetic intended for extradural injection, the effect of lung uptake on blood concentrations will be greatly reduced. It is likely then that towards the end of the intravenous injection, arterial local anaesthetic concentrations will be directly related to the rate of drug injection and cardiac output, i.e., the faster the drug is injected, the greater the resultant blood concentrations. However, in the initial stages of the injection, the brain will be protected from high blood concentrations of these drugs.

Recent studies with children receiving bupivacaine for intercostal nerve blocks (ROTHSTEIN et al. 1983) have indicated lung uptake of this drug. This may afford some degree of protection against toxic concentrations of bupivacaine during this procedure.

Displacement of local anesthetics from lung tissue gives some indication as to how drug interactions may affect kinetics in the body. The tricyclic antidepressant nortriptyline was shown to displace lidocaine from an isolated perfused rat lung preparation (POST et al. 1979). Bupivacaine competition with lidocaine for binding sites was also demonstrated by this study. In vivo, this displacement of lidocaine from lung and other tissues, would cause an increase in blood concentrations.

II. Age

Studies quoting values of pharmacokinetic parameters for various drugs frequently base their observations on healthy, young male volunteers. Use of drugs is obviously not restricted to this age group and local anesthetics are frequently administered to humans of all ages. Due to the obvious ethical restrictions when working with children, pharmacokinetic information in this age group has been limited to data obtained from blood and urine samples acquired during procedures requiring local anesthesia. A major problem arises when comparing the pharmacokinetic parameters of children and adults. Correlation between body weight and clearance, or body weight and volume of distribution, is poor in a group of normal healthy adults so to compare these terms on a per kilogram basis between children and adults is not entirely adequate.

Limited blood sampling from neonates given mepivacaine subcutaneously, revealed a much longer half life of elimination than in adults, 8.69 h and 3.17 h respectively (MOORE et al. 1978). Clearance values for this drug based on body weight were approximately half those found in adults, but more than 6 times the amount of unmetabolized mepivacaine was excreted in the urine of neonates. It was suggested that this was due to a greatly reduced hepatic enzyme metabolic capability in neonates. Similarly, the half life of elimination of etidocaine in neonates was shown to be greater than in adults, 6.42 h and 2.6 h respectively (MORGAN et al. 1978). However, it was implied that neonatal metabolism of etidocaine was not impaired and the differences were due to increased volume of distribution in neonates. In agreement with this study, MIHALY et al. (1978) reported that the increased half-life of elimination of lidocaine in neonates (3.16 h) compared to adults (1.6 h) was also due to an increased volume of distribution. This apparent increase in volume of distribution was related to decreased plasma protein binding of these drugs in neonates, which would make a greater proportion of the drug in blood available for tissue uptake. Using the sheep as an experimental model, no difference in elimination half-life was seen between adults and neonates (PEDERSEN et al. 1982) which is not in agreement with the data of MORGAN et al. (1978). However, neonatal sheep did demonstrate greater volume of distribution and total body clearance than the adult. Earlier work with lidocaine in sheep showed a larger volume of distribution in adults than in newborns (MORISHIMA et al. 1979). Here, the half-life of elimination was greater in newborns than adults as was total body clearance.

In infants, there is a higher percentage of well perfused tissues in the body and a smaller percentage of fat and muscle in relation to young adults. On the other hand, the elderly person has a greater percentage of adipose tissue and less muscle (GREENBLATT et al. 1982). As the amide type local anesthetics are lipid soluble, this would suggest that there is a possibility of a greater apparent volume of distribution in the elderly. This was shown to be the case for lidocaine by TRIGGS et al. (1975) and CUSACK et al. (1980) found a similar trend. Also, hepatic blood flow can be significantly reduced in the elderly (GREENBLATT et al. 1982), implying that those drugs for which clearance is limited by hepatic blood flow would have a reduced clearance. Lidocaine, which falls into this category of drugs, exhibits unchanged clearance values in the elderly although the half-life of elimination is prolonged somewhat (TRIGGS et al. 1975; CUSACK et al. 1980).

Data obtained from infants and children regarding the pharmacokinetics of bupivacaine is conflicting. CALDWELL et al. (1976) determined that the half-life of elimination for bupivacaine in infants immediately after birth was 25 h as opposed to 1.3 h in adults. Conversely, MAGNO et al. (1976) showed that for bupivacaine there was no difference between the half-life of elimination between infant and adult. In both these studies, drug was "administered" to the infant by placental transfer from the mother after bupivacaine had been given epidurally during childbirth. In both cases, data was based on a small number of blood samples. Using an older group of children, age 3–192 months, receiving bupivacaine for intercostal nerve block, it was found that the half-life of elimination for bupivacaine in this group of subjects was very similar to that reported for adults (ROTHSTEIN et al. 1982). The total body clearance of bupivacaine however, was over twice that reported for adults (16.2 ml min^{-1} kg^{-1} and 6.7 ml min^{-1} kg^{-1} respectively). This could partially have been due to a greater hepatic blood flow, related to body weight, in this group of children.

III. Other Drugs

As the clearance of the amide type local anesthetics is generally limited by hepatic blood flow, any agent increasing hepatic blood flow will cause an increase in clearance of these drugs. The least affected clearance value with increased hepatic blood flow would be that for bupivacaine, it has the lowest hepatic extraction and hence, would be more affected by increased hepatic enzyme activity. TUCKER et al. (1977) reported an increase in hepatic blood flow in subjects receiving prolonged local anesthetic infusions. Thus, lidocaine and etidocaine clearance values increased over a 150-min infusion period.

Using phenobarbitone treated dogs to study the effects of increased hepatic enzyme activity and increased hepatic blood flow on the disposition of lidocaine and warfarin, the systemic clearance of lidocaine increased from 31–55 ml min^{-1} kg^{-1} after phenobarbitone treatment (ESQUIVEL et al. 1978). The phenobarbitone treated animals had an increase in hepatic blood flow from 52 ml min^{-1} kg^{-1} to 113 m min^{-1} kg^{-1}, but this difference was not found to be statistically significant. This increase in hepatic blood flow combined with an increase in liver weight to 1.8 times normal, satisfactorily accounts for the increased lidocaine clearance. Studying the opposite effect, OCHS et al. (1980) found that the co-administration of propranolol to volunteers for 3 days prior to an intravenous lidocaine infusion changed the kinetics of this drug both after short and long infusions. After a short infusion, the half-life of elimination of lidocaine increased from 65–101 min in association with a significant decrease in the clearance from 18–11 ml min^{-1} kg^{-1}. However, the total apparent volume of distribution of lidocaine was unaffected. When steady state lidocaine concentrations were attained after prolonged drug infusion, blood concentrations were significantly increased and clearance values significantly decreased in propranolol treated subjects. These changes could be partially explained by a reduced hepatic blood flow caused by a decrease in cardiac output which is a direct effect of propranolol. Also, propranolol may reduce the hepatic metabolic capacity of the liver for lidocaine.

Another drug which reduces liver blood flow is cimetidine. This agent, when administered for some time prior to an intravenous lidocaine infusion in volunteers, was found to reduce lidocaine clearance (0.77 l min^{-1} – normal, 0.58 l min^{-1} – with cimetidine. FEELY et al. (1982 b). Although cimetidine administration increased the amount of free lidocaine in plasma, a decrease in the volume of distribution was noted.

In a more clinically related study, effects relating to the use of diazepam (0.1 mg kg^{-1}), prior to the epidural injection of either etidocaine or bupivacaine to adult patients, were investigated (GIASI et al. 1980). In the groups receiving epidural bupivacaine, a significant decrease in the half-life of elimination was seen in those patients in the diazepam treatment group. It was proposed that a reduction in plasma protein binding of bupivacaine due to direct competition for binding sites with diazepam could explain the shorter half-life. If the free fraction of bupivacaine were increased, this would probably enhance its hepatic extraction, as bupivacaine has the lowest hepatic extraction of the amide type local anesthetic drugs and hence is most likely to be affected by an increased free fraction of drug.

IV. Disease

Any disease state reducing or increasing hepatic blood flow is likely to alter pharmacokinetic parameters of the amide type local anesthetics. Of this group of drugs, lidocaine has been the most extensively studied mainly because of its intravenous use as an antiarrhythmic agent. Under these circumstances, most recent studies have shown a reduced clearance of lidocaine in patients with heart failure, when compared to normal values. BAX et al. (1980) reported a clearance of 7.2 ml min^{-1} kg^{-1} in a group of patients with heart failure as opposed to 11.8 ml min^{-1} kg^{-1} in patients without heart failure, and SAWYER et al. (1981) reported clearances of 5.8 ml min^{-1} kg^{-1} in patients with heart failure as opposed to 8.4 ml min^{-1} kg^{-1} in normal subjects.

In patients with cirrhosis of the liver, due to alcoholism, a reduced capacity to clear lidocaine has been demonstrated (THOMPSON et al. 1971). This was associated with increases in the volume of distribution and elimination half-life. Patients with renal failure were also included in this study, but no significant changes in lidocaine pharmacokinetics were noted. However, in a study of a smaller group of patients with renal failure, a slightly prolonged half-life of elimination for lidocaine was noted although clearance values were similar to normal (COLLINSWORTH et al. 1975). A more important fact illustrated by this study was the accumulation of GX, which may have some bearing on toxic reactions during long term lidocaine blocks. However, the primary metabolite of lidocaine (MEGX) was shown to exist at normal concentrations. Although only 2%–3% of an administered dose of lidocaine is excreted in the urine of man as GX, (BOYES 1975) in renal failure this substance will tend to accumulate in the blood. This data is not in keeping with observations made by BROMAGE and GERTEL (1972), who reported that brachial plexus blocks for patients with renal failure, using lidocaine, mepivacaine and bupivacaine, were consistently shorter in duration (38% less) than normal. This they attributed to increased cardiac output observed in patients with renal failure resulting in greater drug clearance and hence faster wash out of drug from tissue.

FEELY et al. (1982a) determined pharmacokinetic parameters of lidocaine in 5 patients with orthostatic hypotension in both the supine position (blood pressure normal) and in the sitting position (blood pressure reduced). In the hypotensive condition, clearance of drug was significantly reduced as was volume of distribution; half-life of elimination remaining unchanged. These effects were most likely due to reduced hepatic perfusion caused by hypotension.

The increase of α_1-acid glycoprotein due to cancer and other factors discussed earlier, can increase the amount of drug delivered to the liver and thus increase the clearance of those agents whose hepatic metabolism is dependent on the rate of drug delivery to the liver. Similarly, tolerance to what may be regarded as toxic concentrations of local anesthetics may be greater with increased plasma protein binding.

It is unlikely that many disease states will greatly affect the quality or duration of local anesthetic block, as drug is generally administered directly at the site of action. However, some concern may be necessary regarding toxicity of these local anesthetic agents under certain conditions, e.g., toxicity of ester agents in subjects with abnormal pseudocholinesterase activity. In the case of lidocaine use as an antiarrhythmic, effects of disease states and other factors on its pharmacokinetics are more fully discussed in the review of BENOWITZ and MEISTER (1978).

V. Other Factors

A high protein meal has been shown to increase the clearance of lidocaine and it was suggested that this was due to stimulation of hepatic blood flow (ELVIN et al. 1981). In an investigation limited to the elimination phase of lidocaine in man, no difference in pharmacokinetic parameters was observed between groups of young adult Caucasian, Oriental or Black subjects (GOLDBERG et al. 1982). Also, there was no significant difference in lidocaine plasma protein binding among these three different racial groups.

Studies using the isomers of mepivacaine, bupivacaine (ABERG 1972) and prilocaine (AKERMAN and ROSS 1970) revealed distinct differences between the D- and L-forms of these drugs. The D-isomer of mepivacaine was found to be more rapidly absorbed from the site of injection than the L-isomer in guinea pigs and results obtained with the D- and L-isomers of bupivacaine suggested that the same relationship existed. After intravenous administration of mepivacaine isomers to rabbits, significantly greater amounts of the L-isomer were found in the lung and kidney. However, significantly greater concentrations of the D-isomer were detected in the cerebellum of rabbits which probably explains the observation that D-mepivacaine was more toxic than L-mepivacaine. In the study of the isomers of prilocaine (AKERMAN and ROSS 1970), different animal liver preparations were shown to hydrolyze D-prilocaine at a higher rate than L-prilocaine.

Direct pharmacokinetic studies of local anesthetics in pregnant humans are obviously limited for ethical reasons. However, it has been demonstrated in sheep

Table 5. Pharmacokinetic parameters of lidocaine in pregnant and nonpregnant sheep (BLOEDOW et al. 1980)

	Nonpregnant	Pregnant
Clearance ($ml\,min^{-1}\,kg^{-1}$)	38	42
$t_{1/2}\beta$ (min)	42	62[a]
V_c ($l\,kg^{-1}$)	0.24	0.48[a]
V_Dss ($l\,kg^{-1}$)	1.30	2.74[a]
Hepatic extraction (%)	69	57
Hepatic blood flow ($ml\,min^{-1}\,kg^{-1}$)	55	65

[a] Statistical difference between two groups.

that pregnancy significantly alters the pharmacokinetics of lidocaine administered as an intravenous bolus (BLOEDOW et al. 1980). Although total body clearance values appeared to be unaltered, the hepatic extraction of lidocaine was apparently reduced in pregnancy thus compensating for an increase in hepatic blood flow (Table 5).

F. Pharmacokinetics in Experimental Animals

The use of animals as experimental models to study local anesthetic action poses some problems regarding the suitability of the chosen model. However, because local anesthetics are administered directly to the site of action, i.e., at the nerve, minor differences in pharmacokinetic parameters between species will have less effect on drug action than in other drugs administered by other routes (intravenously, orally, etc). Differences in local anesthetic action between man and animals are more likely to be affected by the physiology and anatomy of the nerves blocked than by differences in rate of drug metabolism and excretion.

Table 6 is a comparison of pharmacokinetic parameters for some of the amide type local anesthetics between man and some animal species. Again, lidocaine has been most extensively studied and it is apparent that man has the lowest total body clearance of this drug, approximately 9 times less than that found in the rat. The total body clearance of lidocaine in rats ($115 \text{ ml min}^{-1} \text{ kg}^{-1}$) was found to be in excess of hepatic blood flow (DEBOER et al. 1980). The hepatic extraction value of 100% is in agreement with the data of LENNARD et al. (1978) and marginally greater than the 95% value determined by SHAND et al. (1975) from isolated perfused rat liver preparations. It was suggested by DEBOER et al. (1980) that lidocaine may be excreted to a great enough extent in the urine to account for the extrahepatic clearance of drug, but KEENAGHAN and BOYES (1972) reported very low urinary excretion values for lidocaine in the rat ($< 1\%$). It is apparent that there is some degree of extrahepatic metabolism of lidocaine in the rat which is not the case in man. 2 of the major metabolites of lidocaine excreted in the urine of rats are hydroxylated products of the parent drug and MEGX. As these two metabolites represent only a very small percentage of excreted metabolites in man (KEENAGHAN and BOYES 1972) not only do they represent a different emphasis on metabolic pathway, but may possibly be the product of extrahepatic metabolism.

A very close agreement between the data of BLOEDOW et al. (1980) and MORISHIMA et al. (1979) for the pharmacokinetic parameters of lidocaine in sheep is in sharp contrast to the vast differences for the same data in two groups of Rhesus monkeys (BENOWITZ et al. 1974; DENSON et al. 1981). The higher clearance, lower volume of distribution and shorter half-life of elimination in the earlier set of monkey data were ascribed to a shorter sampling time and possibly the use of younger animals for the experiment (DENSON et al. 1981).

With the exception of prilocaine, the total body clearance of the amide type local anesthetics is greater in animals than in man. This is related in most cases to a greater hepatic extraction of these drugs in the different animal species and/or a greater hepatic blood flow per kilogram body weight.

Table 6

	Lidocaine Man[a]	Dog[g]	Rat[e]	Sheep[d]	Sheep[h]	Monkey[i]	Monkey[j]	Prilocaine Man[c]	Dog[k]	Rabbit[k]	Bupivacaine Man[a]	Dog[l]	Etidocaine Man[a]	Sheep[m]
Cl (ml min⁻¹ kg⁻¹)	13.2	31	115	38	41	65	28	35.5	35.1	28.2	8.1	24	15.4	30
$t_{1/2\beta}$ (min)	96		33	42	31	15	114	97	80	134	162		162	35
V_c (l kg⁻¹)	0.12			0.24	0.9	0.4	1.1	1.3	1.1	2.4	0.19		0.17	0.52
$V_{D\beta}$ (l kg⁻¹)	1.3[b]			2.13	1.84	0.94	4.5	4.9	4.1	5.6	1.0[b]		1.9[b]	1.52
HE (%)	72	79		69					59		40	60	72	–
HBF (ml min⁻¹ kg⁻¹)	24[p]	52[f]	100	55				24[p]	38[n]	28[o]	24[p]		24[p]	–

a TUCKER and MATHER (1979) – based on a 72 kg body weight.
b Value quoted is V_{DSS}.
c ARTHUR et al. (1979).
d BLOEDOW et al. (1980).
e DEBOER et al. (1980).
f ESQUIVEL et al. (1978).
g LELORIER et al. (1977).
h MORISHIMA et al. (1979).

i BENOWITZ et al. 1974).
j DENSON et al. (1981).
k ARTHUR (1981).
l IRESTEDT et al. (1978).
m PEDERSEN et al. (1982).
n KETTERER et al. (1960).
o WYLER (1974).
p 72 kg man with a total hepatic blood flow of 1700 ml min⁻¹ (PRICE et al. 1960).

Although the clearance values for both bupivacaine and lidocaine are much greater in dog than man, the duration of motor blockade during spinal anesthesia is only marginally shorter in the dog (FELDMAN and COVINO 1981). In this study of spinal anesthesia in the dog, durations of motor blockade for dibucaine, tetracaine and chloroprocaine were also found to be similar to that in man, with mepivacaine showing the greatest interspecies difference. Duration of epidural anesthesia, using lidocaine and bupivacaine in dogs and bupivacaine in sheep, has also been shown to be very similar to values obtained in man (LEBEAUX 1973, 1975).

The data obtained for prilocaine in man (ARTHUR et al. 1979), rabbit and dog (ARTHUR 1981) appears quite similar, but when the clearance values are compared to the relative hepatic blood flow, it is apparent that differences in the metabolism and excretion of these drugs exist.

References

Aberg G (1972) Toxicological and local anaesthetic effects of optically active isomers of two local anaesthetic compounds. Acta Pharmacol Toxicol 31:273–286

Akerman B, Ross S (1970) Stereospecificity of the enzymatic biotransformation of the enantiomers of prilocaine. Acta Pharmacol Toxicol 28:445–453

Akerman B, Astrom A, Ross S, Telc A (1966a) Studies on the absorption, distribution and metabolism of labelled prilocaine and lidocaine in some animal species. Acta Pharmacol Toxicol 24:389–403

Akerman B, Petersson SA, Wistrand P (1966b) Methemoglobin forming metabolites of prilocaine. Third International Pharmacological Congress: Abstracts of Communications, Lectures and Symposia, Juli 24–30, 1966, Sao Paolo, Brazil, p 237

Arthur GR (1981) Distribution and elimination of local anesthetic agents: the role of lung, liver and kidneys Ph D thesis, University of Edinburgh

Arthur GR, Scott DHT, Boyes RN, Scott DB (1979) Pharmacokinetic and clinical pharmacological studies with mepivacaine and prilocaine. Br J Anaesth 51:481–485

Bax ND, Tucker GT, Woods HF (1980) Lignocaine and indocyanine green kinetics in patients following myocardial infarction. Br J Clin Pharmacol 10:353–361

Benowitz NL, Meister W (1978) Clinical pharmacokinetics of lignocaine. Clin Pharmacokinet 3:177–201

Benowitz N, Forsyth RP, Melmon KL, Rowland M (1974) Lidocaine disposition kinetics in monkey and man. I. Prediction by a perfusion model. Clin Pharmacol Ther 16:87–98

Bertler A, Lewis DH, Lofstrom JB, Post C (1978) In vivo lung uptake of lidocaine in pigs. Acta Anaesthesiol Scand 22:530–536

Bloedow DC, Ralston DH, Hargrove JC (1980) Lidocaine pharmacokinetics in pregnant and nonpregnant sheep. J Pharm Sci 69:32–37

Boyes RN (1975) A review of the metabolism of amide local anaesthetic agents. Br J Anaesth 47:225–230

Brodie BB, Lief PA, Poet R (1948) The fate of procaine in man following its intravenous administration and methods for the estimation of procaine and diethylaminoethanol. J Pharmacol Exp Ther 94:359–366

Bromage PR, Gertel M (1972) Brachial plexus anaesthesia in chronic renal failure. Anesthesiology 36:488–493

Brown JE, Kitchell BB, Bjornsson TD, Shand DG (1981) The artifactual nature of heparin-induced drug protein binding alterations. Clin Pharmacol Ther 30:636–643

Burney RG, Difazio CA, Foster JA (1978) Effects of pH on protein binding of lidocaine. Anesth Analg 57:478–480

Caldwell J, Moffatt JR, Smith RL, Lieberman BA, Cawston MO, Beard RW (1976) Pharmacokinetics of bupivacaine administered epidurally during childbirth. Br J Clin Pharmacol 3:956P–957P

Collinsworth KA, Strong JM, Atkinson AJ, Winkle RA, Pelroth F, Harrison DC (1975) Pharmacokinetics and metabolism of lidocaine in patients with renal failure. Clin Pharmacol Ther 18:59–64

Covino BG, Vassallo HG (1976) Local anesthetics. Mechanisms of action and clinical use. Grune and Stratton, New York

Coyle DE, Denson DD (1982) Plasma protein binding of bupivacaine in the dog. Anesthesiology 5:A 209

Cusack B, Kelly JG, Lavan J, Noel J, O'Malley K (1980) Pharmacokinetics of lignocaine in the elderly (Proceedings). Br J Clin Pharmacol 9:293–294

De Boer AG, Breimer DD, Pronk J, Gubbens Stibbe JM (1980) Rectal bioavailability of lidocaine in rats. Absence of significant first pass elimination. J Pharm Sci 69:804–807

Denson DD, Ritschel WA, Turner PA, Ohlweiler DF, Bridenbaugh PO (1981) A comparison of the intravenous and subarachnoid lidocaine pharmacokinetics in the rhesus monkey. Biopharm Drug Dispos 2:367–380

DuSouich P, Erill P (1977) Altered metabolism of procainamide and procaine in patients with pulmonary and cardiac disease. Clin Pharmacol Ther 21:101–102

Edwards DJ, Lalka D, Cerra F, Slaughter RL (1982) Alpha 1 – acid glycoprotein concentration and protein binding in trauma. Clin Pharmacol Ther 31:62–67

Effros RM, Chinard P (1969) The in vivo pH of the extravascular space of the lung. J Clin Invest 48:1983–1996

Elvin AT, Cole AF, Pieper JA, Rolbin SH, Lalka D (1981) Effect of food on lidocaine kinetics: mechanism of food-related alteration in high intrinsic clearance drug elimination. Clin Pharmacol Ther 30:455–460

Eriksson E (1966) Prilocaine. An experimental study in man of a new local anesthetic with special regard to efficacy, toxicity and excretion. Acta Chir Scand (Suppl) 358:1–82

Esquivel M, Blaschke TF, Snidow GH, Meffin PJ (1978) Effect of phenobarbitone on the disposition of lignocaine and warfarin in the dog. J Pharm Pharmacol 30:804–805

Feely J, Wade D, McAllister CB, Wilkinson GR, Robertson D (1982a) Effect of hypotension on liver blood flow and lidocaine disposition. N Engl J Med 307:866–868

Feely J, Wilkinson GR, McAllister CR, Wood AJJ (1982b) Increased toxicity and reduced clearance of lidocaine by cimetidine. Ann Intern Med 96:592–594

Feinstein MB, Paimre M (1969) Pharmacological action of local anesthetics on excitation-contraction coupling in striated and smooth muscle. Fed Proc 28:1643–1648

Feldman HS, Covino BG (1981) A chronic model for investigation of experimental spinal anesthesia in the dog. Anesthesiology 54:148–152

Foldes FF, Davidson GM, Duncalf D, Kunabara S (1965) The intravenous toxicity of local anesthetic agents in man. Clin Pharmacol Ther 6:328–335

Friedman GA, Rowlingson JC, Difazio CA, Donegan MF (1982) Evaluation of the analgesic effect and urinary excretion of systemic bupivacaine in man. Anesth Analg 61:23–27

Geddes IC (1965) Studies on the metabolism of Citanest ^{14}C. Acta Anaesthesiol Scand (Suppl) 16:37–44

Giasi RM, D'Agostino E, Covino BG (1980) Interaction of diazepam and epidurally administered local anesthetic agents. Reg Anesth 5:8–11

Goehl TJ, Davenport JB, Stanley MJ (1973) Distribution, biotransformation and excretion of bupivacaine in the rat and the monkey. Xenobiotica 3:761–772

Goldberg MJ, Spector R, Johnson GF (1982) Racial background and lidocaine pharmacokinetics. J Clin Pharmacol 22:391–394

Greenblatt DJ, Sellers EM, Shader RI (1982) Drug disposition in old age. N Engl J Med 306:1081–1088

Grossman SH, Davis D, Kitchell BB, Shand DG, Routledge PA (1982) Diazepam and lidocaine plasma protein binding in renal disease. Clin Pharmacol Ther 31:350–357

Halkin H, Meffin P, Melmon KL, Rowland M (1975) Influence of congestive heart failure on blood levels of lidocaine and its active monodeethylated metabolite. Clin Pharmacol Ther 17:669–676

Hansson E (1971) Absorption, distribution and excretion of local anesthetics. Int Encycl Pharmacol Ther 8:239–260

Hollunger G (1960) Some characteristics of an amide-hydrolysing microsomal enzyme before and after its solubilization. Acta Pharmacol Toxicol 17:384–389

Irestedt L, Andreen M, Belfrage P, Fagerstrom T (1978) The elimination of bupivacaine (Marcaine®) after short intravenous infusion in the dog: with special reference to the role played by the liver and lungs. Acta Anaesthesiol Scand 22:413–422

Jackson PR, Tucker GT, Woods HF (1982) Altered plasma drug binding in cancer: role of α_1-acid glycoprotein and albumin. Clin Pharmacol Ther 32:295–302

Jorfeldt L, Lewis DH, Lofstrom JB, Post C (1979) Lung uptake of lidocaine in healthy volunteers. Acta Anaesthesiol Scand 23:567–574

Keenaghan JB, Boyes RN (1972) The tissue distribution, metabolism and excretion of lidocaine in rats, guinea pigs, dogs and man. J Pharmacol Exp Ther 180:454–463

Ketterer SG, Wiegand BD, Rapaport E (1960) Hepatic uptake and biliary excretion of indocyanine green and its use in estimation of hepatic blood flow in dogs. Am J Physiol 199:481–484

Lalka D, Vicuna N, Burrow SR, Jones DJ, Ludden TM, Haegele KD, McNay JL (1978) Bupivacaine and other amide local anesthetics inhibit the hydrolysis of chloroprocaine by human serum. Anesth Analg 57:534–539

Lanks KW, Sklar GS (1980) Pseudocholinesterase levels and rates of chloroprocaine hydrolysis in patients receiving adequate doses of pholine iodide. Anesthesiology 52:434–435

Le Lorier J, Moisan R, Gagne J, Caille G (1977) Effect of the duration of infusion on the disposition of lidocaine in dogs. J Pharmacol Exp Ther 203:507–511

Lebeaux MI (1973) Experimental epidural anesthesia in the dog with lignocaine and bupivacaine. Br J Anaesth 45:549–555

Lebeaux M (1975) Sheep: a model for testing spinal and epidural anesthetic agents. Lab Anim Sci 25:629–633

Lennard MS, Bax NDS, Tucker GT, Woods HF (1978) Product-inhibition of hepatic lignocaine metabolism. Clin Sci Mol Med 55:5 p

Magno R, Berlin A, Karlsson K, Kjellmer I (1976) Anesthesia for cesarean section IV. Placental transfer and neonatal elimination of bupivacaine following epidural analgesia for elective cesarean section. Acta Anaesthesiol Scand 20:141–146

Mather LE, Thomas J (1978) Bupivacaine binding to plasma protein fractions. J Pharm Pharmacol 30:653–654

Mather LE, Tucker GT (1978) Pharmacokinetics and biotransformation of local anesthetics. Anesthesiol Clin 16:23–51

McNamara PJ, Slaughter RL, Visco JP, Elwood CM, Siegel JH, Lalka D (1980) Effect of smoking on binding of lidocaine to human serum proteins. J Pharm Sci 69:749–751

McNamara PJ, Slaughter RL, Pieper JA, Wyman MG, Lalka D (1981) Factors influencing serum protein binding of lidocaine in humans. Anesth Analg 60:395–400

Meffin P, Thomas J (1973) The relative rates of formation of the phenolic metabolites of mepivacaine in man. Xenobiotica 3:625–632

Meffin P, Robertson AV, Thomas J, Winkler J (1973) Neutral metabolites of mepivacaine in humans. Xenobiotica 3:191–196

Mihaly GW, Moore RG, Thomas J, Triggs EJ, Thomas D, Shanks CH (1978) The pharmacokinetics of the anilide type local anesthetics in neonates: I. Lignocaine. Eur J Clin Pharmacol 13:143–152

Moore RG, Thomas J, Triggs EJ, Thomas DB, Burnard ED, Shanks CA (1978) The pharmacokinetics and metabolism of the anilide local anesthetics in neonates: III. Mepivacaine. Eur J Clin Pharmacol 14:203–212

Morgan DH, McQuillan D, Thomas J (1978) Pharmacokinetics and metabolism of the anilide type local anesthetics in neonates: II. Etidocaine. Eur J Clin Pharmacol 13:365–371

Morgan DJ, Smyth MP, Thomas J, Vine J (1977) Cyclic metabolites of etidocaine in humans. Xenobiotica 7:365–375

Morgan DJ, Koay BB, Paull JD (1982) Plasma protein binding of etidocaine during pregnancy and labor. Eur J Clin Pharmacol 22:451–458

Morishima HO, Finster M, Pedersen AL, Fukunaga A, Ronfeld RA, Vassallo HG, Covino BG (1979) Pharmacokinetics of lidocaine in fetal and neonatal lambs and adult sheep. Anesthesiology 50:431–436

Nation RL, Triggs EJ, Selig M (1977) Lignocaine kinetics in cardiac patients and aged subjects. Br J Clin Pharmacol 4:439–448

O'Brien JE, Abbey V, Hinsvark O, Perel J, Finster M (1979) Metabolism and measurement of chloroprocaine, an ester-type local anesthetic. J Pharm Sci 68:75–78

Ochs HR, Carstens G, Greenblatt DJ (1980) Reduction in lidocaine clearance during continuous infusion and by co-administration of propranolol. N Engl J Med 303:373–377

Pedersen H, Morishima HO, Finster M, Arthur GR, Covino BG (1982) Pharmacokinetics of etidocaine in fetal and neonatal lambs and adult sheep. Anesth Analg 61:104–108

Piafsky KM, Knoppert D (1978) Binding of local anesthetics to α_1-acid glycoprotein. Clin Res 26:836 A

Post C, Andersson RGG, Rynfeldt A, Nilsson E (1979) Physico-chemical modification of lidocaine uptake in rat lung tissue. Acta Pharmacol Toxicol 44:103–109

Price HL, Kovnat PJ, Safer JM, Conner EH, Price ML (1960) The uptake of thiopental by body tissues and its relation to the duration of narcosis. Clin Pharmacol Ther 1:16–22

Raj PP, Ohlweiler D, Hitt BA, Denson DD (1980) Kinetics of local anesthetic esters and the effects of adjuvant drugs on 2-chloroprocaine hydrolysis. Anesthesiology 53:307–314

Reidenberg MM, James M, Dring LG (1972) The rate of procaine hydrolysis in serum of normal subjects and diseased patients. Clin Pharmacol Ther 13:279–284

Reynolds F (1971) Metabolism and excretion of bupivacaine in man: a comparison with mepivacaine. Br J Anaesth 43:23–37

Rothstein P, Arthur GR, Feldman H, Barash PG, Kopf G, Sudan N, Covino BG (1982) Pharmacokinetics of bupivacaine in children following intercostal block. Anesthesiology 5:A 426

Rothstein P, Arthur GR, Feldman HS, Covino BG (1983) The lung modifies arterial concentrations of bupivacaine in humans. Reg Anesth 8:44

Routledge PA, Barchowsky A, Bjornsson TD, Kitchell BB, Shand DG (1980) Lidocaine plasma protein binding. Clin Pharmacol Ther 27:347–351

Routledge PA, Shand DG, Barchowsky A, Wagner G, Stargel WW (1981 a) Relationship between alpha 1-acid glycoprotein and lidocaine disposition in myocardial infarction. Clin Pharmacol Ther 30:154–157

Routledge PA, Stargel WW, Kitchell BB, Barchowsky A, Shand DG (1981 b) Sex-related differences in the plasma protein binding of lignocaine and diazepam. Br J Clin Pharmacol 11:245–250

Sawyer DR, Ludden TM, Crawford MH (1981) Continuous infusion of lidocaine in patients with cardiac arrhythmias. Unpredictability of plasma concentrations. Arch Intern Med 141:43–45

Scott DB, Jebson PJR, Braid DP, Ortengren B, Frisch P (1972) Factors affecting plasma levels of lignocaine and prilocaine. Br J Anaesth 44:1040–1049

Seifen AB, Ferrari AA, Seifen EE, Thompson DS, Chapman J (1979) Pharmacokinetics of intravenous procaine infusion in humans. Anesth Analg 58:382–386

Shand DG, Kornhawer DM, Wilkinson GR (1975) Effects of route of administration and blood flow on hepatic drug elimination. J Pharmacol Exp Ther 195:424–432

Thomas J, Meffin P (1972) Aromatic hydroxylation of lidocaine and mepivacaine in rats and humans. J Med Chem 15:1046–1049

Thomas J, Morgan D, Vine J (1976) Metabolism of etidocaine in man. Xenobiotica 6:39–48

Thompson PD, Rowland M, Melmon K (1971) Influence of heart failure, liver disease and renal failure on the disposition of lidocaine in man. Am Heart J 82:417–421

Triggs EJ, Nation RL, Long A, Ashley JJ (1975) Pharmacokinetics in the elderly. Eur J Clin Pharmacol 8:55–62

Tucker GT, Boas RA (1971) Pharmacokinetic aspects of intravenous regional anesthesia. Anesthesiology 34:538–549

Tucker GT, Mather LE (1975) Pharmacokinetics of local anesthetic agents. Br J Anaesth 47:213–224

Tucker GT, Mather LE (1979) Clinical pharmacokinetics of local anesthetics. Clin Pharmacokinet 4:241–278

Tucker GT, Boyes RN, Bridenbaugh PO, Moore DC (1970) Binding of anilide-type local anesthetics in humans plasma: I. Relationships between binding, physicochemical properties anesthetic activity. Anesthesiology 33:287–303

Tucker GT, Wiklund L, Berlin-Wahlen A, Mather LE (1977) Hepatic clearance of local anesthetics in man. J Pharmacokinet Biopharm 5:111–122

Vine J, Morgan D, Thomas D (1978) The identification of eight hydroxylated metabolites of etidocaine by chemical ionization mass spectrometry. Xenobiotica 8:509–513

Wiklund L (1977a) Human hepatic blood flow and its relation to systemic circulation during intravenous infusion of lidocaine. Acta Anaesthesiol Scand 21:148–160

Wiklund L (1977b) Human hepatic blood flow and its relation to systemic circulation during intravenous infusion of bupivacaine and etidocaine. Acta Anaesthesiol Scand 21:189–199

Wood M, Wood AJ (1981) Changes in plasma drug binding and alpha 1 acid glycoprotein in mother and newborn infant. Clin Pharmacol Ther 29:522–526

Wyler F (1974) Effect of general anesthesia on distribution of cardiac output and organ blood flow in the rabbit: halothane and chloralose-urethane. J Surg Res 17:381–386

CHAPTER 6

Toxicity and Systemic Effects of Local Anesthetic Agents

B. G. COVINO

The primary pharmacological action of local anesthetic agents is the inhibition of the excitation conduction process in peripheral nerves. However, the ability of these agents to stabilize membranes is not limited to peripheral nerves. Any excitable membranes such as exist in heart, brain, neuromuscular junction will be altered by local anesthetic agents if they achieve a sufficient tissue concentration. Regional anesthesia which is properly performed usually does not result in blood levels of local anesthetics which are sufficient to cause systemic effects. However, the accidental intravascular injection or the use of an excessive extravascular amount of local anesthetics can result in blood and tissue levels which will cause profound systemic effects. Most of the systemic effects of local anesthetic agents are considered to be undesirable and toxic in nature. However, some actions have proven to be of therapeutic value. For example, the effect of lidocaine on cardiac membranes is responsible for the efficacy of this agent in the treatment of ventricular dysrhythmias (ROSEN et al. 1975). The effect of various local anesthetics on membrane structures in the brain have also proven to be of therapeutic value in the treatment of epilepsy (BERNHARD and BOHN 1965). In general, the primary systemic effects of local anesthetic agents are manifest in the central nervous system and the cardiovascular system.

A. Effects on the Central Nervous System

The central nervous system appears to be particularly susceptible to the systemic actions of local anesthetic agents (SCOTT 1981). Since these agents are relatively small molecular compounds, they readily cross the blood brain barrier and can effect neuronal structures in the brain. A detailed description of the CNS effects of local anesthetic agents has been presented in another chapter in this text (p. 253). The following is a description of the general CNS effects of local anesthetics in animals including man and the comparative effects of various local anesthetic agents on the central nervous system (COVINO and VASSALLO 1976). Initially, local anesthetic agents produce signs of CNS excitation. Human volunteers receiving intravenous infusions of local anesthetics describe feelings of lightheadedness and dizziness followed frequently by visual and auditory disturbances such as difficulty in focusing, and tinnitus. Other subjective CNS symptoms include disorientation and occasional feelings of drowsiness. Objective signs of an excitatory CNS effect include shivering, muscular twitching and tremors initially involving muscles of the face and distal parts of the extremities. Ultimately, generalized convulsions of a tonic-clonic nature occur. If a sufficiently large dose of a local anesthetic agent is administered systemically, the initial signs of CNS excitation are rapidly followed by a state of generalized CNS depression. Seizure activity ceases and respiratory depression and ultimately respiratory arrest occur.

Attempts have been made to correlate electroencephalographic changes with the subjective and objective signs of CNS activity following administration of local anesthetic agents. In some subjects, the appearance of slow waves on the EEG and increased amount of delta theta-activity and a decreased alpha-activity have been correlated with early signs of CNS stimulation (DE JONG 1977). In general, however, there does not appear to be a good correlation between changes in EEG-activity and subjective symptoms of CNS excitation. Animals studies have been carried out to determine the effect of local anesthetics on the EEG. The amygdala shows the most consistent changes in activity following the administration of local anesthetic agents in doses sufficient to cause CNS effects. Lidocaine has been shown to produce an electrical pattern described as rhythmic spindling prior to the development of overt convulsions (WAGMAN et al. 1968). Slow, high voltage cortical activity appears after the onset of changes in the amygdala. At the time of generalized convulsions in animals, amygdaloid spike-spindle complexes, spiking, and finally ictal episodes of a generalized nature have been observed on the EEG (WAGMAN et al. 1968). As the effect of the local anesthetic on the CNS passes from an excitatory to a depressant phase, electroencephalographic evidence of seizure activity disappears and a flat brain wave pattern consistent with generalized central nervous system depression is observed. SEO et al. (1982) have described a tetraphasic action of intravenous lidocaine on CNS electrical activity and behavior in awake cats. An inital phase of diffuse EEG slowing and a decrease of reticular neuronal firing was associated with signs of behavior depression. This was followed by a second stage of low-voltage fast-wave EEG changes and an increase of reticular neuronal firing which correlated with symptoms of agitation and/or catatonic behavior. Next, slow-waves were again observed on the EEG and a decrease in reticular neuronal firing which was associated with behavior depression. Finally, an epileptiform EEG pattern occurred with increased reticular neuronal firing at the time of tonic-clonic convulsions.

The mechanism by which local anesthetic agents produce an initial state of CNS excitation followed by generalized CNS depression has been elucidated by several investigators (TANAK and YAMASAKI 1966; DE JONG et al. 1967; HUFFMAN and YIM 1969). As indicated previously, electroencephalographic studies have indicated that the amygdala appears to be particularly sensitive to the excitatory effect of local anesthetic agents. Unilateral focal discharges have been observed in the amygdala following administration of lidocaine or prilocaine into the common carotid artery of the dog (ENGLESSON et al. 1962). Moreover, bilateral ablation of the amygdaloid areas in rats prevented the development of seizures following the injection of cocaine (EIDELBERG et al. 1965). As a result of these studies, several authors have postulated that local anesthetic agents may concentrate in the amygdala due either to enhanced vascular perfusion of this area, or due to the selective uptake of local anesthetics by small neurons in this area. The more commonly accepted mechanism for the excitatory effect of local anesthetics in the brain involves the selective blockade of inhibitory pathways in the cerebral cortex. The specific sites of action may involve either inhibitory cortical synapses or inhibitory cortical neurons. The CNS effect of local anesthetics is not believed to be related to inhibitory neurohumoral agents such as gamma-aminobutyric acid since lidocaine did not block the inhibitory effects of gamma-aminobutyric acid, nor the release of this agent in cortical neurons obtained from the brain of cats (WARNICK et al. 1971). The possible interaction of local anesthetics and other biogenic amines in the brain has also been investigated. Cocaine has the ability to increase the level of norepinephrine stores in brain tissue by blocking the reuptake of norepinephrine by storage granules (GORDON 1968). However, none of the other local anesthetic agents appear to possess this property. Thus, the possibility that elevated levels of norepinephrine in the brain are responsible for the excitatory effect of local anesthetic agents does not appear tenable. The initial inhibition of inhibitory pathways by local anesthetic agents would allow facilatory neurons to function in an unopposed fashion which would result in an increase in excitatory activity leading to convulsions. Following an increase in the dose of local anesthetics administered, these agents would then tend to inhibit both inhibitory and facilatory pathways resulting in a generalized state of CNS depression.

Considerable quantitative differences exist in terms of the dose of different local anesthetic agents required for excitation of the central nervous system followed by depression. In general, the dose of a local anesthetic agent administered intravenously and the blood level of this agent at which signs and symptoms of CNS excitation and overt convulsions occur is directly related to the intrinsic anesthetic potency of the particular agent (Table 1). For example, in cats procaine was least potent in terms of CNS activity. A dose of approximately 35 mg/kg was required to cause convulsions (ENGLESSON 1973). On the other hand, bupivacaine was the most potent agent studied in terms of CNS activity with convulsions occurring at a mean dose of 5 mg/kg. Lidocaine, mepivacaine, and prilocaine were agents of intermediate potency with regard to the dose required to produce con-

Table 1. Relative in vivo local anesthetic potency and intravenous convulsant dose (CD_{100}) of various agents in animals

Agents	Relative anesthetic potency	CD_{100} (mg/kg)			
		Cats[a]	Dogs[b]	Monkey[c]	Rabbit[d]
Procaine	1	35	–	–	15
Chloroprocaine	1	–	–	–	–
Mepivacaine	2	18	–	18	–
Prilocaine	2	22	–	18	–
Lidocaine	2	15	22	14–22	6
Etidocaine	6	–	8	5	–
Bupivacaine	8	5	5	4	–
Tetracaine	8	–	4	–	3

[a] ENGLESSON (1973).
[b] LIU et al. (1982).
[c] MUNSON et al. (1970, 1975).
[d] SOREL and LEJEUNE (1955).

vulsive activity. Comparison of the intrinsic anesthetic potency of these local anesthetics indicates that a correlation does exist between the ability of the compound to suppress conduction in peripheral nerve and the ability to cause CNS excitation (see Table 1). Bupivacaine is approximately 8 times more potent than procaine when used for production of regional anesthesia and approximately 7 times more toxic than procaine with regard to the dose required to produce convulsive activity in cats. A similar study in dogs indicated that a dose of approximately 20 mg/kg of lidocaine was required to produce convulsions compared to doses of 8 mg/kg for etidocaine and 5 mg/kg of bupivacaine (LIU et al. 1983). Thus, the relative CNS toxicity of bupivacaine, etidocaine and lidocaine is approximately 4:2:1 which is similar to the relative potency of these agents for the production of regional anesthesia in man.

A comparison of the blood level of various local anesthetic agents associated with CNS excitation and convulsions and the relative anesthetic potency of the various compounds again reveals that a correlation exists between CNS toxicity and local anesthetic activity (Fig. 1). Studies in monkeys have shown that bupivacaine produces convulsions at a blood level of approximately 4.5 µg/ml whereas lidocaine induced convulsions were observed at a mean blood level of 25 µg/ml (MUNSON et al. 1975). Studies in man in which blood levels of local anesthetics have been determined at the time of subjective symptoms of CNS excitation in volunteers or frank convulsions occurring during the accidental intravenous injection of local anesthetics in patients have also shown that a correlation exists between the local anesthetic activity of these agents and their effect on the CNS (Table 2).

Some qualitative differences in CNS activity may exist between the various local anesthetic agents. Although all of the agents can cause convulsions, the type of CNS event that precedes convulsive activity may vary depending on the specific local anesthetic agent. For example, lidocaine and procaine have been reported

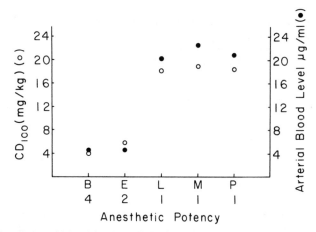

Fig. 1. Dose (mg/kg) and blood level (µg/kg) of various local anesthetics required for production of convulsions in monkeys. *B* bupivacaine, *E* etidocaine, *L* lidocaine, *M* mepivacaine, *P* prilocaine. Data derived from MUNSON et al. (1970, 1975)

to cause sedative like symptoms of drowsiness and temporary loss of consciousness prior to the onset of convulsive activity. Electroencephalographic recordings in monkeys treated with lidocaine have indicated that a characteristic preconvulsive pattern of diffuse slowing and irregular appearance of large spontaneous spikes and slow waves leading directly into general seizure activity may occur (MUNSON et al. 1975). Other local anesthetic agents such as mepivacaine, bupivacaine and etidocaine have not been reported to cause drowsiness in patients prior to the onset of CNS excitation. These agents did not produce any distinctive preconvulsive EEG changes in monkeys. The only EEG alteration observed following the administration of mepivacaine, bupivacaine and etidocaine was a generalized seizure pattern at the time of overt convulsions. The results indicate that the potential use of an electroencephalograph to detect impending central nervous system toxicity due to local anesthetics is of limited value since little or no EEG alterations occur prior to the onset of convulsive activity.

The acid base status of animals and patients can markedly effect the CNS activity of local anesthetic agents (ENGLESSON 1973). Studies in cats have shown that the convulsive threshold of various local anesthetics is inversely related to the arterial pCO_2 level (Table 3). The convulsive threshold dose of procaine was de-

Table 2. Comparative anesthetic potency of various local anesthetic agents and dose to produce symptoms of CNS toxicity in man

Agent	In vivo anesthetic potency	IV dose for CNS symptoms (mg/kg)	
		Data from FOLDES et al. (1965)	Data from SCOTT et al. (1975)
Procaine	1	19.2	–
Chloroprocaine	1	22.8	–
Lidocaine	2	6.4	>4
Mepivacaine	2	9.8	–
Prilocaine	2	–	>6
Etidocaine	6	–	3.4
Bupivacaine	8	–	1.6
Tetracaine	8	2.5	–

Table 3. Effect of pCO_2 on the convulsive threshold (CD_{100}) of various local anesthetics in cats. Data derived from ENGLESSON (1973)

Agent	CD_{100} (mg/kg)		% change in CD_{100}
	pCO_2 25–40 Torr	pCO_2 65–81 Torr	
Procaine	35	17	51
Mepivacaine	18	10	44
Prilocaine	22	12	45
Lidocaine	15	7	53
Bupivacaine	5	2.5	50

creased from approximately 35 mg/kg–17 mg/kg when the pCO_2 was elevated from 25–40 Torr to 65–81 Torr. Similarly, the convulsive threshold of mepivacaine, prilocaine, lidocaine, and bupivacaine were decreased to a similar extent when the pCO_2 was elevated. A direct relationship exists between arterial pH and the convulsive threshold of local anesthetic agents. A decrease in arterial pH is associated with a decrease in the convulsive threshold of these agents. The relationship between pCO_2, pH and the CNS activity of local anesthetic agents has been evaluated (ENGLESSON 1973). Respiratory acidosis with a resultant increase in pCO_2 and a decrease in arterial pH will consistently decrease the convulsant threshold of local anesthetic agents. However, and increase in pCO_2 in response to an elevated arterial pH as may occur during metabolic alkalosis exerts less of a potentiating effect on the CNS activity of local anesthetic agents. The relationship between pCO_2 and the effect of local anesthetics on the CNS may be due to several factors. An elevation of pCO_2 will enhance cerebral blood flow so that more anesthetic agent is delivered to the brain. In addition, the diffusion of CO_2 across the nerve membrane may result in a fall in intracellular pH. Local anesthetic agents which diffuse across the nerve membrane will then encounter an area of decreased pH which will tend to favor the conversion of the base form of local anesthetic agents to the cationic form. This will result in an increase in the intraneuronal level of the cationic form of the local anesthetic agent. The cationic form of local anesthetics does not diffuse well across the nerve membrane so that ionic trapping will occur, which will tend to potentiate the effect of local anesthetic agents on the central nervous system.

The effect of local anesthetic agents on the central nervous system is usually considered to be undesirable in nature. However, under certain conditions the depressant action of local anesthetics on the CNS has proven to be of therapeutic value. Studies in animals have demonstrated that procaine, lidocaine, and prilocaine are capable of preventing various forms of experimentally induced convulsions. Infiltration of exposed scalp wound margins with 30 mg of lidocaine or 60 mg of procaine significantly increases the threshold for electrically induced cortical afterdischarges in cats (JULIEN and DEMETRESCU 1974; DEMETRESCU and JULIEN 1974). Penicillin induced convulsive activity in cats has also been inhibited by infiltration of the scalp with lidocaine (JULIEN 1973). Production of audiogenic seizures or electrically induced cvonvulsions in mice have been successfully aborted with intraperitoneal injections of lidocaine and procaine (ESSMAN 1966). In general, local anesthetic agents are capable of suppressing hyperexcitable cortical neurons. The blood level of local anesthetics associated with suppression of hyperexcitable neurons is generally lower than the dose required to produce convulsive activity (DEMETRESCU and JULIEN 1974). For example, blood levels of 0.5–4 µg/ml of lidocaine have been shown to be effective in terminating seizures in cats in which epileptiform activity was produced by intracortical injections of penicillin. Lidocaine blood levels to 4.5–7 µg/ml produced an increase in EEG activity and frank seizures reoccurred when blood levels in excess of 7.5 µg/ml of lidocaine were achieved. The anticonvulsive properties of local anesthetics have been utilized clinically to terminate or decrease the duration of electrically induced seizures in patients (BERNHARD and BOHN 1965). Both procaine and lidocaine have been reported to be effective in terminating grand mal or petit mal seizures.

Again, in man the anticonvulsive dose of lidocaine was found to be significantly lower than the dose which caused seizure activity.

In summary, the local anesthetic agents are indeed capable of producing marked effects on the central nervous system. Under normal conditions signs of initial CNS excitation followed by CNS depression are considered to be toxic effects of local anesthetic drugs. However, in the presence of hyperexcitable cortical neurons such as may occur in an epileptic patient, the depressant effect of local anesthetics on these irritable foci may be therapeutic.

B. Effects on the Cardiovascular System

Local anesthetic agents can produce profound effects on the cardiovascular system. The systemic administration of these agents can exert a direct action both on cardiac muscle and on peripheral vascular smooth muscle. In general, the cardiovascular system appears to be more resistant to the effects of local anesthetic agents than the central nervous system (SCOTT 1981) (Table 4). Studies in dogs and sheep have indicated that doses of local anesthetic agents which cause significant cardiovascular effects are approximately 3 times higher than the dose of these agents which will have distinct effects on the central nervous system. For example, the blood level of lidocaine associated with convulsive activity in adult sheep was approximately 12 µg/ml (MORISHIMA et al. 1981). However, a blood level of approximately 30 µg/ml of lidocaine was required to produce significant transient hypotension. A comparison of the dose of various local anesthetic agents to cause convulsions in dogs and the dose required to cause irreversible cardiovascular changes indicated that the ratio of cardiovascular toxicity to CNS toxicity varied from 3.5–6.7 for lidocaine, etidocaine, tetracaine, and bupivacaine (LIU et al. 1982a, b). Although the studies presented above indicate a greater resistance of the cardiovascular system as compared to the central nervous system, they also show that local anesthetic agents administered systemically can cause profound effects on the cardiovascular system.

Table 4. Intravenous dose of local anesthetic agents required for convulsive activity (CD_{100}) and irreversible cardiovascular collapse (LD_{100}) in dogs. Data derived from LIU et al. (1982)

Agent	CD_{100}	LD_{100}	$LD_{100}/$ CD_{100} ratio
	mg/kg		
Lidocaine	22	76	3.5
Etidocaine	8	40	5.0
Bupivacaine	4	20	5.0
Tetracaine	5	27	5.4

I. Cardiac Effects

Electrophysiological studies on cardiac muscle have been carried out with various local anesthetics but particularly lidocaine due to the use of this agent for the treatment of ventricular arrhythmias (GETTES 1981, Table 5). A detailed description of the cardiac electrophysiological effects of local anesthetics is presented in Chap. 7.

Electrical conduction in the isolated whole rabbit heart has been determined following infusion of a variety of local anesthetic agents (BLOCK and COVINO 1982). All the agents produce a similar effect on conduction through various parts of the heart. A dose related decrease in atrial conduction velocity, atrio-ventricular conduction velocity, and ventricular conduction velocity has been observed. The AV node appears to be more resistant to the depressant effect of local anesthetics than atrial and ventricular tissue. A correlation exists between the potency of the various local anesthetic agents with regard to their anesthetic activity and the depression of cardiac conduction (Table 6). Thus, bupivacaine, etidocaine, and tetracaine, which are highly potent local anesthetics, tend to decrease conduc-

Table 5. Cardiac electrophysiological effects of lidocaine

	Sinus node	Atrial tissue	A-V node	Purkinje fiber ventricular muscle
Resting potential	–	–	–	–
Slow phase IV depolarization	–	–	–	–
Rapid phase 0 depolarization	–↓	–↓	–↓	↓↓
Action potential duration (APD)	–↓	–↓	–↓	↓↓
Effective refractory period (ERP)	–↑	–↑	–↑	↑↑
ERP/APD	–	–	–	↑
Conduction velocity	–↓	–↓	–↓	–↓

Table 6. Relationship between anesthetic potency of various local anesthetic agents and depression of conduction velocity (CV) in the isolated rabbit heart. Data derived from BLOCK and COVINO (1982)

Agent	Relative anesthetic potency	LA concentration (µg/ml)		
		50% ↓ Intra-atrial CV	25% ↓ AV nodal CV	50% ↓ His-Purkinje CV
Lidocaine	1	6.5	26.4	9.4
Prilocaine	1	10.4	24.8	27.5
Mepivacaine	1	8.9	25.8	6.9
Etidocaine	3	1.1	1.4	1.1
Bupivacaine	4	0.7	0.9	0.9
Tetracaine	4	0.4	0.9	0.5

tion velocity through various parts of the heart at relatively low concentrations. Whereas mepivacaine, lidocaine, and prilocaine require higher concentrations before significant decreases in cardiac conductivity are seen.

Electrophysiological studies in intact dogs and in man essentially reflect the findings observed in isolated cardiac tissue (LIEBERMAN et al. 1968; SUGIMOTO et al. 1969). As the dose and blood levels of lidocaine are increased, a prolongation of conduction time through various parts of the heart occurs. These are reflected in the electrocardiogram as an increase in the PR interval and QRS duration. Extremely high concentrations of local anesthetics will depress spontaneous pacemaker activity in the sinus node resulting in sinus bradycardia and sinus arrest. A similar depression at the AV node also occurs resulting in prolonged PR intervals and partial and complete AV dissociation.

In summary, the effect of local anesthetics on the electrophysiological properties of cardiac tissue are consistent with the action of these drugs on the electrophysiological events occurring in peripheral nerve. The inhibitory effect of these agents both on impulses in cardiac membrane and nerve membrane is related to a decrease in the rate of depolarization secondary to their blockade of sodium channels.

Local anesthetic agents also exert profound effects on the mechanical activity of cardiac muscle in addition to their effect on electrical activity. Detailed investigations on isolated cardiac tissues, isolated whole hearts, and intact animals have been carried out to elucidate the inotropic action of local anesthetic drugs. Studies on isolated atria from guinea pigs have shown that all local anesthetics essentially exert a dose dependent negative inotropic action (FELDMAN et al. 1982). The ability of local anesthetic agents to depress the contractility of cardiac muscle is proportional to their ability to suppress conduction in peripheral nerves. Thus, the more potent local anesthetic agents tent to depress cardiac contractility

Table 7. Comparative effect of various local anesthetic agents on cardiac contractility

Agent	LA concentrations (µg/ml) to produce 25%–50% Decrease in cardiac contractility	
	Isolated rabbit heart[a] (25%↓)	Isolated guinea pig atria[b] (50%↓)
Procaine	–	277
Chloroprocaine	–	102
Cocaine	–	56
Lidocaine	16.4	67
Prilocaine	11.7	42
Mepivacaine	9.9	55
Etidocaine	1.3	–
Bupivacaine	1.4	6
Tetracaine	0.9	6

[a] Data derived from BLOCK and COVINO (1982).
[b] Data derived from FELDMAN et al. (1982).

at lower doses and concentrations than the less potent local anesthetic agents (Table 7). In general, recent studies have suggested that local anesthetics can be divided into 3 groups in terms of their myocardial depressant effect. The more potent agents, bupivacaine, tetracaine, and etidocaine depress cardiac contractility at the lowest concentrations. The agents of moderate anesthetic potency, i.e., lidocaine, mepivacaine, prilocaine, chloroprocaine, and cocaine form an intermediate group of compounds in terms of their potency as myocardial depressants. Finally, procaine, which is the least potent of the local anesthetics, is also the least depressant in terms of decreasing contractility of atrial tissue. Studies on the isolated whole rabbit heart have essentially confirmed the results observed on isolated atria (BLOCK and COVINO 1982). Again, the more potent local anesthetics, bupivacaine, tetracaine, and etidocaine depress vetricular contractility by 25% at concentrations of approximately 1–1.5 µg/ml. On the other hand, lidocaine, mepivacaine, and prilocaine require concentrations of approximately 10–15 µg/ml to cause a similar decrease of 25% in the maximum rate of tension development (see Table 7).

Blood levels of local anesthetics which usually obtain following various regional anesthetic procedures rarely are associated with signs of myocardial depression and/or a decrease in cardiac output. However, following the accidental rapid intravenous administration of local anesthetics, or the administration of excessive doses decreases in myocardial contractility can occur. Studies in dogs in which a strain gauge arch was sutured to the right ventricle revealed that all local anesthetic agents evaluated were capable of exerting a negative inotropic action (STEWART et al. 1963). As in the isolated atrial and ventricular muscle studies, a relationship appeared to exist between the local anesthetic potency of various agents and their ability to decrease myocardial contractility in intact animals. For example, tetracaine is approximately 8–10 times more potent than procaine in man as a local anesthetic and similarly tetracaine was found to be approximately 8 times more potent as a depressant of myocardial contractility than procaine in intact dogs. Additional investigations have been conducted in closed-chest anesthetized dogs in which cardiac output has been measured by means of a thermodilution technique. The hemodynamic effect of the various clinically useful ester

Table 8. Effect of various local anesthetics on cardiac output in dogs. Data derived from LIU et al. (1982a, b)

Agent	Dose (mg/kg)		
	25%↓	50%↓	100%↓
Procaine	80	100	240
Chloroprocaine	20	30	60
Lidocaine	20	30	75
Mepivacaine	25	40	80
Prilocaine	25	40	80
Etidocaine	10	20	40
Bupivacaine	5	10	20
Tetracaine	10	20	26

and amide local anesthetics were compared (LIU et al. 1982 a, b). Statistically significant decreases in cardiac output were observed at doses of approximately 20 mg/kg of tetracaine, 40 mg/kg of chloroprocaine, and 100 mg/kg of procaine (LIU et al. 1982 a, Table 8). A similar study involving the amide local anesthetics revealed that the more potent amino-amides, bupivacaine and etidocaine, caused a marked decrease in cardiac output at doses of approximately 5–10 mg/kg, while the less potent local anesthetics, mepivacaine, prilocaine and lidocaine required doses of 10–30 mg/kg to cause a significant depression of cardiac output (LIU et al. 1982 b; see Table 8). The direct effect of lidocaine on myocardial contractility in patients under general anesthesia was evaluated by HARRISON et al. (1963) during thoracic surgical procedures. A strain gauge was sutured to the right ventricle for the recordcing of ventricular contractility. The intravenous administration of 2–4 mg/kg of lidocaine was associated with minimal change in right ventricular contractile force.

The mechanism by which local anesthetics depress myocardial contractility is not precisely known. The decrease in myocardial contractility may be secondary to the depressant effect on cardiac membranes. A more probable explanation for the negative inotropic action of local anesthetics is the interaction of local anesthetics with calcium. For example, it has been demonstrated that both procaine and tetracaine can increase the release of calcium from isolated skeletal muscle preparations (KUPERMAN et al. 1968). The relative potency of tetracaine and procaine in terms of their ability to increase the rate of calcium efflux from sartorius muscle was proportional also to their local anesthetic activity. A similar displacement of calcium from cardiac muscle would result in a decrease in myocardial contractility.

II. Peripheral Vascular Effects

Local anesthetic agents can exert significant effects on peripheral vascular smooth muscle. Both in vitro and in vivo studies have demonstrated that these agents have a biphasic action on smooth muscle of peripheral blood vessels (BLAIR 1975). In vitro preparations such as the isolated rat portal vein have been employed to demonstrate that local anesthetic drugs stimulate spontaneous myogenic contractions and augment basal tone at low concentrations. There did not appear to be a correlation between the anesthetic potency of various agents and their ability to stimulate vascular smooth muscle. For example, prilocaine produced the greatest enhancement of myogenic activity, while etidocaine was least effective. Prilocaine, mepivacaine, and procaine also caused the greatest increase in basal tone whereas minimal changes were seen with lidocaine, tetracaine, bupivacaine, and etidocaine. In vivo studies have confirmed this initial stimulatory effect of local anesthetic agents on vascular smooth muscle. For example, the intra-arterial administration of mepivacaine in human volunteers resulted in a decrease in forearm blood flow without any change in arterial pressure, which suggests that mepivacaine caused vasoconstriction which increases peripheral vascular resistance (JORFELDT et al. 1970). Similar studies with lidocaine also showed an increased tone in capacitance vessels with less consistent effect on resistance vessels. Animal studies in which vascular tone was reduced by alpha adrenergic blockade or by spinal cord section showed that hind limb vascular resistance increased following administration of mepivacaine and procaine.

An increase in contractility of vascular smooth muscle following the administration of local anesthetics is most apparent in the pulmonary vascular system. WOLLENBERGER and KRAYER (1948) originally reported that procaine markedly increased pulmonary vascular resistance in their Starling heart-lung preparation. This observation went relatively unnoticed until recent studies in intact dogs employing pulmonary artery catheters also showed that both the ester and amide agents can cause marked increases in pulmonary artery pressure and pulmonary vascular resistance (LIU et al. 1982 a, 1982 b). Increases in pulmonary artery pressure achieved statistical significance at doses of approximately 10–15 mg/kg of procaine, chloroprocaine, and tetracaine. Peak increases in pulmonary vascular resistance of approximately 300% were observed after administration of these 3 ester agents. Similar studies with the amide agents also revealed significant increases in pulmonary artery pressure at doses varying from 3–10 mg/kg of bupivacaine, etidocaine, mepivacaine, lidocaine, and prilocaine. Marked increases in pulmonary vascular resistance were observed with the various amide local anesthetics. Increases of 100%–200% in pulmonary vascular resistance were observed after the administration of 3 mg/kg of bupivacaine and etidocaine. The administration of 10 mg/kg doses of mepivacaine, lidocaine, and procaine resulted in increases in pulmonary vascular resistance of approximately 50%–100%.

As the dose of local anesthetic agent adminstered and the concentration of the agent to which the vascular smooth muscle is exposed increases, the stimulatory or vasoconstrictor action of these agents changes to one of inhibition and vasodilation. In vitro studies have shown that as the dose of local anesthetic agents is increased an inhibition of myogenic activity occurs. Studies of hind limb blood flow in dogs and cats following intraarterial administration of lidocaine, mepivacaine, prilocaine, and tetracaine reveal that an increase in blood flow occurs as the dose of these agents is increased (BLAIR 1975). Similar studies in man again have shown that lidocaine, mepivacaine, and bupivacaine can cause vasodilation and an increase in forearm blood flow, depending on the amount of drug administered (ABERG and DHUNER 1972). A comparison of the peripheral vascular effects of local anesthetic agents has failed to demonstrate a good correlation between the relative anesthetic potency of these agents and their ability to cause peripheral vasodilation. However, a correlation does appear to exist between the duration of action of these agents as local anesthetics and their duration of vasodilation. Thus, lidocaine, mepivacaine, and prilocaine cause a duration of peripheral vasodilation of approximately 5 min following intraarterial injection into the femoral artery of dogs. On the other hand, agents such as bupivacaine, etidocaine, and tetracaine which are long acting local anesthetics produce a prolonged period of vasodilation. The pulmonary vascular tree also will change from a state of vasoconstriction to one of vasodilation as the dose of local anesthetics is markedly increased. Thus, at doses of local anesthetics which approach lethal levels, decreases in pulmonary artery pressure and pulmonary vascular resistance were seen with both the ester and amide type local anesthetic agents (LIU et al. 1982 a, b).

The biphasic peripheral vascular effect of local anesthetic agents may be related to changes in smooth muscle concentrations of calcium. A competitive antagonism exists between local anesthetic drugs and calcium ions in smooth muscle (ABERG and ANDERSSON 1972). Local anesthetic compounds may displace calcium from membrane binding sites resulting in diffusion of this ion into the smooth muscle cytoplasm. Such an increase in cytoplasmic calcium concentration should stimulate the interaction between contractile proteins leading to an increase in myogenic tone which would produce a state of vasoconstriction. However, as the concentration of local anesthetic agent at the smooth muscle membrane is increased, the displacement of calcium by these agents will ultimately decrease both the cytoplasmic calcium concentration and the interaction between the contractile protein elements of smooth muscle, which will then result in a state of muscle relaxation leading to vasodilation. All of the local anesthetic agents which have been studied to date with the exception of cocaine appear to exert this biphasic effect on vascular smooth muscle. Cocaine is the only agent which produces a state of vasoconstriction at most doeses. Although direct blood flow studies in dogs have shown that the initial effect of cocaine is one of vasodilation, this is then followed by a long period of vasoconstriction regardless of the dose of cocaine administered (NISHIMURA et al. 1965). This unique property of cocaine is not related to a direct effect of cocaine itself on vascular smooth muscle, but is basically an indirect action of this agent. Cocaine has been shown to inhibit the uptake of norepinephrine by tissue binding studies. Thus, following the release of norepinephrine from postganglionic sympathetic fibers, the decrease in the reuptake of norepinephrine by tissue binding sites will result in an excess amount of free norepinephrine which will lead to a prolonged and profound state of vasoconstriction. This property of cocaine to inhibit the reuptake of norepinephrine has not been demonstrated to occur with other local anesthetics such as lidocaine and bupivacaine.

In summary, the sequence of cardiovascular events that usually occurs following the systemic administration of local anesthetic agents is as follows (Fig. 2): At relatively nontoxic blood levels of these agents, either no change in blood pressure or a slight increase in blood pressure may be observed. The slight increase in blood pressure may be related to a slight increase in cardiac output and heart rate which have been seen in some animal preparations and is believed due to an enhancement of sympathetic activity by these agents (KAO and JALAR 1959). In addition, the direct vasoconstrictor action of local anesthetics on certain peripheral vascular beds at low concentrations may be responsible in part for a slight increase in systemic blood pressure. As the blood level of local anesthetic agents approaches toxic concentrations, a fall in blood pressure is usually the first sign of a systemic effect on the cardiovascular system. Studies with both the ester and amide agents in intact dogs have demonstrated that the initial hypotension observed is probably not related to peripheral vasodilation and a subsequent decrease in peripheral vascular resistance. The initial hypotension appears to be correlated to the negative inotropic action of these agents which results in a decrease in cardiac output and stroke volume. The initial depression in blood pressure related primarily to a fall in cardiac output, is transient in nature and spontaneously reversible in most patients. However, if the amount of local anesthetic adminis-

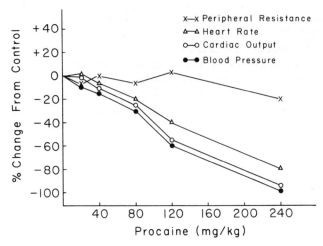

Fig. 2. Cardiovascular changes following progessive increases in dose of procaine in dogs. Data derived from Liu et al. (1982)

tered is excessive or if additional local anesthetic agent continues to be administered, then a profound and irreversible state of cardiovascular depression occurs. The profound hypotension and cardiovascular collapse seen prior to death is related not only to the negative inotropic action of the local anesthetics, but also to the profound peripheral dilation that these agents can produce due to their direct relaxant effect on vascular smooth muscle. At high concentrations the depressant effect of these agents on the excitability of cardiac tissue will also become evident as a decrease in sinus rate and AV conduction block. Ultimately, the combined peripheral vasodilation, decreased myocardial contractility and depressant effect on rate and conductivity will lead to cardiac arrest and circulatory collapse.

Most investigations have shown that a general relationship exists between the potency of various agents as local anesthetic drugs, and their depressant effect on the cardiovascular system. In recent years there has been some suggestion that the more potent highly lipid soluble and highly protein bound local anesthetic agents such as bupivacaine may be relatively more cardiotoxic than the less potent, less lipid soluble and protein bound local anesthetics, such as lidocaine (ALBRIGHT 1979). Several case reports have appeared in the literature in which bupivacaine and etidocaine were associated with rapid and profound cardiovascular depression (PRENTISS 1979; EDDE and DEUTSCH 1977). These cases differed from the usual cardiovascular depression seen with local anesthetics in several respects. The onset of cardiovascular depression occurred relatively early. In some cases severe cardiac arrhythmias were observed, and the cardiac depression appeared resistant to various therapeutic modalities. Studies in intact animals to evaluate the relative cardiovascular effects of various local anesthetics have been somewhat contradictory (Table 9). LIU et al. (1982a, b) have reported that cardiovascular depression produced by local anesthetic agents in anesthetized dogs is related to the potency of the various drugs. On the other hand, DEJONG and

Table 9. Comparative CNS (CD_{100}) and cardiovascular toxicity (LD_{100}) of lidocaine and bupivacaine or etidocaine in various animal species

Agent	Dogs[a]			Mice[b]			Sheep[c, d]		
	mg/kg		LD/CD ratio	mg/kg		LD/CD ratio	mg/kg		LD/CD ratio
	CD	LD		CD	LD		CD	LD	
Lidocaine	22	76	3.5	111	133	1.3	5.8	36.7	7.13
Bupivacaine	4	20	5.0	57	58	1.0	2.7	8.9	3.7
Etidocaine	8	40	5.0	–	–	–	2.21	9.36	4.44

[a] From LIU et al. (1983).
[b] From DE JONG et al. (1980).
[c, d] From MORISHIMA et al. (1983a, b)

Table 10. Effect of hypoxia, acidosis, and hypoxia-acidosis on rate and contractility of isolated guinea pig atria exposed to lidocaine ($50 \mu g/ml$) and bupivacaine ($5 \mu g/ml$). Data derived from SAGE et al. (1982)

Normal	Lidocaine		Bupivacaine	
	Rate	Contractile force	Rate	Contractile force
	% change		% change	
pO_2, pCO_2, pH	34	39	41	57
Hypoxia	45	62	36	47
Acidosis	44	47	65	65
Hypoxia and acidosis	27	45	66	71

BONIN have indicated that a narrow margin of safety exists in mice between the dose of bupivacaine to cause CNS toxicity and the dose to cause cardiovascular toxicity, as compared to lidocaine (DEJONG 1980, 1981). Studies in sheep have also suggested that less difference exists between the dose of etidocaine and bupivacaine required for production of CNS and cardiovascular toxicity as compared to an agent such as lidocaine (MORISHIMA et al. 1983a, b).

In 1982, DEJONG et al. reported that bupivacaine can induce cardiac arrhythmias in awake but paralyzed cats, whereas no such changes were observed with lidocaine. Studies in unanesthetized sheep have also demonstrated that severe cardiac arrhythmias occur following the rapid intravenous administration of bupivacaine while no cardiac irregularities were observed when lidocaine was given intravenously (KOTELKO et al. 1984). No cardiac arrhythmias were observed in the anesthetized dogs studied by LIU et al. (1982b). However, in unanesthetized dogs, convulsant or supraconvulsant intravenous doses of bupivacaine caused ventricular fibrillation in approximately 25% of the animals while no arrhythmias were seen with lidocaine (SAGE et al. 1983). The etiology of the bupivacaine induced ventricular arrhythmias remains to be clarified.

Changes in acid-base status will alter the potential cardiovascular toxicity of local anesthetic agents. As shown previously, hypercarbia and acidosis will decrease the threshold of local anesthetic agents for convulsive activity. Similarly, hypercarbia, acidosis and hypoxia will tend to increase the cardiodepressant effect of local anesthetic agents (SAGE et al. 1984). Studies on isolated atrial tissues have shown that hypercarbia, acidosis and hypoxia will tend to potentiate the negative chronotropic and inotropic action of lidocaine and bupivacaine. In particular, the combination of hypoxia and acidosis appear to markedly potentiate the cardiodepressant effects of bupivacaine (Table 10). It has been observed in some patients that marked hypercarbia, acidosis and hypoxia occurs very rapidly following seizure activity due to the rapid accidental intravascular injection of local anesthetic agents (MOORE et al. 1980). Thus, it has been postulated that the cardiovascular depression observed with the more potent agents such as bupivacaine may be related in part to the severe acid-base changes that occur following the administration of toxic doses of these agents.

C. Effects on the Neuromuscular Junction

As indicated previously, local anesthetic agents tend to exert a generalized stabilizing action on all excitable membranes. Therefore, it is not surprising that this class of agents has also been shown to exert discernable effects on the neuromuscular junction. Procaine, lidocaine, mepivacaine, prilocaine, and bupivacaine have all been shown to inhibit in vitro myoneural junction preparations and to block neuromuscular transmission in man at certain dosages (KATZ and GISSEN 1969; HIRST and WOOD 1971; GALINDO 1971). Although localized neuromuscular paralysis occurs following the intraarterial injection of local anesthetic drugs in man, minimal alterations in neuromuscular activity have been observed when these agents were administered intravenously. The inhibitory effect of local anesthetics at the neuromuscular junction may involve either pre- or postjunctional structures. GALINDO (1971) ascribed the depressant action of procaine at the myoneural junction to inhibition of the prejunctional motor nerve terminal. Other investigators have reported that local anesthetic agents either decrease the sensitivity of the postjunctional motor endplate to acetylcholine or block the depolarizing action of acetylcholine on the motor endplate (KATZ and GISSEN 1969; HIRST and WOOD 1971). Measurements of ionic conductances across the endplate membrane have demonstrated that procaine exerts a profound inhibitory effect on sodium flux suggesting that the basic action of local anesthetic agents is similar at all excitable membranes, i.e., a block of sodium channels in the cell membrane (DEGUCHI and NARAHASHI 1971). Local anesthetic agents do not appear to be sufficiently potent in terms of their neuromuscular blocking activity to represent a potential problem when they are used properly. A clinically significant degree of neuromuscular blockade may occur when local anesthetics are administered in the presence of classical neuromuscular blocking agents. For example, it has been shown that procaine and lidocaine can significantly enhance the action of both depolarizing and nondepolarizing types of myoneural blockers (KATZ and GISSEN 1969; TELIVUO 1967). The duration of apnea produced by succinylcholine or

curare can be considerable prolonged by lidocaine both in dogs and man (DE-
KORNFELD and STEINHAUS 1959; HALL et al. 1972). Since the depolarizing neuromuscular blocking agent, succinylcholine and the procaine-like amino ester local
anesthetics are both hydrolyzed by plasmacholinesterases, the combined use of
these agents may produce clinically significant effects. It has been observed in animals that prolonged apnea can occur following the combined administration of
succinylcholine and procaine (FOLDES et al. 1963). Thus, the interaction of local
anesthetics and neuromuscular blocking agents may be related to a combined effect at the myoneural junction and may also represent a competition for the same
enzyme system responsible for the hydrolysis of succinylcholine and amino-ester
local anesthetics.

D. Miscellaneous Effects

A variety of miscellaneous systemic actions have been ascribed to local anesthetic
drugs, most of which are related to the generalized membrane stabilizing property
of this class of drugs. For example, local anesthetics have been reported to possess
ganglionic blocking, anticholinergic, antihistaminic, and antibacterial activity.
There is little evidence to suggest that any of these miscellaneous effects are clinically significant under normal conditions.

Local anesthetics can influence respiration in a significant manner due to a direct effect on tracheo-bronchial smooth muscle. The action of local anesthetics
on airway smooth muscle is biphasic in nature similar to the effect on vascular
smooth muscle. WEISS et al. (1975) have reported that low concentrations of lidocaine produced contractures of isolated guinea pig trachealis muscle. Higher concentrations of lidocaine causes smooth muscle relaxation. In this preparation lidocaine in appropriate doses reversed histamine, acetylcholine and depolarizing
hypertonic potassium contractures (Fig. 3). Pretreatment of tracheal muscle in vitro shifted in a nonparallel fashion the dose response curves of histamine, acetylcholine, depolarizing potassium, and electrical stimulation. The authors suggested that the action of lidocaine represented a non-specific, reversible antagonism on smooth muscle that may involve an effect on calcium. A similar study
involving a comparison of procaine and lidocaine indicated that procaine exerted
a more potent spasmolytic effect than lidocaine which suggests that this action
of local anesthetics on airway smooth muscle does not correlate with the anesthetic potency of various agents (WANNA and GEIGIS 1978). Lidocaine also can

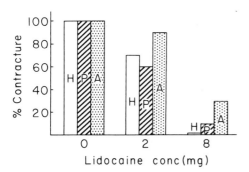

Fig. 3. Effect of lidocaine on tracheal
muscle. Histamine (*H*), potassium (*P*),
and accetylcholine (*A*) induced
contracture of isolated guinea pig
trachealis muscle before and after
treatment with lidocaine. Data derived
from WEISS et al. (1975)

inhibit anaphylactic-induced contractures in guinea pig tracheal muscle due to the blockade of histamine release. A bimodal effect of lidocaine was again observed. Low concentrations caused a slight release of histamine while higher concentrations inhibited histamine release (WEISS et al. 1978). On the basis of these in vitro studies, the potential use of lidocaine as a bronchodilator has been evaluated in man (WEISS and PATWARDHAN 1977). Little effect on various pulmonary function parameters was observed following the administration of 40 mg of lidocaine to normal volunteers. Subsequent attempts to utilize the spasmolytic property of local anesthetic agents in asthmatic subjects met with limited success. The aerosol administration of 40–100 mg of lidocaine in asthmatic patients caused a 20% fall in expiratory flow rates initially. In some subjects the initial response was followed by a further deterterioration in pulmonary function. On the other hand, approximately 50% of the patients manifested a significant improvement in airway resistance. The reason for this differential response of asthmatic patients to lidocaine ist not known.

The effect of local anesthetics on the respiratory center and the brain have already been described as part of the discussion concerning the effects of local anesthetics on the central nervous system. During the phase of CNS excitation prior to development of frank convulsions, an increased respiratory rate may be observed in patients. During the convulsive episode itself respiration appears to be severely depressed as indicated by the marked fall in pO_2, pH, and increase in pCO_2 observed by Moore. This may be related in part to the inability of convulsive patients to ventilate properly. The production of excess lactic acid due to contracting muscles, may also contribute to the rapid development of acidosis. Animal studies in dogs and sheep have shown that these animals tend to hyperventilate during convulsive activity such that little change in pO_2 and pCO_2 is seen. At doses of local anesthetic agents that cause complete CNS depression the respiratory center is significantly inhibited and respiratory arrest occurs prior to the advent of cardiovascular collapse.

E. Other Toxicological Effects

Reports of allergic reactions, hypersensitivity, or anaphylactic responses to local anesthetic agents appear periodically. Unfortunately, systemic toxic reactions to local anesthetic agents are frequently misdiagnosed as representing allergic or hypersensitivity type reactions. The amino-ester agents such as procaine have been shown to produce allergic type reactions. Since these agents are derivatives of paraminobenzoic acid which is known to be allergenic in nature, it is not unusual that a certain percentage of the population will demonstrate allergic reactions to this class of local anesthetics. The advent of the amino-amide local anesthetics which are not derivatives of parminobenzoic acid markedly changed the incidence of allergic type reactions to local anesthetic drugs. Toxic reactions of an allergic type to the amino-amides are extremely rare, although several cases have been reported in the literature in recent years which suggest that this class of agents can on rare occasions produce an allergic type phenomenon (BROWN et al. 1981). ALDRETE et al. (1970, 1971) employed a technique of intradermal injections to study

Table 11. Frequency of dermal reactions in patients exposed to various local anesthetic agents[a]

Agent	Non-allergic[a] patients (N = 60)	Allergic patients (N = 11)
NaCl	0	0
Procaine	20	8
Chloroprocaine	11	8
Tetracaine	25	8
Lidocaine	0	0
Mepivacaine	0	0
Prilocaine	0	0
Methylparaben	8 (16)	–

[a] From ALDRETE and JOHNSON (1970).

the frequency of allergic type responses to both amino-ester and amino-amide local anesthetics in patients with and without a presumptive history of local anesthetic allergy. Positive skin reactions were observed in 25 of 60 patients who did not describe any previous allergic symptomatology (Table 11). In all cases the cutaneous reactions occurred following the injection of an amino-ester type of agent such as procaine, tetracaine, and chloroprocaine. No cutaneous reactions occurred following the use of the amino-amide agents, namely lidocaine, mepivacaine, or prilocaine. 11 patients were studied who had a history of alleged local anesthetic allergy. 8 of these patients showed a positive skin reaction to procaine, tetracaine, or chloroprocaine. However, no positive cutaneous response was seen following the administration of lidocaine, mepivacaine, or prilocaine. No signs of systemic anaphylaxis occurred in any of the subjects. It should be remembered that although the amino-amide agents appear to be relatively free from allergic type reactions, solutions of these agents may contain a preservative, methylparaben, whose chemical structure is similar to that paraminobenzoic acid. It has been shown that patients in whom methylparaben was administered intradermally demonstrated a positive skin reaction (ALDRETE and O'HIGGINS 1971).

F. Treatment of Systemic Toxicity

Adverse reactions are usually due to an accidental intravascular injection of a local anesthetic agent. The severity and duration of the toxic reaction varies depending on the amount of drug administered and the specific agent which was employed. Convulsions which represent the most common adverse reaction associated with the local anesthetic agents are usually transient in nature. Convulsive activity in dogs developed within 2–3 min following the intravenous administration of a potent local anesthetic such as etidocaine (LIU et al. 1983). In contrast, approximately 20 min transpired before convulsions occurred in lidocaine treated dogs. The duration of convulsive activity was relatively short in these canine experiments, varying from 2.9 min in the etidocaine treated animals, to 5.2 min in the dogs in which tetracaine was administered. The onset and duration of toxic reactions is probably related to the physical-chemical and pharmacokinetic properties of the different drugs. Etidocaine is the most lipid soluble local anesthetic agent which may suggest a rapid penetration of brain tissue by this agent. On the other hand, local anesthetics which possess relatively short pharmacokinetic half-lives, such as prilocaine, lidocaine, chloroprocaine and etidocaine, will produce toxic reactions of shorter duration compared to agents such as bupivacaine which has a relatively long pharmacokinetic half-life.

The primary treatment of CNS toxicity is directed towards maintaining adequate ventilation. Therefore, every effort should be made to establish and maintain a patent airway. Ventilation should then be assisted or controlled with oxygen in order to prevent the development of hypoxia and acidosis. Frequently, no additional therapy is required since the convulsions are self-limiting. If CNS toxicity persists, the use of a central nervous system depressant drug is indicated. Intravenous diazepam (0.1–0.2 mg/kg) or a short-duration rapid-acting barbiturate such as thiopental (1–2 mg/kg) are most commonly employed to terminate persistent signs of CNS excitation. A rapid-acting short-duration neuromuscular blocking agent such as succinylcholine may also be employed to abort a state of generalized convulsions. In such a situation, the patient should be intubated in order to control respiration adequately.

Signs of cardiovascular depression require immediate therapy. Hypotension should be initially treated with intravenous fluids. Persistent hypotension requires the use of vasopressor agents. Phenylephrine or epinephrine are usually effective in reversing hypotension due to the administration of excessive doses of local anesthetic agents. Severe circulatory depression should be treated with agents which exert a positive inotropic action as well as a peripheral vasoconstrictor effect.

In those rare situations in which signs of dermal allergic reactions occur, administration of an intravenous antihistamine such as diphenylhydramine (50 mg) may prove useful. Immediate therapy should be applied if signs of anaphylaxis occur. Hypotension again requires the administration of vasopressor agents which possess a positive inotropic and a perpheral vasoconstrictor action. Bronchoconstriction may be treated with adrenergic bronchodilators such as epinephrine or terbutaline or xanthine derivatives like aminophylline. Steroids such as hydrocortisone may also be of value in the treatment of anaphylactic reactions.

Toxic reactions are best avoided by the use of proper precautions regarding dosage of the local anesthetic agent administered and avoidance of intravascular injections. Moreover, resuscitative-type equipment should always be readily available during the performance of regional anesthetic techniques in order to treat the occasional unavoidable adverse reaction that may occur.

G. Local Tissue Toxicity

Although the primary toxic effect of local anesthetic agents involves the systemic administration of excessive doses of these drugs, the potential local irritant action of this class of compounds has also been the subject of considerable interest. Local anesthetic agents which are employed clinically rarely produce localized nerve damage. Studies on isolated frog sciatic nerve revealed that concentrations of pro-

Table 12. Neurotoxicity of local anesthetics animal studies

Type of study	Investigator	Toxicity			
		2-CP	LIDO	BUP.	Other solns.
Rabbit	Barsa	+++	0	–	–
Rabbit sciatic nerve	Pizzolato	0	0	–	–
Rabbit vagus nerve	Gissen	0	–	–	+++
Spinal dog	Ravindran	+++	–	0	0
Spinal rabbit	Wang	+++	–	–	+++, 0
Spinal sheep	Rosen	+	+	0	+
Spinal monkey	Rosen	+	–	+	–

0 = No effect; + = Mild toxicity; +++ = Severe toxicity; – = Not studied

caine, cocaine, tetracaine, and dibucaine required to produce irreversible conduction blockade are far in excess of the concentration of these agents used clinically (SKOU 1954). A comparison of lidocaine, tetracaine, or etidocaine administered subdurally in rabbits revealed histopathological spinal cord changes following the use of 2% tetracaine which is considerably greater than the maximum concentration of 1% employed for spinal anesthesia in man (ADAMS et al. 1974). Recently, however, some concern has been expressed regarding the potential neurotoxicity of chloroprocaine. The possibility that this agent can cause localized neural damage is based on the report of prolonged sensory motor deficits in four patients following the epidural or subarachnoid injection of large doses of this particular drug (RAVINDRAN et al. 1980; REISNER et al. 1980). Subsequent studies in animals have proven somewhat contradictory regarding the potential neurotoxicity of chloroprocaine (Table 12). BARSA et al. (1982), employing an isolated rabbit vagus nerve preparation, reported that chloroprocaine was associated with signs of neural irritation, whereas the use of lidocaine under similar conditions failed to cause local toxic effects. However, histological examination of rabbit sciatic nerves exposed to chloroprocaine for a period of 6 h did not reveal any signs of histological damage (PIZZALATO and RENEGAR 1959). Investigations in dogs in which chloroprocaine and bupivacaine were administered intrathecally in doses sufficient to cause total spinal anesthesia demonstrated that chloroprocaine produced total paralysis in approximately 30% of the animals, whereas none of the bupivacaine treated dogs showed evidence of permanent neurological sequelae (RAVINDRAN et al. 1982). Studies of a similar nature in sheep and monkeys have failed to show any difference in neurotoxicity between chloroprocaine and other local anesthetics or control solutions (ROSEN et al. 1982). More recently, it has been reported that paralysis has been observed in rabbits in whom intrathecal chloroprocaine solutions were administered intrathecally (WANG et al. 1984). However, the paralysis was believed to be related to the sodium bisulfite which is employed as a antioxidant in chloroprocaine solutions. The use of pure solutions of chloroprocaine without sodium bisulfite did not cause paralysis whereas the sodium bisulfite alone was associated with paralysis. Detailed studies on isolated nerves indicate that the low pH and sodium bisulfite are probably responsible for the neurotoxicity associated with the use of chloroprocaine solutions. Cloroprocaine itself does not appear to be neurotoxic (GISSEN et al. 1984).

Skeletal muscle appears to be more sensitive to the local irritant properties of local anesthetic agents than other tissues. Skeletal muscle changes have been observed with most of the clinically used local anesthetic agents such as lidocaine, mepivacaine, prilocaine, bupivacaine, and etidocaine (BENOIT and BELT 1972; LIBELIUS et al. 1970). In general, the more potent longer acting agents such as bupivacaine and etidocaine appear to cause a greater degree of localized skeletal muscle damage than the less potent, shorter acting agents such as lidocaine and prilocaine. This effect on skeletal muscle is reversible and muscle regeneration occurs rapidly and is complete within 2 weeks following injection of local anesthetic agents. These changes in skeletal muscle have not been correlated with any overt clinical signs of local irritation. However, an increase in blood levels of creatinine phosphokinase have been reported following the intramuscular administration of lidocaine which is indicative of skeleton muscle damage (ZENER and HARRISON 1974).

H. Summary

The toxicity of local anesthetic agents can be divided into basically 3 categories. (1) Systemic toxic reactions due usually to accidental intravascular injections or the administration of excessive doses of these agents. (2) Allergic or hypersensitivity type reactions (3) Local tissue toxicity. The systemic toxicity of local anesthetic agents is primarily related to the effect of this class of compounds on excitable membranes. In general, local anesthetic agents tend to stabilize excitable membranes. The primary clinical utility of these agents is related to their ability to stabilized membranes of peripheral nerve leading to conduction blockade and a localized state of analgesia. However, the administration of excessive doses resulting in high blood and tissue levels of these agents can cause similar effects on neuronal membranes in the brain. Inhibition of inhibitory fibers occurs initially resulting in signs of CNS excitation and convulsive activity. An increase in the dose and concentration of local anesthetics will result in a depressant effect on facilitory neurons which ultimately leads to a generalized state of CNS depression. Local anesthetic agents also can exert toxic effects on the cardiovascular system. In general, the cardiovascular system is more resistant to the toxic actions of local anesthetics than is the central nervous system. However, if sufficient doses and blood levels of local anesthetics are achieved, signs of profound cardiovascular depression may be observed. Local anesthetics can depress the rate of depolarization of cardiac membranes and can exert a negative chronotropic and inotropic action on the heart. In addition, these agents can cause profound peripheral vascular dilation resulting in profound irreversible circulatory collapse.

Allergic reactions to local anesthetic agents are relatively rare. They tended to occur more frequently when the amino-ester agents were used almost exclusively, and were related to the formation of paraminobenzoic acid following the hydrolysis of the amino-ester local anesthetics. The amino-amide local anesthetic agents are not derivatives of paraminobenzoic acid and are rarely associated with allergic type phenomena.

Finally, local tissue toxicity can occur following the administration of these agents. Skeletal muscle appears to be particularly susceptible to the local irritant properties of local anesthetic agents. However, the skeletal muscle damage observed following the administration of local anesthetics is transient and reversible in nature. Of greater concern is the potential local neurotoxicity of local anesthetic agents. In general, neural tissue appears to be relatively resistant tot the irritant effects of local anesthetic drugs. However, if employed in sufficiently large concentrations or administered in large dosages, local anesthetics may cause evidence of neural damage.

In general, the incidence of toxic reactions to local anesthetic agents is extremely low considering the fact that this class of drugs actually possesses a therapeutic ratio which is lower than would normally be considered clinically desirable. However, since these drugs are administered into a circumscribed area of the body usually by a trained physician, the frequency of adverse reactions is quite low. Epidemiological studies have been reported involving large numbers of patients in whom regional anesthesia has been performed. For example, studies of epidural and spinal anesthesia in which more than 10,000 patients per study were evaluated, demonstrated a frequency of complications associated with the anesthetic procedure of 0.3%–1.5% (LUND 1962; MOORE and BRIDENBAUGH 1966). A review of the world literature on epidural anesthesia by Dawkins in 1969 showed that the frequency of toxic reactions was 0.2% of 60,000 patients included in the study. Thus, local anesthetic agents are a relatively safe and efficacious group of chemical compounds provided that the individual administering the drug is aware of the pharmacological properties of these agents and is skilled in the performance of regional anesthetic techniques.

References

Aberg G, Andersson R (1972) Studies on mechanical actions of mepivacaine (Carbocaine) and its optically active isomers on isolated smooth muscle: role of Ca^{2+} and cyclic AMp. Acta Pharmacol Toxicol 31:321–336

Aberg G, Dhuner KG (1972) Effects of mepivacaine (Carbocaine) on femoral blood flow in the dog. Acta Pharmacol Toxicol 31:267–272

Adams HJ, Mastri AR, Eichholzer A, Kilpatrick G (1974) Morphologic effects of intrathecal etidocaine and tetracaine on the rabbit spinal cord. Anesth Analg 53:904–908

Albright GA (1979) Cardiac arrest following regional anesthesia with etidocaine or bupivacaine. Anesthesiology 51:285–287

Aldrete JA, Johnson DA (1970) Evaluation of intracutaneous testing for investigation of allergy to local anesthetic agents. Anesth Analg 49:173–181

Aldrete JA, O'Higgins JW (1971) Evaluation of patients with history of allergy to local anesthetic drugs. South Med J 64:1118–1121

Barsa JE, Batra M, Fink BR, Sumi SM (1982) Prolonged neural blockade following regional analgesia with 2-chloroprocaine. Anesth Analg 61:961–967

Benoit PW, Belt WD (1972) Some effects of local anesthetic agents on skeletal muscle. Exp Neurol 345:264–278

Bernhard CG, Bohn E (1965) Local anaesthetics as anticonvulsants. A study on experimental and clinical epilepsy. Almqvist and Wiksell, Stockholm

Blair MR (1975) Cardiovascular pharmacology of local anaesthetics. Br J Anaesth 47:247–252

Block A, Covino BG (1982) Effect of local anesthetic agents on cardiac conduction and contractility. Reg Anesth 6:55–61

Brown DT, Beamish D, Wildsmith JAW (1981) Allergic reaction to an amide local anaesthetic. Br J Anaesth 53:435–437

Covino BG, Vassallo HG (1976) Local anesthetics. Mechanism of action and clinical use. Grune and Stratton, New York

Dawkins CJM (1969) An analysis of the complications of extradual and caudal block. Anaesthesia 24:554–563

Deguchi T, Narahashi T (1971) Effects of procaine on ionic conductances of end-plate membranes. J Pharmacol Exp Ther 176:423–433

DeJong RH (1977) Local anesthetics, 2nd ed. Thomas, Springfield

DeJong JA, Bonin JD (1980) Deaths from local anesthetic-induced convulsions in mice. Anesth Analg 59:401–405

DeJong JA, Bonin JD (1981) Mixtures of local anesthetics are no more toxic than the parent drugs. Anesthesiology 54:177–181

DeJong RH, Wagman IH, Prince DA (1967) Effect of carbon dioxide on the cortical seizure threshold to lidocaine. Exp Neurol 17:221–232

DeJong RH, Ronfeld RA, DeRosa RA (1982) Cardiovascular effects of convulsant and supraconvulsant doses of amide local anesthetics. Anesth Analg 61:3–9

DeKornfeld TJ, Steinhaus JE (1959) The effect of intravenously administered lidocaine and succinylcholine on the respiratory activity of dogs. Anesth Analg 38:173

Demetrescu M, Julien RM (1974) Local anesthesia and experimental epilepsy. Epilepsia 15:235

Edde RR, Deutsch S (1977) Cardiac arrest after interscalene brachial plexus block. Anesth Analg 55:446–447

Eidelberg E, Neer HM, Miller MK (1965) Anticonvulsant properties of some benzodiazepine derivatives. Neurology (Minneap) 15:223–230

Englesson S (1973) The influence of acid-base changes on central nervous system toxicity of local anaesthetic agents. Dissertation, Faculty of medicine, University of Uppsala

Englesson S, Eriksson E, Wahlqvist S, Ortengren B (1962) Differences in tolerance to intravenous Xylocaine and Citanest (L67), a new local anesthetic. A double blind study in man. Proc 1st Eur Congr Anesthesiol 2:206–209

Essman WB (1966) Anticonvulsive properties of Xylocaine in mice susceptible to audiogenic seizures. Arch Int Pharmacodyn Ther 164:376

Feldman HS, Covino BM, Sage DJ (1982) Direct chronotropic and inotropic effects of local anesthetic agents in isolated guinea pig atria. Reg Anaesth 7:149–156

Foldes FF, Foldes VM, Smith JC, Zsigmond EG (1963) The relation between plasma cholinesterase and prolonged apnea caused by succinylcholine. Anesthesiology 24:208–216

Foldes FF, Davidson GM, Duncalf D, Kuwabara J (1965) The intravenous toxicity of local anesthetic agents in man. Clin Pharmacol Ther 6:328–335

Galindo A (1971) Procaine, pentobarbital and halothane: effects on the mammalian myoneural junction. J Pharmacol Exp Ther 177:360–368

Gettes LS (1981) Physiology and pharmacology of antiarrhythmic drugs. Hosp Pract 16:89–101

Gissen AJ, Datta S, Lambert D (1984) The chloroprocaine controversy: II. Is chloroprocaine neurotoxic? Reg Anesth 9:135–145

Gordon HR (1968) Fetal bradycardia after paracervical block. Correlation with fetal and maternal blood levels of local anesthetic (mepivacaine). N Engl J Med 279:910–914

Hall DR, McGibbon DH, Evans CC, Meadows GA (1972) Gentamicin, tubocuraine, lignocaine and neuromuscular blockade. Br J Anaesth 44:1329–1332

Harrison DC, Sprouse JH, Morrow AG (1963) The antiarrhythmic properties of lidocaine and procaine amide; clinical and physiologic studies of their cardiovascular effects in man. Circulation 28:486–491

Hirst GDS, Wood Dr (1971) On the neuromuscular paralysis produced by procaine. Br J Pharmacol 41:94–104

Huffman RD, Yim GKW (1969) Effects of diphenylaminoethanol and lidocaine on central inhibition. Int J Neuropharmacol 8:217–225

Jorfeldt L, Lofstrom B, Pernow B, Wahren J (1970) The effect of mepivacaine and lidocaine on forearm resistance and capacitance vessels in man. Acta Anaesthesiol Scand 14:183–201

Julien RM (1973) Lidocaine in experimental epilepsy. Correlation of anticonvulsant effect with blood concentration. Electroencephalogr Clin Neurophysiol 34:639–645

Julien RM, Demetrescu M (1974) A neutral local anesthetic for research in experimental epilepsy. J Life Sci 4:27–30

Kao FF, Jalar UH (1959) The central action of lignocaine and its effect on cardiac output. Br J Pharmacol 14:522–526

Katz RL, Gissen AJ (1969) Effects of intravenous and intraarterial procaine and lidocaine on neuromuscular transmission in man. Acta Anaesthesiol Scand [Suppl] 36:103–113

Kotelko DM, Shnider SM, Dailey PA, Brizgys RV, Levinson G, Shapiro A, Koike M, Rosen MA (1984) Bupivacaine-induced cardiac arrhythmias in sheep. Anesthesiology 60:10–18

Kuperman AS, Altura BT, Chezar JA (1968) Action of procaine on calcium efflux from frog nerve and muscle. Nature 217:673

Libelius R, Sonesson B, Stamenovic BA, Thesleff S (1970) Denervationlike changes in skeletal muscle after treatment with a local anesthetic (Marcaine). J Anat 106:297–309

Lieberman NA, Harris RS, Katz RI, Lipschutz HM, Dolgin M, Fisher VJ (1968) The effects of lidocaine on the electrical and mechanical activity of the heart. Am J Cardiol 22:375–380

Liu P, Feldman HS, Covino BM, Giasi R, Covino BG (1982a) Acute cardiovascular toxicity of procaine, chloroprocaine and tetracaine in anesthetized ventilated dogs. Reg Anaesth 7:14–19

Liu P, Feldman HS, Covino BM, Giasi R, Covino BG (1982b) Acute cardiovascular toxicity of intravenous amide local anesthetics in anesthetized ventilated dogs. Anesth Analg 61:317–322

Liu PL, Feldman HS, Giasi R, Patterson MK, Covino BG (1983) Comparative CNS toxicity of lidocaine, etidocaine, bupivacaine and tetracaine in awake dogs following rapid IV administration. Anesth Analg 62:375–379

Lund PC (1962) Peridural anesthesia: a review of 10,000 administrations. Acta Anaesthesiol Scand 6:143–159

Moore DC, Bridenbaugh LD (1966) Spinal (subarachnoid) block: a review of 11,574 cases. JAMA 195:907–912

Moore DC, Crawford RD, Scurlock JE (1980) Severe hypoxia and acidosis following local anesthetic-induced convulsions. Anesthesiology 53:259–260

Morishima HO, Pedersen H, Finster M, Sakuma K, Bruce SL, Gutsche BB, Stark RI, Covino BG (1981) Toxicity of lidocaine in adult, newborn and fetal sheep. Anesthesiology 55:56–61

Morishima HO, Pederson H, Finster M, Feldman HS, Covino BG (1983a) Etidocaine toxicity in the adult, newborn and fetal sheep. Anesthesiology 58:342–346

Morishima HO, Pederson H, Finster M, Tsuji A, Hiraoka H, Feldman HS, Arthur RA, Covino BG (1983b) Is bupivacaine more cardiotoxic than lidocaine? Anesthesiology 59:A409

Munson ES, Gutnick MJ, Wagman IH (1970) Local anesthetic druginduced seizures in rhesus monkeys. Anesth Analg 49:486–494

Munson ES, Tucker WK, Ausinsch B, Malagodi H (1975) Etidocaine, bupivacaine, and lidocaine seizures thresholds in monkeys. Anesthesiology 42:471–478

Nishimura N, Morioka T, Sato S, Kuba T (1965) Effects local anesthetic agents on the peripheral vascular system Anesth Analg 44:135

Pizzalato D, Renegar OJ (1959) Histopathologic effects of long exposure to local anesthetics on peripheral nerves. Anesth Analg 38:138–141

Prentiss JE (1979) Cardiac arrest following caudal anesthesia. Anesthesiology 50:51–53

Ravindran RS, Bond VK, Tasch MD, Gupta CD, Luerssen TG (1980) Prolonged neural blockade following regional analgesia with 2-chloroprocaine. Anesth Analg 59:447–451

Ravindran RS, Turner MS, Muller I (1982) Neurological effects of subarachnoid administration of 2-chloroprocaine-CE, bupivacaine and low pH normal saline in dogs. Anesth Analg 61:279–283

Reisner LS, Hochman BN, Plumer MH (1980) Persistent neurologic deficit and adhesive arachnoiditis following intrathecal 2-chloroprocaine injection. Anesth Analg 59:452–454

Rosen MR, Wit AL, Hoffman BF (1975) Electrophysiology and pharmacology of cardiac arrhythmias: V. Cardiac antiarrhythmic effects of lidocaine. Am Heart J 89:526–536

Rosen MA, Baysinger CL, Shnider SM, Dailey DA, Norton M, Levinson G, Curtis JD, Collins W, Davis RL (1982) Evaluation of neurotoxicity of local anesthetics following subarachnoid injection. Anesthesiology 57:A196

Sage D, Feldman HS, Arthur GA, Covino BG (1983) Cardiovascular effects of lidocaine and bupivacaine in the awake dog. Anesthesiology 59:A210

Sage DJ, Feldman HS, Arthur GR, Datta S, Ferretti AM, Norway SM, Covino BG (1984) Influence of lidocaine and bupivacaine on isolated guinea pig atria in the presence of acidosis and hypoxia. Anesth Analg 63:1–7

Scott DB (1975) Evaluation of the toxicity of local anaesthetic agents on man. Br J Anaesth 47:56–61

Scott DB (1981) Toxicity caused by local anaesthetic drugs. Br J Anaesth 53:553–554

Seo N, Oshima E, Steven J, Mori K (1982) The tetraphasic action of lidocaine on CNS electrical activity and behavior in cats. Anesthesiology 57:451–457

Skou JC (1954) Local anaesthetics. II. The toxic potencies of some local anaesthetics and of butyl alcohol, determined on peripheral nerves. Acta Pharmacol Toxicol 10:292–296

Sorel L, Lejeune R (1955) Modifications de l'EEG du Lapin sons l'action de divers succedanes de la cocaine injectes par voie intraveineuse. Arch Int Pharmacodyn Ther 102:314–334

Stewart DM, Rogers WP, Mahaffey JE, Witherspoon S, Woods EF (1963) Effect of local anesthetics on the cardiovascular system in the dog. Anesthesiology 24:620–624

Sugimoto T, Schaal SF, Dunn NM, Wallace AG (1969) Electrophysiological effects of lidocaine in awake dogs. J Pharmacol Exp Ther 166:146–150

Tanaka K, Yamasaki M (1966) Blocking of cortical inhibitory synapses by intravenous lidocaine. Nature 209:207–208

Telivuo L (1967) Effects of intra-arterial mepivacaine and bupivacaine on neuromuscular transmission in man. Acta Anaesthesiol Scand 11:327–332

Wagman IH, deJong RH, Prince DA (1968) Effects of lidocaine on spontaneous cortical and subcortical electrical activity: Production of seizure discharges. Arch Neurol 18:277–290

Wang BC, Hillman DE, Spiedholz NI, Turndorf H (1984) Chronic neurological deficits and Nesacaine-CE – An effect of the anesthetic, 2-chloroprocaine, or the antioxidant, sodium bisulfite. Anesth Analg 63:445–447

Wanna HT, Geigis SD (1978) Procaine, lidocaine, and ketamine inhibit histamine-induced contracture of guinea pig tracheal muscle in vitro. Anesth Analg 57:25–27

Warnick JE, Kee RD, Yim GKW (1971) The effects of lidocaine on inhibition in the cerebral cortex. Anesthesiology 34:327–332

Weiss EB, Patwardhan AV (1977) The response to lidocaine in bronchial asthma. Chest 72:429–438

Weiss EB, Anderson WH, O'Brien KP (1975) The effect of a local anesthetic, lidocaine, on guinea pig trachealis muscle in vitro. Am Rev Resp Dis 112:393–400

Weiss EB, Hargraves WA, Viswanath S (1978) The inhibitory action of lidocaine in anaphylaxis. Am Resp Dis 117:859–869

Wollenberger A, Krayer O (1948) Experimental heart failure caused by central nervous system depressants and local anesthetics. J Pharmacol Exp Ther 94:439–443

Zener JC, Harrison DC (1974) Serum enzyme values following intramuscular administration of lidocaine. Arch Intern Med 134:48–49

CHAPTER 7

The Role of Local Anesthetic Effects
in the Actions of Antiarrhythmic Drugs

G. A. GINTANT and B. F. HOFFMAN

A. Introduction

Pharmacologic therapy is the most common therapeutic approach towards the control and treatment of cardiac arrhythmias. The therapeutic efficacy of antiarrhythmic drugs may derive from any number (or combination) of actions, including effects on the central nervous system, sympatholytic effects, as well as direct and/or indirect effects on active and passive properties of cardiac membranes (including sodium, calcium, and potassium channels, gap junctions, and exchange mechanisms). A majority of antiarrhythmic drugs have demonstrated local anesthetic effects, in that they reduce the fast inward sodium current of cardiac fibers. It is the purpose of this review to briefly discuss the contributions of local anesthetic effects to the actions of antiarrhythmic agents.

B. Electrophysiology of Cardiac Fibers

I. Description of the Cardiac Action Potential

Before considering the antiarrhythmic effects of local anesthetic-type antiarrhythmic drugs, we shall briefly review some relevant aspects of normal cardiac cellular electrophysiology. We shall emphasize the electrical activity of canine cardiac Purkinje fibers (Fig. 1 a) which comprise the specialized conduction system within the ventricles. In physiologic Tyrode's solution ($[K^+]_o = 4$ mM), the resting membrane potential (RMP) is approximately -90 mV, and follows the Goldman-Hodgkin-Katz equation with the constant field permeability ratio (P_{Na}/P_K) of 0.01 for potassium concentrations greater than 4 mM (GADSBY and CRANEFIELD 1977). The action potential upstroke (termed phase 0) is fast and large (typical maximum rate of rise of 600 V/s, amplitude of 130 mV), with an overshoot of 30–40 mV, and is due to sodium ions flowing through fast inward sodium channels. Sodium channels in cardiac and nerve preparations show many similarities, including the sigmoid voltage dependence of the inactivation mechanism (WEIDMANN 1955a), the relationship between membrane potential and sodium conductance, and the linear instantaneous I–V relationship between sodium conductance and membrane potential [BROWN et al. 1981; see also HONDEGHEM and KATZUNG (1977) and FOZZARD et al. (1985) for reviews]. As a consequence, cardiac sodium channels have been modeled as Hudgkin-Huxley type channels. However, cardiac sodium channels differ from nerve sodium channels in the more hyperpolarized range over which inactivation occurs, and in their in-

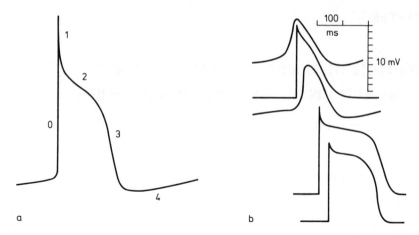

Fig. 1. a The five phases of the cardiac action potential of a sheep Purkinje fiber labeled according to Woodbury, Hecht, and Christopherson (1951) (from Coraboeuf and Weidmann 1954, with permission). **b** Comparisons of action potentials from different regions of the heart including (starting from top) sinoatrial node, atrium, atrioventricular node, Purkinje fiber (false tendon), and ventricular muscle fiber. Action potentials displayed on times axis according to sequence of activation during normal sinus rhythm. [Original records by Hoffman and Cranefield (1960), adapted from Gadsby and Wit (1980) with permission]

teractions with local anesthetics and neurotoxins. For example, reduction of fast inward sodium current by tetrodotoxin (TTX) is enhanced by repetitive stimulation (use-dependent block, see below) in cardiac fibers (Reuter et al. 1978; Cohen et al. 1981) but not in nerve or skeletal muscle. Furthermore, cardiac sodium channels are several orders of magnitude less sensitive to TTX (dissociation constant for block of $I_{Na} > 1$ uM, Dudel et al. 1967; Reuter et al. 1978; Brown et al. 1981 b; Cohen CJ et al. 1981) and are more sensitive to lidocaine and other local anesthetics (Hille 1978). Little work has been done investigating the selectivity of cardiac sodium channels.

After the action potential upstroke there is an initial rapid repolarization (phase 1), followed by a relatively prolonged period of very slow repolarization, termed phase 2 or the plateau. The plateau is maintained by a fine balance between inward and outward currents due to the high resistance of the membrane during this period. The time-dependent inward currents include an inward current carried predominantly by calcium ions (i_{Ca}), and a residual sodium current likely due to the slow or incomplete inactivation of fast inward channels (TTX-sensitive "window" current; Attwell et al. 1979; Coraboeuf et al. 1979; Colatsky and Gadsby 1980; Carmeliet and Saikawa 1982; Gintant et al. 1984). The outward currents include a slowly-activating potassium current carried mainly by potassium ($i_{x,1}$) and a time-independent K^+ current in $i_{K,1}$ (see Carmeliet and Vereecke 1979). Inactivation of calcium current and delayed activation of potassium currents lead to the more rapid final repolarization (termed phase 3) that returns membrane potential to the resting value.

A slow diastolic depolarization may follow the action potential and may lower the transmembrane potential to the threshold potential and initiate another action potential. This slow depolarization, termed phase 4 depolarization, is responsible for the normal automaticity of cardiac Purkinje fibers. Phase 4 depolarization was thought to result from the time- and voltage-dependent inactivation of an outward K^+ current ($i_{K,2}$) (VASSALLE 1966; NOBLE and TSIEN 1968), but recent evidence indicates that it more likely is caused by the activation of an inward current (i_f) carried by sodium and potassium ions (DIFRANCESCO and OJEDA 1980; DIFRANCESCO 1981).

Ventricular fibers and Purkinje fibers differ in that in the former 1) the maximum rate of rise of the upstroke is lower (approx. 200 V/s), 2) the plateau is shorter and occurs at more depolarized potentials, 3) the action potential duration (APD) is shorter, and 4) phase 4 depolarization is not seen in normally polarized fibers (see Fig. 1 b). The action potential configuration of atrial muscle fibers is similar to that of ventricular fibers; the major difference is that the plateau phase in atrium is usually not as prominent so that the action potential is triangular in shape. The ionic basis for electrical activity in other types of cardiac fibers [sinus (SA) node, specialized atrial fibers, atrioventricular (AV) node] will be commented on in subsequent sections. The action potential duration of Purkinje fibers (and to a lesser extent, ventricular and atrial muscle cells) is modulated by the stimulation rate and the interval between action potentials. More rapid or premature stimulation typically causes action potential shortening due primarily to abbreviation of the plateau.

II. Fast Responses and Slow Responses

Action potentials of normally polarized fibers with rapid upstrokes (> 50 V/s) and large amplitude (120 mV) have been termed "fast-response" action potentials (CRANEFIELD et al. 1972; CRANEFIELD 1975). Under normal conditions, action potentials of atrial and ventricular myocardial fibers and Purkinje fibers are fast responses (maximum upstroke velocity may attain 1000 V/s in Purkinje fibers). The magnitude of the fast inward current under physiologic conditions [estimated at 0.5–0.8 mA/cm² in Purkinje fibers (CARMELIET and VEREECKE 1979)] ensures rapid, non-decremental conduction. Ischemic, infarcted or otherwise damaged Purkinje fibers and ventricular and atrial muscle may be partially depolarized (RMP more positive than -70 mV) and their action potentials upstrokes reduced in amplitude (< 100 mV) and maximum rate of rise (10–100 V/s) (FRIEDMAN et al. 1973a, b; LAZZARA et al. 1973, 1975; DOWNAR et al. 1977). Such action potentials have been called depressed fast responses (BRENNAN et al. 1978). It is uncertain whether depressed fast responses result entirely from increased sodium channel inactivation due to membrane depolarization or also from derangements of channel gating or selectivity characteristics.

Action potentials generated by severely depolarized cells (RMP < -55 mV) which have slow and prolonged upstrokes (< 10 V/s) are called "slow responses" (ROUGIER et al. 1969; CRANEFIELD et al. 1972; CRANEFIELD 1975). Slow response upstrokes are caused by inward current (i_{Ca}) through kinetically slow calcium-selective channels (REUTER and SCHOLZ 1977, but see also ISENBERG and KLOCKNER

1982; MITCHELL et al. 1983; NOBLE 1984). The small magnitude of the calcium current [estimated at 35 uA/cm^2 (ARONSON and CRANEFIELD 1973)] is primarily responsible for the slow rate of rise, low amplitude, low conduction velocity (0.01–0.1 M/s) and low safety factor for propagation of slow responses. The threshold for activation of i_{Ca} is approximately -50 mV, and all channels are inactivated at approximately 0 mV (CORABOEUF 1980; ISENBERG and KLOCKNER 1982). i_{Ca} is augmented by catecholamines and other agents that increase cyclic-AMP (see REUTER 1983) as well as some dihydropyridine derivatives (SCHRAMM et al. 1983; HESS et al.. 1984). Whereas Mn, D-600 and verapamil reduce i_{Ca}, (KOHLHARDT et al. 1972, 1973; KASS and TSIEN 1975), tetrodotoxin does not.

Cells in the sinus node and the center (N-region) of the atrioventricular node normally generate slow responses that are dependent on i_{Ca} and are blocked by slow channel blockers (CRANEFIELD 1975). Slow responses can be generated by any type of cardiac fiber if the resting potential is reduced sufficiently and i_{Ca} is enhanced relative to outward background currents. When partially depolarized by high $[K^+]_o$, atria, Purkinje fibers, and ventricular muscle fibers develop slow responses during superfusion with catecholamines (CARMELIET and VEREECKE 1969; PAPPANO 1970; CRANEFIELD et al. 1972; BRENNAN et al. 1978). Isolated preparations of diseased human atrium often generate slow responses (HORDOF et al. 1976; MARY-RABINE et al. 1980) as do tissues from infarcts (FRIEDMAN et al. 1973 a; LAZZARA et al. 1973). However, the action potential characteristics of tissues damaged by ischemia vary with the type of infarct, the anatomical location of the tissue and age of the infarct (FRIEDMAN et al. 1973 a; FENOGLIO et al. 1979; SPEAR et al. 1983).

III. Excitability, Refractoriness, and Responsiveness

The cardiac action potential has been divided into different periods based upon the response to electrical stimuli applied at various times during and after the action potential (Fig. 2 a). The absolute refractory period (ARP, also known as the effective refractory period, ERP) refers to the time during which a supramaximal stimulus fails to elicit an active membrane response. The absolute refractory period normally extends from phase 0 through Phase 3 repolarization until transmembrane potential is more negative than -50 mV. During this period, a premature stimulus can initiate only a decrementally propagating response. The period following the effective refractory period when responses to strong stimuli propagate is termed the relative refractory period (RRP). Early during the relative refractory period the stimulus requirement is increased over the diastolic value; later there is a period of supernormal excitability (with reduced stimulus requirement) when transmembrane potential is between the control threshold potential and maximum diastolic potential. During this supernormal period (SNP) responses are still depressed. The full recovery time (FRT, LEWIS and DRURY 1926) signals the moment when both electrical excitability and responses attain their control values; usually this coincides with attainment of the normal resting or maximum diastolic potential. Full recovery time is determined by the plateau length and the time required for sodium channel reactivation during and follow-

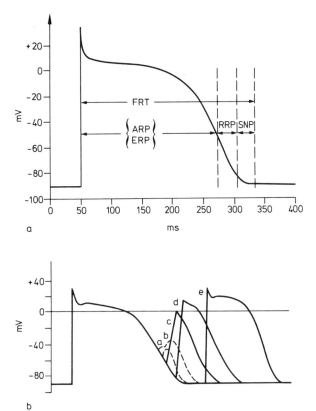

Fig. 2. a The excitability of a Purkinje fiber to cathodal stimulation during the action potential. *ARP*, absolute refractory period; *ERP*, effective refractory period; *RRP*, relative refractory period; *SNP*, supernormal period; *FRT*, full recovery time. See text for further discussion. From HOFFMAN and CRANEFIELD (1960) with permission. **b** Schematically represented are responses to premature stimuli applied at various times during repolarization to illustrate responsiveness in Purkinje fibers. Responses arising early during repolarization (*a* and *b*) are graded or local responses which propagate decrementally. The earliest propagated action potential (*c*) propagates slowly because of its low upstroke velocity and amplitude. Response (*d*) propagates more rapidly as a result of the increased rate of rise and amplitude, but not as rapidly as response (*e*) elicited after complete repolarization with a rate of rise and amplitude similar to a nonpremature upstroke. After SINGER and TEN EICK (1969) by permission

ing phase 3 repolarization. In contrast to fast responses, full recovery time for slow responses may extend significantly beyond fiber repolarization [(post-repolarization refractoriness), HOFFMAN and CRANEFIELD 1960; STRAUSS and BIGGER 1972] due in part to the slower reactivation kinetics of the calcium channel.

Action potential upstrokes elicited during phase 3 are slower and smaller than upstrokes evoked during phase 4 (Fig. 2 b) because there is more steady-state inactivation at membrane potentials less than the resting potential and, because time is required for sodium channel reactivation at each potential during phase 3 repolarization. This results in slowing of conduction of premature impulses (KAO and HOFFMAN 1958). If the resting potential is reduced, reactivation will also be slowed (GETTES and REUTER 1974; CHEN et al. 1975) and full recovery of excitability and responsiveness delayed significantly beyond the end of phase 3.

The relationship of the maximum upstroke velocity of premature upstrokes to the membrane potential during phase 3 repolarization is known as a "membrane responsiveness" curve. Owing to difficulties in voltage clamping the fast inward sodium current in syncytial cardiac preparations, membrane responsiveness has traditionally been used as a gross measure of the voltage- and time-dependent reactivation kinetics of cardiac sodium channels and changes in these parameters caused by drugs.

C. The Effects of Local Anesthetics on Cardiac Fibers

I. Effects on Fast Inward Sodium Current

The first study of the effects of local anesthetics on heart fibers using microelectrode techniques demonstrated that cocaine, procaine amide, quinidine, and diphenylhydramine decreased the maximum upstroke velocity and overshoot of sheep cardiac Purkinje fibers (WEIDMANN 1955 b). Considering the "antifibrillatory actions" of some of these agents, Weidmann commented

"Possibly it is of importance that they decrease the 'safety factor' for impulse propagation... More probably their tendency to suppress spontaneous firing is of some value. Even the slight dissociation between membrane repolarization and the return of excitability may be beneficial."

Since that time, studies of the local anesthetic effects of various antiarrhythmic agents on all types of cardiac preparations have been published. Until recently, nearly all have used changes in the maximum rate of rise of the action potential upstroke ($\dot{V}_{max}$) to assess changes of peak inward sodium current, because of difficulties and uncertainties inherent in voltage-clamping fast time-dependent currents in multicellular cardiac preparations under physiologic conditions (see JOHNSON and LIEBERMAN 1971; BEELER and McGUIGAN 1978; ATTWELL and COHEN 1977; COLATSKY and TSIEN 1979; BROWN et al. 1981 a, b; FOZZARD 1985). Although interpretation of results derived from studies using $\dot{V}_{max}$ recently have been debated (HUNTER et al. 1975; COHEN and STRICHARTZ 1977; WALTON and FOZZARD 1979; COHEN IS et al. 1981; COHEN CJ et al. 1981; COHEN CJ et al. 1984), this measure has proven valuable in understanding the interactions of local anesthetic agents with cardiac sodium channels. Recently, voltage clamp studies on rabbit Purkinje fibers (BEAN et al. 1983), disaggregated rat ventricular cells (LEE et al. 1981; SANCHEZ-CHAPULA et al. 1983) human atrial cells (BUSTAMANTE and McDONALDS 1983) and other cell types have begun to provide data on the effects of local anesthetics on fast inward current and conductance mechanisms. Patch clamp techniques have also been applied to record single channel cardiac sodium currents (CACHELIN et al. 1983; GRANT et al. 1983; TEN EICK et al. 1984).

Studies of local anesthetic effects in nerve and cardiac muscle have characterized the reduction of fast inward current on the basis of tonic and use-dependent block of sodium channels (STRICHARTZ 1973; COURTNEY 1975; HILLE 1977; HONDEGHEM and KATZUNG 1977). We also have found it convenient to consider the antiarrhythmic actions of local anesthetic-type antiarrhythmic drugs in terms of their tonic and use-dependent blocking effects. We define use-dependent block as the drug-induced reduction of fast inward sodium current that is reversibly enhanced by rapid stimulation or activity. We define tonic block as the drug-induced reduction of fast inward sodium current that remains during very slow or infrequent stimulation. We have assumed that changes in $\dot{V}_{max}$ provide a reasonable qualitative index of changes in peak inward sodium current in cardiac fibers.

1. Use-Dependent Block

The first report of use-dependent block in cardiac fibers investigated the effect of stimulation rate on changes in the action potential upstroke by quinidine (JOHNSON and McKINNON 1957). Subsequently, many observations demonstrating use-dependent block of cardiac sodium channels by local anesthetic-type antiarrhythmic agents have appeared. We have found it convenient to classify antiarrhythmic agents in terms of their recovery kinetics (Table 1).

On a molecular level, many aspects of use-dependent block may be understood using the "modulated receptor hypothesis" postulated independently by HILLE (1977) and HONDEGHEM and KATZUNG [1977; see HONDEGHEM and KATZUNG (1984) and GRANT et al. (1984) for a review pertaining to this hypothesis and antiarrhythmic agents]. According to this hypothesis, there exists a single receptor for local anesthetics presumably located within the pore of the sodium channel (see Fig. 3). Receptor affinity for local anesthetics changes (i.e., is modulated) as the channel cycles through the resting, open, and inactivated states. It is generally believed that the affinity of the inactivated channel receptor for drug is greater than the affinity of either the resting or open channel receptor. This requires that the voltage-dependence of the inactivation gating mechanism of drug-bound channels differ from those of drug-free channels (see HILLE 1978). Furthermore, drug access to the receptor site (via either hydrophilic or hydrophobic pathway) may be limited by the state of the channel. Once drug has bound to receptor, the channel is thought to be in a drug-blocked, non-conducting state, although transitions between the blocked forms of the resting, open, and inactivated states are allowed.

Table 1. Effects of therapeutic concentrations of local anesthetic-type antiarrhythmic agents on electrical activity of cardiac Purkinje fibers

Drug	Tonic block	Recovery kinetics, use-dependent block	Action potential duration	Effective refractory period	Normal automaticity
Lidocaine	Yes	Fast	Shorten	Shorten	Decrease
Tocainide	Yes	Fast	Shorten	Shorten	Decrease
Phenytoin	Yes	Fast	Shorten	Shorten	Decrease
Quinidine	Yes	Slow	Prolong	Prolong	Decrease
Procainamide	Yes	Slow	Prolong	Prolong	Decrease
Disopyramide	Yes	Slow	Prolong	Prolong	Decrease

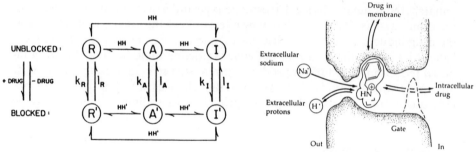

Fig. 3. *Left panel:* The modulated receptor hypothesis represented as a kinetic scheme. Channel blockade is attributed to drug association to a single sodium channel receptor which changes conformations (and therefore, affinity for drugs) as the channel cycles through the resting (R), open (or activated, A) and inactivated (I) states according to Hoodgkin-Huxley (*HH*) kinetics. Drugs combine with different conformations of the receptor according to association (k_R, k_A, k_I) and dissociation (l_R, l_A, l_I) rate constants for the different conformations. Drug-associated sodium channels (R', A', I') may still undergo state transitions, although the voltage-dependence of these transitions (*HH'*) appear to be shifted in a hyperpolarized direction. Drug-associated channels are considered as blocked, nonconducting channels, even when in the activated state. From HONDEGHEM and KATZUNG (1980) with permission of the American Heart Association, Inc. *Right panel:* A cartoon illustrating some physical aspects of the modulated receptor hypothesis. Drug may gain access to the intrachannel receptor site either via the hydrophilic pathway (formed when the gating structure allows channel opening) or via the hydrophobic pathway (via passage through the membrane). Hydrogen ions may be able to exchange with the intrachannel drug molecule via passage through the channels selectivity filter. From HILLE (1984) with permission

It is assumed that use-dependent block results from the accumulation of drug-bound, nonconducting channels which occurs when the rate of drug association exceeds drug dissociation during stimulation. Accordingly, for any drug, drug concentration, and stimulation rate, the rate constants for both drug association and dissociation will determine the magnitude of use-dependent block. If the dissociation rate constant is much greater than the association rate constant, little or no use-dependent block may be evident at very rapid stimulation rates. If the dissociation rate constant is much less than the association rate constant, prominent use-dependent block may be observed at very slow stimulation rates. Indeed, use-dependent block is much more prominent for quinidine [with slow recovery kinetics (HEISTRACHER 1971; GRANT et al. 1982; WELD et al. 1982)] than for lidocaine [with fast recovery kinetics (WELD and BIGGER 1975; GRANT et al. 1980; SANCHEZ-CHAPULA et al. 1983)].

A number of attempts have been made to correlate the physicochemical properties of local anesthetic-type antiarrhythmic agents with their use-dependent kinetics. COURTNEY (1980) found that both size and solubility affect the rate of channel unblock of 15 prospective antiarrhythmic compounds in guinea pig myocardium (the size/solubility hypothesis). Using multiple regression analysis, he reported that both drug size (log Mol. wt.) and estimated distribution coefficient of neutral drug form in the membrane (log Q, based upon octanol/water partition coefficients) could reasonably predict the measured half-times for recovery from use-dependent block (measured at normally polarized potentials following rapid stimulus trains using $\dot{V}_{max}$ as an index of sodium current). In general, recovery is faster for drugs of lower molecular weight and higher lipid solubility, although exceptionally high lipid solubility does not appear to speed recovery kinetics (COURTNEY 1983 b). More recently, he has found (using recovery kinetics data compiled from a number of different laboratories) that the recovery characteristics of 34 of 40 drugs (molecular weights ranging from 178–344) could be predicted using a linear combination of drug size and lipid distribution coefficient, with drug size as the most important parameter (K. Courtney, personal communication). For the six remaining drugs which did not reasonably fit, steric factors were postulated to play a role. Fairly good correlations have also been reported between molecular weight and the recovery kinetics for other local anesthetic-type antiarrhythmic agents (CAMPBELL 1983) and for a series of beta-blocker analogues (BAN et al. 1985).

Differences in the unblocking kinetics of local anesthetics will determine a drugs' effect on membrane responsiveness. Under drug-free conditions, recovery of responsiveness is determined primarily by the time course of phase 3 repolarization and the time- and voltage-dependent kinetics of sodium channel reactivation. Following equilibration with local anesthetic agents (and assuming no changes in the action potential configuration), recovery of responsiveness will depend on the above parameters as well as the number of drug-blocked channels and their recovery kinetics. A drug showing recovery kinetics comparable to the duration of phase 3 will slow recovery of responsiveness during phase 3 and prolong the process into the initial part of phase 4 without depressing maximum responsiveness during diastole. A drug showing slower recovery kinetics may prolong recovery of responsiveness throughout most of diastole. Drugs with much slower kinetics will not effect recovery of responsiveness during phase 3, but will reduce the maximum responsiveness throughout all of diastole. In such circumstances, full recovery of responsiveness will not be observed since it extends into the next action potential, and membrane responsiveness will appear more uniformly reduced throughout phases 3 and 4. Indeed, at physiologic stimulation rates lidocaine depresses membrane responsiveness primarily during phase 3 whereas quinidine appears to depress membrane responsiveness uniformly (CHEN et al. 1975). This effect is consistent with lidocaine's ability to slow intraventricular conduction of early premature impulses without affecting conduction of nonpremature impulses at slow and intermediate heart rates (SAITO et al. 1978; SUGIMOTO et al. 1969; CARSON and DRESEL 1981).

The rates of channel block (association rate) and channel unblock (dissociation rate) determine the time required to attain a new steady-state level of use-dependent block following a change in stimulation rate. If one compares two drugs that differ only in terms of unblocking kinetics, after an increase in the stimulus frequency, the drug with the slower unblocking kinetics will cause a greater increase in use-dependent block; also, block will attain a steady value more slowly. If one compares two drugs that differ only in terms of the association rate constants, the drug with the faster kinetics will cause greater use-dependent block; block will attain a steady value more rapidly. These predictions fail if the drug concentration near the receptor (or within the hydrophilic/hydrophobic pathways) varies with changing stimulation protocols (see below).

The rate of channel block during an action potential by amide-linked local anesthetics appears to increase with increasing lipid solubility (COURTNEY 1983 b). This observation suggests that access to the receptor site of lipid soluble drugs is less limited than for more lipid-insoluble drugs, and is consistent with the postulated hydrophobic pathway. Such an effect probably plays an important role in determining the extent of use-dependent block in fibers with different action potential durations.

Use-dependent block may play an important role in determining the clinical effects of antiarrhythmic drugs by modifying impulse conduction. Drugs with slow recovery kinetics may reduce sodium current and slow conduction at both fast and slow heart rates, whereas drugs with fast recovery kinetics may slow conduction only during rapid rhythms or with premature beats. Indeed, intraventricular conduction at basal physiologic heart rates is not slowed by therapeutic concentrations of lidocaine, whereas the slowing of intraventricular conduction by quinidine has been used clinically as an indicator of the therapeutic concentration of quinidine (HEISSENBUTTEL and BIGGER 1970; BIGGER 1980). The preferential slowing of conduction at rapid heart rates by kinetically fast drugs may be antiarrhythmic or arrhythmogenic, depending upon the physiologic state of different regions in the heart (see below).

Although it has generally been assumed that use-dependent block results from drug binding to a "receptor" site associated with the sodium channel, direct evidence in favor of a classical "receptor" or of a single type/class of receptors is weak. The different molecular structures for local anesthetic-type antiarrhythmic agents tend to suggest that a classical "receptor" (i.e., lock-key or induced fit type binding) may not mediate use-dependent block. However, YEH (1980) found that use-dependent block of fast inward sodium current in squid giant axons by stereoisomers of the local anesthetic RAC 109 was stereospecific. Similar evidence with cardiac sodium channels is not available.

Taking a different approach, CLARKSON and HONDEGHEM (1985) investigated the effects of kinetically dissimilar local anesthetics on use-dependent block, to determine if competitive antagonism was evident. Using guinea-pig papillary muscles, they found that the application of lidocaine (rapid dissociation kinetics) reduced the extent of use-dependent block caused by bupivacaine (slow dissociation kinetics, stim. rates 1–3.3 Hz), while having no effect on use-dependent block caused by quinidine (very slow dissociation kinetics, stim. rates 0.05–3.3 Hz). Evidence for displacement of quinidine by lidocaine was demonstrated by the changes in post-stimulation recovery kinetics in the presence of the drug mixture compared to either drug alone. These results are consistent with the notion of competitive antagonism of these three local anesthetic agents at a common receptor site. (An alternative explanation, however, is that the competitive interaction involves the final common access pathway to the receptor site, rather than binding to the receptor.) Such competitive interactions may be clinically valuable in situations where it is desirable to rapidly attenuate use-dependent block (and associated impaired conduction) caused by an agent with moderately slow unblocking kinetics; the application of an agent with rapid unblocking kinetics may displace the slower drug and thereby lessen the extent of use-dependent block.

An alternative hypothesis which successfully mimics many of the local anesthetic effects of charged anesthetics is the "guarded receptor" hypothesis (STARMER et al. 1984). This hypothesis differs from the modulated receptor hypothesis in that the postulated channel binding site for local anesthetics is a constant affinity binding site. Use-dependent block within the guarded receptor hypothesis results not from modulation of receptor affinity, but rather from modulation of drug access to receptor site. Drug access to binding site is viewed as being restricted by the channel gating mechanism, and, for charged drug forms, further influenced by the potential energy difference between the source pool of drug (cytoplasm) and channel receptor. One prediction of the model is the acceleration of recovery from block by cationic drugs caused by hyperpolarization should not be limited at very negative potentials. $\dot{V}_{max}$ studies suggest that this may not be the case (GINTANT and HOFFMAN 1984; see Figs. 7 and 9). Studies using voltage clamp techniques would be helpful in further clarifying this new hypothesis.

a) Modulation of Use-Dependent Block

Use-dependent block by antiarrhythmic drugs in the heart is modulated by a number of factors; such modulation may significantly influence therapeutic efficacy through effects on impulse conduction. Knowledge of these modulating factors and the physiological differences between normal and diseased regions of the heart should make it possible to target a drug to specifically affect conduction in different regions of the heart, thereby removing conditions necessary for arrhythmogenesis.

One factor which modulates use-dependent block is drug concentration. Greater drug concentrations cause greater use-dependent block presumably by increasing the association rate of drug with receptor, thereby increasing the steady-state level of use-dependent block and decreasing the time required to attain a steady-state level following an increase in the stimulation rate. Although similar concentration changes do not affect the rate of recovery from use-dependence during post-stimulation recovery (HEISTRACHER 1971; COURTNEY 1980; SADA and BAN 1981; GINTANT et al. 1983; BEAN et al. 1983), higher drug concentrations may further depress membrane responsiveness by increasing the number of drug-blocked channels prior to repolarization.

Another factor to consider when assessing use-dependent block is the species, age, and type of fiber studied. For example, amiodarone causes appreciable use-dependent block with guinea-pig papillary muscle (MASON et al. 1983), but not in rabbit fibers (SINGH and VAUGHAN-WILLIAMS 1970). It has been suggested that this difference results from differences in the action potential configuration of guinea-pig and rabbit preparations which affect the time during which channel receptors are in the high-affinity (inactivated) form (MASON et al. 1983). Drugs that preferentially bind to inactivated sodium channels would be expected to cause greater use-dependent block in regions of the heart with long compared to short action potentials. (This assumes that a hydrophobic pathway for drug access to receptor is available during the plateau and repolarization phases of the action potential.) Similarly, if there is a voltage-dependent component of drug association to inactivated channels (WELD et al. 1982), differences in the height and duration of the action potential plateau may modulate use-dependent block. The age of the animal may also affect use-dependent block. It has recently been reported that use-dependent block with lidocaine is greater in adult then in young Purkinje fibers (MORIKAWA and ROSEN 1984).

Use-dependent block in the heart is also modified by changes in either intracellular or extracellular pH. Since many antiarrhythmic agents are tertiary amines with pKa values generally ranging between 6 and 8, varying proportions of charged and uncharged drug forms are present for different drugs. Consequently, changes in pH of the aqueous environment will change the proportion of charged and uncharged drug forms according to the Henderson-Hasselbach equation. These changes will affect the partitioning, diffusion and equilibration of drugs across cell membranes.

Experiments in nerve (NARAHASHI et al. 1970; FRAZIER et al. 1970; HILLE 1977), skeletal muscle (SCHWARZ et al. 1977) and cardiac muscle (FRAME et al. 1981; GINTANT et al. 1983) suggest that intracellular, charged, hydrophilic drug molecules are responsible for use-dependent block. Decreasing intracellular pH will increase the ratio of charged to uncharged intracellular drug species, and changing extracellular pH may affect the protonation of tertiary amines while they are bound to receptor (SCHWARZ et al. 1977; BROUGHTON et al. 1984). As a consequence, changes in pH as occur during ischemia and infarction (GERBERT et al. 1971; GARLICK et al. 1979; TAIT et al. 1982) may directly alter the characteristics of use-dependent block of antiarrhythmic agents. (These effects may be confounded by pH-dependent effects on resting membrane potential and action potential configuration.) Decreasing the extracellular or intracellular pH prolongs recovery from use-dependent block by lidocaine (GRANT et al. 1980; BEAN et al. 1983) and quinidine (GRANT et al. 1982), a finding consistent with the rate- and interval-dependent slowing of conduction (CARSON and DRESEL 1983) and the prolongation of the effective refractory period (KUPERSMITH et al. 1975) by lidocaine in ischemic as compared to normal myocardium. However, additional effects of ischemia on sodium channels (which may affect drug-channel interactions) may be involved.

The effects of resting membrane potential on use-dependent block are inconsistent and complex, and result from effects on the blocking and unblocking kinetics of different local anesthetic-type agents. It has been demonstrated that moderate depolarization slows recovery from use-dependent block (CHEN et al. 1975; GRANT et al. 1980; OSHITA et al. 1980; WELD et al. 1982). Assuming moderate depolarization of the resting membrane potential affected only the recovery kinetics, use-dependent block would be augmented. However, moderate depolarization (as occurs with slight elevations of $[K^+]_o$) will shorten the action potential duration. At constant stimulation rates, this shortening will cause prolongation of the diastolic interval, which may offset the direct effect of membrane potential on recovery kinetics by providing more time for channel unblock. Abbreviation of the action potential may also reduce the rate of drug association to inactivated channels during the plateau and repolarization phases of the action potential, thereby attenuating use-dependent block. Decreasing the resting membrane potential will increase sodium channel inactivation during diastole, thereby decreasing the number of sodium channels available to open during an upstroke. Consequently, for drugs which gain access to the receptor primarily through the hydrophilic pathway, depolarization will reduce drug access, thereby reducing the rate of drug association and relieving use-dependent block. This later effect is seen with the quarternary lidocaine analogues QX-314 and QX-222 (GINTANT et al. 1983) which use the hydrophilic pathway for drug-receptor interactions (STRICHARTZ 1973; GINTANT et al. 1984).

The net effect of moderate depolarization will therefore depend upon the fiber type, action potential configuration, as well as the stimulation rate, drug, and characteristics of the drug-receptor interaction. Use-dependent block by lidocaine and quinidine (HONDEGHEM and KATZUNG 1980; OSHITA et al. 1980), procainamide (SADA et al. 1979) and disopyramide (KOJIMA 1981; FRAME and HOFFMAN 1981) is increased by depolarization of the resting membrane potential from -100 to -75 mV. However, use-dependent block by lidocaine is diminished when the resting membrane potential is reduced further towards -65 mV (GINTANT et al., unpublished observations). In any event, even slight modulation of use-dependent block in partially depolarized fibers (where the safety factor for conduction is lowered) may be sufficient to slow or block conduction.

Yet another factor which modulates use-dependent block is the stimulation protocol. The kinetics of onset of use-dependent block in cardiac fibers have traditionally been characterized by monitoring the exponential decline of $\dot{V}_{max}$ during trains of rapid stimulation preceeded by pauses in stimulation (rest recovery periods) sufficiently long to ensure maximal recovery from use-dependent block (HEISTRACHER 1971). We have found that the time course of block onset with quaternary local anesthetics is affected by the duration of the preceeding rest recovery period. Figure 4 illustrates typical results obtained with a canine cardiac Purkinje fiber equilibrated with the lidocaine analogue QX-222. Following the shorter rest

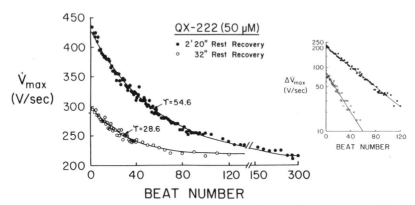

Fig. 4. Effect of stimulation protocol on the kinetics of onset of use-dependent block. *Left panel:* Following equilibration with QX-222, rapid stimulation was interrupted for 2′20″ (*closed circles*) and 32″ (*open circles*) to vary recovery from use-dependent block. The time course of the exponential decline of $\dot{V}_{max}$ upon resumption of stimulation was much faster following the shorter pause in stimulation ($\tau = 28.6$ bts) than following the longer pause in stimulation ($\tau = 54.6$ bts). *Right panel:* Same data as on left, plotted using semilogarithmic coordinates. Fiber was superfused with QX-222 for over 1 h prior to start of experiment; in contrast to nerve, appreciable use-dependent block develops following extracellular application of this quaternary lidocaine analogue. Resting membrane potential (RMP) range -87 to -90 mV, stimulus basic cycle length (BCL) = 500 ms

recovery period of 32 sec, the relaxation of $\dot{V}_{max}$ towards steady-state was fit to
an exponential with a time constant of 28.6 beats (stim. rate = 2 Hz). Following
a longer rest recovery period of 2 min–20 sec, the relaxation of $\dot{V}_{max}$ was fit to a
much slower exponential with a time constant of 54.6 beats. We observed qualitatively similar results with the quarternary lidocaine analogue QX-314. This effect can also be seen by comparing the decline of $\dot{V}_{max}$ during rapid stimulation
trains in which there are inserted brief pauses in stimulation (Fig. 5). This "memory effect", by which the kinetics of block onset "remembers" the previous stimulation history, is not due to the proposed nonlinear relationship between $\dot{V}_{max}$
and maximal sodium conductance (g_{Na}, see COHEN et al. 1984), since lowering the
range of values over which $\dot{V}_{max}$ declines during stimulus trains (by the addition
of low concentrations of TTX) does not affect the time constant for the exponential decline of $\dot{V}_{max}$. This memory effect is also not due to changes in the action
potential duration during rapid stimulus trains (which could affect the rate of
drug association), since block onset with QX-222 is minimally affected by changes
in the action potential duration (GINTANT and HOFFMAN 1984).

   We postulate that this memory effect is due to a transient increase of drug concentration near the receptor caused by newly dissociated drug molecules which
slowly diffuse away from the receptor site (possibly within the limiting pathways

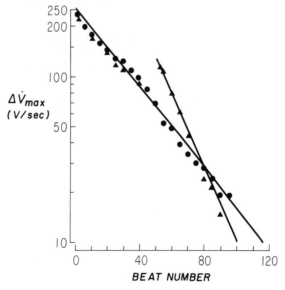

Fig. 5. Effect of a pause in stimulation on the onset kinetics of use-dependent block. Plotted
on semilogarithmic coordinates are the declining $\dot{V}_{max}$ values during rapid stimulation
trains preceeded by 2'30" rest recovery periods. *Circles* represent the changing $\dot{V}_{max}$ values
during an uninterrupted stimulus train, while the *triangles* represent the decline of $\dot{V}_{max}$ during a stimulus train in which a brief (10 s) interruption in stimulation occurred (at beat 40).
The time constant characterizing the exponential decline of $\dot{V}_{max}$ following the brief inter-
ruption ($\tau = 19.8$ beats) was much faster than during the uninterrupted stimulus train ($\tau = 36.7$ bts). Lines represent fits generated using least squares exponential regression analysis.
Fiber was superfused with QX-222 for over 1 h prior to start of experiment. [QX-222] =
6×10^{-5} M, RMP = -84 mV, asymptotic $\dot{V}_{max}$ value of 225 V/s

for drug access to the receptor). If rapid stimulation is resumed prior to dissipation of this drug pulse, more drug is transiently available for binding to receptor and the rate of block onset is accelerated. With longer recovery periods the drug pulse would be minimized since 1) less drug is dissociating from the receptor (per unit time) as the recovery period progresses (exponential recovery kinetics) and 2) those drug molecules which earlier had dissociated from the receptor have had time to diffuse away from the receptor site. Thus, with longer recovery periods, the development of use-dependent block attains a maximal, slower rate. Of course, the final level of block for either long or short rest recovery periods remains unaltered. These results indicate that the stimulation protocols must be considered when assessing the kinetics of block onset of quaternary analogues. It is unknown whether similar results are found with tertiary amine local anesthetics. Preliminary results suggest that this memory effect is not seen with quinidine.

2. Tonic Block

We define tonic block as the drug-induced reduction of fast inward current that remains during very slow or infrequent stimulation. Tonic block is manifest as a dose-dependent displacement to more negative potentials of the "inactivation" curve relating either $\dot{V}_{max}$ or peak inward sodium current to membrane potential

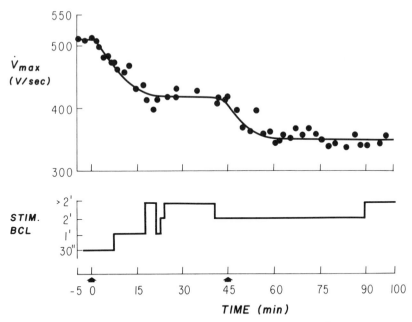

Fig. 6. The time course of equilibration of tonic block with 6×10^{-5} M (*first arrow*) and 1.2×10^{-4} M (*second arrow*) QX-222. To enhance tonic block, the preparation was partially depolarized (RMP range -66–-68 mV) by elevating $[K^+]_o$ to 9 mM. Stimulation basic cycle length (*BCL*) was varied (maximum duration = 5 min) to ensure the absence of use-dependent block. Steady-state tonic block was achieved within 20 min of exposure to either drug concentration. Curves drawn by eye

(CHEN et al. 1975; LEE et al. 1981; GINTANT et al. 1983; SANCHEZ-CHAPULA et al. 1983; BEAN et al. 1983). This displacement results in the greater depression of fast inward current of partially depolarized fibers compared to normally polarized fibers (i.e., tonic block increases as the resting membrane potential is depolarized through the voltage range of sodium channel inactivation). As a consequence, tonic block causes the preferential impairment of propagation and block in partially depolarized fibers independent of stimulation rate. Also as a result of tonic block, the fast inward current of upstrokes from any given potential during phase 3 repolarization is reduced, and membrane responsivenes is thereby depressed. This acts to prolong both the effective and relative refractory periods, and undoubtedly decreases the likelihood of the initiation and propagation of premature impulses. Correlations between the physicochemical properties of antiarrhythmic agents and their tonic blocking effects are inconsistent. Whereas a good correlation is obtained between tonic block and log P (log n-octanol/water partition coefficient) for similar concentrations of a series of beta-adrenergic blocking agents (BAN et al. 1985), a poor correlation is obtained for other local anesthetic-type antiarrhythmic agents (CAMPBELL 1983).

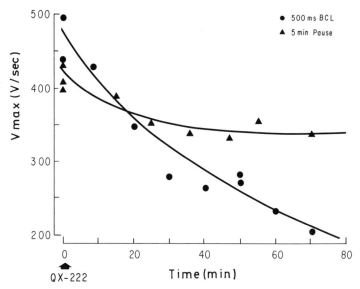

Fig. 7. A comparison of the time course for equilibration of tonic and use-dependent block with QX-222 in the same preparation. The preparation was alternately rested (5 min pauses) and stimulated (BCL = 500 ms) to demonstrate (respectively) tonic and use-dependent block during the 80 min equilibration period. The drug induced reduction of $\dot{V}_{max}$ obtained upon termination of 5 min pauses (representing use-dependent block) attains a steady-state value within 20–30 min. In contrast, $\dot{V}_{max}$ values during rapid stimulus trains (representing use-dependent block) continue to decline even after 1 h of drug superfusion. Periods of rapid stimulation were of sufficient duration to attain quasi-steady-state $\dot{V}_{max}$ values. Resting membrane potentials ranged from -73–-75 mV during stimulus trains, and -70–-72 mV during pauses. (The hyperpolarization which occurs during stimulation causes a slight increase in $\dot{V}_{max}$ as a result of a reduction in sodium channel inactivation). [QX-222] = 6×10^{-5} M

It is uncertain whether tonic and use-dependent block result from drug interactions with single or multiple receptor sites or different drug pools associated with the sodium channel. Based upon the principle of microscopic reversibility, HILLE (1978) has postulated that the tighter binding of drug to the inactivated channel receptor causes a shift in equilibrium of sodium channels from the resting towards the inactivated state, reducing the number of resting channels for any given resting membrane potential and causing tonic block. However, it has been suggested that there may exist multiple sites for interactions of local anesthetic-type drugs with cardiac sodium channels based on the different time course for equilibration of tonic and use-dependent block by propafenone (KOHLHARDT and SEIFERT 1980). Since propafenone is a tertiary amine (pKa = 9.0), it is plausible that the charged and uncharged drug forms interact with different receptors on the sodium channel. Alternatively, it is possible that there are 2 drug pools (or access pathways) for the receptor, each with a different rate of equilibration with the superfusing solution.

Table 2. Effect of duration of drug exposure on the time course of development of use-dependent block with QX-222

Drug exposure (min)	τ_{on} (bts.)	r^2	RMP range (−mV)	$\dot{V}_{max}$ (V/s)
40	102.9	0.984	83–85	620–310
80	58.1	0.996	83–84	610–200
60 w/out	56.8	0.989	83–84	645–220
40	94.6	0.957	88–90	650–390
80	52.5	0.982	89–92	640–290
60 w/out	47.3	0.974	89–92	675–310
40	42.9	0.992	79–80	705–325
80	34.0	0.942	79–80	570–230
60 w/out	36.9	0.990	79–80	585–235
40	49.4	0.972	82–83	720–330
80	25.8	0.986	82–83	630–260
−	−	−	−	−
40	49.3	0.989	81–83	476–270
80	34.8	0.987	82–83	508–220
60 w/out	29.3	0.986	81–83	506–230
40	49.9	0.975	81–83	420–190
80	36.6	0.989	82–82	450–270
60 w/out	33.2	0.984	80–84	435–235
40	49.9	0.908	83–87	485–310
80	51.8	0.984	83–86	435–220
60 w/out	63.1	0.975	84–87	420–210

For each maintained impalement τ_{on}, the time constant characterizing the exponential decline of $\dot{V}_{max}$ following a 10 min rest recovery period was determined following 40 and 80 min of drug superfusion, and 60 min of superfusion with drug-free Tyrode's solution (washout, w/out). The 10 min rest recovery period was sufficiently long to produce maximal rest recovery. The maximum and asymptotic $\dot{V}_{max}$ values for each exponential decline are also indicated. $[K^+]_0 = 5$ mM, BCL = 500 ms, [QX-222] = 4 × 10^{-5} M, r^2 = least squares correlation coefficient, RMP range = range of resting membrane potentials during stimulation.

We have conducted studies comparing the time course for equilibration of the tonic and use-dependent blocking effects by the quaternary local anesthetic QX-222 in canine cardiac Purkinje fibers. Whereas equilibration of tonic block occurs within 20 min after starting drug superfusion (Fig. 6), use-dependent block continues to increase even following one hour of drug exposure (Fig. 7). The continuing increase in use-dependent block is a drug-specific effect, since elimination of drug from the superfusate prevents any further increase (Table 2). The time constants characterizing the decline of $\dot{V}_{max}$ during stimulus trains (preceeded by maximal recovery periods) decrease with longer drug exposure, suggesting that the drug pool responsible for use-dependent block equilibrates much more slowly with superfusate than the drug pool responsible for tonic block. Comparable use-dependent block is achieved much more rapidly following intracellular iontophoretic drug injection (GINTANT, unpublished observations; FRAME et al. 1981; also GLIKLICH and HOFFMAN 1978) consistent with the hypothesis that use-dependent block of cardiac sodium channels by QX-222 is caused by drug derived from an intracellular pool. Further investigations are necessary to ascertain if these 2 drug pools supply one or more receptor sites associated with cardiac sodium channels.

II. Effects on Action Potential Duration

The effects of local anesthetic-type agents on action potential duration vary with the drug employed and are modified by stimulation rate, extracellular [K$^+$], resting membrane potential, as well as the physiologic state and type of fibers studied.

In general, since local anesthetics block sodium channels, they may be expected to shorten the action potential by decreasing residual inward ("window") sodium current during the plateau (GADSBY and CRANEFIELD 1977; ATTWELL et al. 1979; COLATSKY 1982; CARMELIET and SAIKAWA 1982; GINTANT et al. 1984b). Lidocaine and a number of other drugs have this effect (DAVIS and TEMTE 1969; ROSEN et al. 1976; GLIKLICH and HOFFMAN 1978). A local anesthetic-type drug might also influence action potential duration by decreasing sodium loading and causing a decrease in the rate of charge transfer by the electrogenic Na$^+$–K$^+$ ATPase exchange pump (see GADSBY and CRANEFIELD 1979; FALK and COHEN 1984). However, other antiarrhythmic drugs that block sodium channels (including procainamide and quinidine) cause significant action potential prolongation (see Table 1), although there appear to be differences in this effect among mammalian species (CARMELIET and SAIKAWA 1982), and quantitative differences among different types of fibers (WITTIG et al. 1973) and various experimental conditions.

Although it has been established that various local anesthetics reduce potassium currents in nerve (HILLE 1966; ARHEM and FRANKENHAEUSER 1974; STRICHARTZ 1973; YEH and NARAHASHI 1976; HILLE 1977; FISHMAN and SPECTOR 1981), little is known of the effects of local anesthetics on potassium currents in the heart. This is due in part to difficulties in identifying and quantifying potassium currents under voltage clamp, as well as because of the numerous overlapping currents during the plateau that influence the action potential duration (CARMELIET and VEREECKE 1979; COHEN et al. 1986). That some antiarrhythmic drugs may act directly on potassium channels is suggested by the finding that N-acetylprocainamide causes marked prolongation of canine Purkinje fiber action potentials even though quite high concentrations have no effect on $\dot{V}_{max}$ and presumably on fast inward and "window" currents (DANGMAN and HOFFMAN 1981). In the case of rabbit Purkinje fibers, voltage clamp data indicate that both lidocaine and quinidine decrease the magnitude of $i_{x,1}$ (COLATSKY 1982). This effect is greater for quinidine than lidocaine, and the action potential prolongation caused by quinidine may arise in this manner. Finally, for drugs that have been studied using voltage clamp it seems that there is little if any effect on the background potassium conductance or inward K^+ rectifier.

Drug-induced changes in the action potential duration and configuration contribute to changes in the effective and relative refractory period independently of changes in membrane responsiveness brought about by sodium channel blockade. Both effects will determine how a drug modifies or blocks conduction of premature impulses. However, the magnitude of change in action potential duration will be minimized during rapid stimulation.

III. Effects on Phase 4 Depolarization and Normal Automaticity

The rate of automatic impulse initiation can be modified by altering the slope of phase 4 depolarization or by changing the threshold potential or maximum diastolic potential (Fig. 8). Quinidine and procainamide suppress normal automaticity in Purkinje fibers by decreasing the slope of phase 4 depolarization as well as shifting the threshold potential towards more positive voltages (BIGGER 1980). Lidocaine suppresses normal automaticity in Purkinje fibers by reducing the slope of phase 4 depolarization (DAVIS and TEMTE 1969; BIGGER and MANDEL 1970). In addition, by blocking sodium channels, local anesthetics may shift the

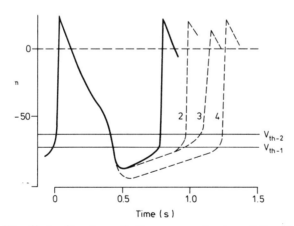

Fig. 8. The possible effects of local anesthetics on normal automaticity of cardiac Purkinje fibers. Normal automatic activity is inscribed as bold transmembrane potentials trace. Rhythm may be slowed by decreasing the slope of phase 4 depolarization (*trace 2*), moving threshold potential ($\dot{V}_{th}$) towards more positive potentials (trace 2 vs. trace 3), increasing the maximum diastolic potential (trace 4 vs. trace 2), or any combination of these effects. From BIGGER JT, Jr (1980) with permission

threshold potential to more positive values and slow automatic rate. The magnitude of this effect would depend strongly on the past and present heart rate and the rate drug dissociation from blocked channels.

However, not all antiarrhythmic drugs modify the slope of phase 4 depolarization even though they decrease $\dot{V}_{max}$ and presumably block fast inward channels. Quaternary lidocaine analogues (Gliklich and Hoffman 1982) and ethmozin (Dangman and Hoffman 1983) are drugs of this sort. It thus appears as though the effect on phase 4 slope is not due merely to a decrease in "background" inward or outward currents (see above). The few voltage clamp studies on this problem have shown that lidocaine and quinidine decrease the inward pacemaker current in Purkinje fibers, whereas procainamide does not (Carmeliet and Saikawa 1982). This latter finding for sheep fibers disagrees with the usual effect of procainamide on automatic canine fibers (Rosen et al. 1973 b). At any rate, there is evidence that some local anesthetic-type agents may interact specifically with the channels that permit normal pacemaker current in Purkinje fibers.

D. Antiarrhythmic Effects of Local Anesthetic Agents

I. Classification of Arrhythmias

It is convenient to consider the antiarrhythmic effects of local anesthetic-type agents using a general scheme for the classification of cardiac arrhythmias in which all disturbances in rhythm are attributed to abnormal impulse initiation, abnormal impulse conduction, or a combination of both (Hoffman 1960; Hoffman and Cranefield 1964; Hoffman and Rosen 1981). Even though it often is not yet possible to identify the mechanism for a specific disturbance of rhythm, we shall consider a number of mechanisms thought to be responsible for the generation of cardiac arrhythmias, and how local anesthetic-type agents may act to modify or prevent these rhythms through specific effects on their mechanisms.

II. Arrhythmias Due to Altered Impulse Initiation

1. Arrhythmias Due to Enhanced Normal Automaticity

Under normal conditions, many parts of the heart can generate spontaneous impulses including the SA node, fibers within the AV node, as well as specialized atrial fibers and the His-Purkinje system. This type of spontaneous impulse generation, termed normal automaticity, results from slow depolarization during phase 4, and is enhanced by β-adrenergic stimulation. Under normal conditions, the SA node is the dominant pacemaker which suppresses all other subsidiary pacemaker regions. If the rate of impulse initiation in the SA node is slower than that in another region of the heart, the subsidiary pacemaker will become the dominant pacemaker and an arrhythmia will result. Enhanced normal automaticity within the ventricles, such as may occur in diseased hearts or through increased regional sympathetic activity, may be responsible for some cardiac arrhythmias.

In general, therapeutic concentrations of local anesthetic-type agents suppress normal automaticity in Purkinje fibers to a greater extent than the SA node. Consequently, local anesthetic-type agents may preferentially slow normal automaticity in the His-Purkinje system and allow the SA node to again become the dominant pacemaker, thereby abolishing the arrhythmia. However, the majority of cardiac arrhythmias probably result from mechanisms other than enhanced normal automaticity.

2. Arrhythmias Due to Abnormal Automaticity

The specialized atrial and ventricular fibers and also atrial and ventricular muscle fibers can demonstrate an abnormal type of automaticity if net outward current during phase 3 is reduced to a value that does not permit the fiber to attain its normal resting or maximum diastolic potential. Characteristic abnormal automatic activity (also termed depolarization-induced automaticity) occurs in Purkinje fibers and ventricular muscle when the diastolic potential is reduced to the range of -55 mV. Automatic impulse generation again results from slow depolarization during phase 4 which is likely due to inactivation of potassium currents and the simultaneous activation of slow inward current (IMANISHI and SURAWICZ 1976; PAPPANO and CARMELIET 1979). The rate of abnormally automatic fibers responds in the usual manner to autonomic mediators. Agents which decrease potassium permeability, including Ba^{2+} (SPERELAKIS et al. 1967), can induce this type of activity (REID and HECHT 1967; DANGMAN and HOFFMAN 1980), as can depolarizing current (REUTER and SCHOLZ 1968; IMINISHI 1971; IMANISHI and SURAWICZ 1976; KATZUNG and MORGENSTERN 1977; FERRIER and ROSENTHAL 1980) and exposures to solution mimicking ischemic conditions (FERRIER et al. 1985). It also is recorded from tissue removed from diseased atria (BUSH et al. 1971; HORDOF et al. 1976) and ischemic and infarcted ventricles (FRIEDMAN et al. 1973 b; LAZZARA et al. 1973; LAZZARA et al. 1975; FENOGLIO et al. 1979). In Purkinje fibers depolarized by infarction (ALLEN et al. 1978) abnormal automaticity may occur in situ as a result of injury currents that partially depolarize nonischemic fibers and enhance normal automaticity early during ischemia and infarction (JANSE and KLEBER 1981). However, it is uncertain whether pacemaker currents other than those responsible for normal automaticity are involved.

a) Effects of Local Anesthetic Drugs

Little is known about the response of abnormal automaticity to local anesthetic-type drugs. In general however, local anesthetics slow abnormal automatic rhythms in concentrations considerably higher than are needed to arrest normally automatic Purkinje fibers. The effects of local anesthetics vary with the model for abnormal automaticity (and probably with the extent of depolarization). Lidocaine reduces the slope of slow diastolic depolarization and thereby slightly slows the automatic rate of guinea-pig fibers depolarized with current (IMANISHI et al. 1978), yet may abolish abnormal automaticity in damaged Purkinje fibers by causing repolarization to more negative resting membrane potentials (ARNSDORF 1977). These later effects may be related to the reduction of the TTX-sensitive "window" current at depolarized potentials by lidocaine. Lidocaine also slows or stops marked spontaneous diastolic depolarization and automaticity in infarcted cardiac preparations (ALLEN et al. 1978).

3. Triggered Activity

a) Definition and Mechanisms

A triggered impulse results from a prior event, usually a prior action potential. Cranefield has restricted the term "triggered activity" to extrasystoles or rhythms that are caused by afterdepolarizations and thus are a sequel of the preceeding action potential (Cranefield 1975, 1977). He has classified afterdepolarizations as either early or delayed; the former appear before the end of phase 3 and the latter after the end of phase 3 (Fig. 9). Early afterdepolarizations (EAD's) have two general forms. In some instances the initial segment of phase 3 is interrupted by a transient depolarization that may or may not initiate a slow response action potential or a series of such action potentials (see Fig. 9 A). In the case of repetitive activity, the second and subsequent action potentials arise from a slow depolarization like that seen during abnormal automatic activity. In other instances the EAD occurs later during phase 3 at a more negative transmembrane potential (see Fig. 9 b). Once again it may initiate one or more action potentials with depressed fast response-type upstrokes.

Early afterdepolarizations can result from a variety of interventions that either diminish outward or augment inward current, including excessive concentration of catecholamines (Brooks et al. 1955), N-acetyl procainamide (Dangman and Hoffman 1981), aconitine (Matsuda et al. 1959), cibenzoline (Dangman 1984), sotalol ([MJ 1999] Strauss et al. 1970), quinidine in the presence of low serum K^+ (Roden and Hoffman 1985) as well as cesium and barium and a reduction in $[K^+]_o$ (Weidmann 1956; Gadsby and Cranefield 1977). EAD's also have been recorded from diseased human atrial fibers (Mary-Rabine et al. 1980). Finally, EAD's can be initiated by depolarizing current clamp (Aronson and Cranefield 1974; Imanishi and Surawicz 1976). EAD's are enhanced by elevated $[Ca^{2+}]_o$ (Katzung 1975) and catecholamines, and are inhibited by the calcium

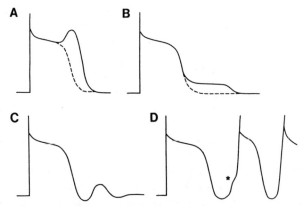

Fig. 9. Schematic examples of afterdepolarizations and triggered activity. Early afterdepolarizations may occur at the beginning (**A**) or prior to termination (**B**) of phase 3. *Dashed lines* represent action potentials without afterdepolarizations. Also illustrated is an example of a delayed afterdepolarization which fails to reach threshold (**C**) and one which attains threshold to initiate triggered activity (**D**, *asterisk*). Early after-depolarizations may also initiate triggered activity. See text for further discussion

channel blockers Mn^{2+} and verapamil (IMANISHI and SURAWICZ 1976; PAPPANO and CARMELIET 1979), suggesting the involvement of the slow inward current during the upstroke. It is generally believed that EAD's result from the interplay of the slow inward current, the time-dependent outward current $i_{K,1}$, and a depolarizing background current under conditions in which outward conductances are reduced. Little is known about the role of triggered activity due to early afterdepolarizations in arrhythmias.

Delayed afterdepolarizations (DAD's) occur after the completion of phase 3; if they lower transmembrane potential to threshold an additional response is initiated (9C,D). Increasing the stimulation rate usually increases DAD amplitude, fostering triggered activity and trains of impulses. Delayed afterdepolarizations have been reported in Purkinje fibers as well as syncytial and single cell ventricular preparations exposed to cardiac glycosides or elevated $[Ca^{2+}]_o$ (ROSEN et al. 1973a; FERRIER and MOE 1973; FERRIER 1976; MATSUDA et al. 1982; LIPSIUS and GIBBONS 1982), in Purkinje fibers superfused with Na^+-free, Ca^{2+}-rich solutions (CRANEFIELD and ARONSON 1974), in coronary sinus preparations exposed to catecholamines (WIT and CRANEFIELD 1977), and in diseased human atrial fibers (MARY-RABINE et al. 1980). Delayed afterdepolarizations apparently result from any intervention or abnormality that increases intracellular calcium activity above a certain value. The elevated $[Ca^{2+}]_i$ apparently causes an oscillatory release of Ca^{2+} from sarcotubular binding sites (FERRIER 1976; KASS et al. 1978a). This, in turn, increases the conductance of a membrane channel for Na^+ and other cations (COLQUHOUN et al. 1981). The resulting transient inward current causes the DAD (LEDERER and TSIEN 1976; KASS et al. 1978a, b). It is generally believed that DAD's may cause a variety of arrhythmias, including repetitive ventricular responses during cardiac glycoside intoxication (REDER and ROSEN 1982) and accelerated AV-junctional escape rhythms (ROSEN et al. 1980).

b) Effects of Local Anesthetic Drugs

The effects of local anesthetic-type antiarrhythmic drugs on triggered activity are quite variable and may be related to the preparations and experimental manipulations employed. Lidocaine, quinidine, procainamide, and TTX reduce the amplitude and upstroke velocity of DAD's induced by cardiac glycosides in Purkinje fibers (ROSEN and DANILO 1980; WASSERSTROM and FERRIER 1982; HEWETT et al. 1983). These results may explain why lidocaine is effective against digitalis-induced ventricular arrhythmias characterized by repetitive ventricular responses and thought to result from DAD's (ZIPES et al. 1974; ROSEN et al. 1975). In contrast, lidocaine has little effect on catecholamine-induced DAD's in human atrial fibers (MARY-RABINE et al. 1980). Quinidine increases DAD amplitude and causes triggering in canine coronary sinus fibers (HENNING and WIT 1984), possibly as a result of drug-induced action potential prolongation modifying $[Ca^{2+}]_i$. The attenuation of DAD's by local anesthetics may be mediated through a reduction of inward sodium current. A reduction of inward sodium current might alter $[Ca^{2+}]_i$ indirectly by affecting $[Na^+]_i$ and sodium-calcium exchange (TSIEN and CARPENTER 1978). In terms of this hypothesis, drug-induced changes in the action potential duration, plateau voltage, or resting membrane potential, as well as reduction of fast inward sodium current and TTX-sensitive "window" current all may effect sodium loading and thereby the generation of DAD's. Although voltage clamp studies indicate that the transient inward current associated with DAD's is insensitive to TTX (KASS et al. 1978 b), it is reduced by lidocaine (EISNER and LEDERER 1979). Local anesthetics may also increase the threshold potential for triggering, as has been shown in glycoside-intoxicated fibers for quinidine (WASSERSTROM and FERRIER 1982).

Discussion of the effects of local anesthetic drugs on triggered rhythms caused by EAD's is complicated by the fact that the triggered impulses may arise either at quite a reduced level of membrane potential and have upstrokes due largely to slow inward current, or at more negative potentials and have upstrokes caused largely by fast inward current. In addition, it is not certain that phase 4 depolarization originating from reduced maximum diastolic potentials (-50 mV) and leading to repetitive impulses has the same ionic mechanism as that occurring at more negative transmembrane potentials (HAUSWIRTH et al. 1969; PAPPANO and CARMELIET 1979). One would expect that EAD's and triggered activity occurring at maximum diastolic potentials of -50 mV to respond to local anesthetic drugs in a manner similar to abnormal automaticity (above; GRANT and KATZUNG 1976). However, if the drug also attenuates $i_{x,1}$ (as does quinidine), it might be expected to increase the likelihood of EAD's and the resulting triggered rhythms.

III. Reentrant Rhythms

1. Mechanisms

Reentrant excitation can result from either circus movement or reflection and can cause extrasystoles or ectopic rhythms. Circus movement occurs when the impulse reexcites some part of the heart after it has recovered from refractoriness. For this to occur there must be a region of one-way block of propagation. Also, if the path over which reentry occurs is short, impulse propagation in it must be slow. Many models of circus movement have been studied (MINES 1914; GARREY 1924; SCHMITT and ERLANGER 1928; WIT et al. 1972 a, b; ALLESSIE et al. 1977) and the subject has been reviewed recently (WIT and CRANEFIELD 1978).

a) Reentry over a Fixed Pathway

Reentry over a short path was modeled by Schmitt and Erlanger (Fig. 10). Here, two branches of a Purkinje fiber insert into ventricular muscle. If, as the impulse propagates towards the ventricle, there is conduction in one branch and block in the other, the impulse can propagate through muscle and enter the unexcited branch in a retrograde direction. If conduction block is unidirectional and retrograde conduction is slow enough for refractoriness to disappear proximal to the area of block, the impulse can circulate around the path. This model can cause either single extrasystoles or sustained rhythms. The conditions causing one-way block and sufficiently slow conduction have been studied in detail (CRANEFIELD et al. 1971; CRANEFIELD and DODGE 1980), and include asymmetry of fiber prop-

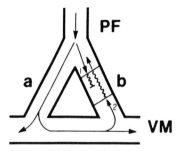

Fig. 10. An example of reentry over a fixed pathway. The diagram schematically illustrates a Purkinje fiber bundle (*PF*) bifurcating into 2 terminal branches (*a* and *b*) leading to ventricular muscle (*VM*). An area of injury and impaired conduction in limb *b* is indicated by the lightly shaded area. Antegrade conduction proceeds through limb *a* to the myocardium but is blocked in limb *b* (at *1*). This allows the impulse to propagate through ventricular muscle to limb *b* (at *2*). If retrograde propagation is sufficiently slow and recovery of excitability occurs in the proximal segment, the impulse may emerge from the injured area to reexcite the Purkinje fiber bundle and cause an extrasystole. Sustained rhythmic activity (circus movement) may result if the impulse continues to circulate around the loop

erties as a function of distance, changes in intercellular coupling, the involvement of depressed fast responses, slow responses, and dispersion of refractoriness.

Reentry over a long path can utilize either an aberrant bypass tract [as in the Wolff-Parkinson-White syndrome (Wellens 1976)] or the right and left bundle branches within the ventricle. In the former case, the atrioventricular node typically provides slow conduction in the orthograde direction and an aberrant atrioventricular bypass tract with prolonged refractoriness provides functional unidirectional block. In the latter case the discrepancy between refractoriness of Purkinje fibers and ventricular muscle permits a properly timed premature impulse to block in regions with prolonged refractoriness and cause reentrant excitation (MOE et al. 1965). Some types of infarction cause marked prolongation of action potentials of subendocardial Purkinje fibers (FRIEDMAN et al. 1973 b) and the resulting dispersion of refractoriness permits one-way block of premature impulses and reentrant excitation.

b) Reentry Around an Anatomical or Functional Barrier

Circus movement also can occur around an antomical barrier (ROSENBLEUTH and GARCIA-RAMOS 1947) or a functional barrier (ALLESSIE et al. 1976, 1977; EL-SHERIF et al. 1977 a, b; JANSE et al. 1980; WIT et al. 1982; ALLESSIE et al. 1984). The basis for the reentrant excitation varies with the model. In the atrium, Allessie has shown that a premature impulse can lead to circus movement around a functional barrier in which the cells are maintained in an inexcitable state by the electrotonic influence from the wavefront propagating around the area of block. In this case, the wavefront propagates in partially refractory tissue. The length of the path for the circus movement, called the leading circle, varies with conduction velocity and duration of effective refractoriness. In the case of circus movement in infarcted ventricles the special properties of the tissues damaged by ischemia may establish the conditions for reentry. Usually one-way block of a premature impulse occurs at the margin of an area damaged by ischemia. The impulse circles around the abnormal area, enters it in a retrograde direction and then propagates slowly through the region of one-way block. Slow conduction may be caused by partial depolarization (and the resulting delayed recovery of responsiveness) or by other mechanisms such as changes in the fine structure of the myocardium. Action potentials in the damaged area may be prolonged or abnormally short. Finally, reentrant excitation may occur over paths that include the atrium or AV and SA nodes; here, block and slow conduction results from the special properties of these tissues.

c) Reentry Caused by Reflection

Reentrant excitation that occurs in an unbranched fiber in which both orthograde and retrograde conduction follow identical pathways, has been termed reflection (WENNEMARK et al. 1968; WIT et al. 1972a; CRANEFIELD 1975; ANTZELEVITCH et al. 1980; ANTZELEVITCH and MOE 1981). In vitro models suggest that an action potential in the proximal region of a fiber may induce an active response in a distal region beyond an inexcitable segment as a result of the electrotonic spread of depolarizing axial current. If the impulse traverses the inexcitable segment sufficiently slowly, the distal action potential may initiate an action potential in the proximal segment where recovery of excitability has already occurred. It is likely that many sites capable of causing reflection are present in ischemic and infarcted myocardium.

2. Effects of Local Anesthetic Drugs on Reentrant Mechanism

Since there are so many mechanisms for circus movement it is difficult to make any specific statement about the manner in which local anesthetic drugs might influence this class of arrhythmias. In spite of this, some generalizations that likely apply to most cases can be offered.

If circus movement requires impulse propagation around a path of fixed length, a drug that significantly prolongs the action potential and refractoriness should slow and ultimately stop the reentrant excitation. Thus, quinidine, procainamide and amiodarone might act in this manner. However, if the drug also slows conduction, the net effect may be small. Drugs like lidocaine, even though they shorten the action potential, still might slow or interrupt the rhythm slowing conduction and by prolonging recovery of responsiveness (KUPERSMITH et al. 1975, EL-SHERIF et al. 1977c; CARSON and DRESEL 1983). A local anesthetic drug also might interrupt this type of circus movement by causing block of some fast inward channels and thus convert the area of one-yway block to an area of bidirectional block. It has been suggested that some drugs act in this manner (HOFFMAN and BIGGER 1971; GIARDINA and BIGGER 1973; WALD et al. 1980). If retrograde conduction through the area of one-way block depends on the slow response, the attenuation of fast inward current (or shortening of action potential duration) might result either in failure to initiate a slow response or failure of the slow response to excite normally polarized fibers downstream (BRENNAN et al. 1978). A local anesthetic-type drug which reduced TTX-sensitive "window" current might cause a net increase in outward repolarizing current sufficient to inhibit the propagation of slow response action potentials (JOSEPHSON and SPERELAKIS 1976; LAMANNA et al. 1982) or alternatively to cause fiber repolarization and the generation of fast responses, thereby improving conduction. If part of the reentrant circuit is partially depolarized, one would expect tonic block to be greater in this area than elsewhere and thus one might selectively interrupt conduction in the depressed segment of the path (WIT et al. 1978; WANG et al. 1979). If the path is not fixed, as when the impulse circulates around an anatomical barrier, one must assume that prolongation of the period of irresponsiveness would merely force the impulse to take a longer path, resulting in a decrease in rate. Of course, impairment of conduction could also be arrhythmogenic, by causing further slowing of conduction and unidirectional block in regions where conduction was minimally depressed.

In regions of impaired conduction, the conversion of unidirectional block to bidirectional block during stable heart rhythms (i.e., constant frequencies) might depend upon the use-dependent blocking characteristics of antiarrhythmic agents. Drugs with slow use-dependent kinetics such as quinidine could reduce the fast inward current sufficiently at all heart rates to cause bidirectional block. Drugs with fast use-dependent kinetics might convert unidirectional block to bidirectional only at rapid heart rates or shorter coupling intervals. In isolated blood perfused dog hearts, antiarrhythmic agents with fast use-dependent block kinetics (tocainide and lidocaine) perferentially slow conduction of closely-coupled premature extrasystoles, whereas drugs with slow use-dependent block kinetics (quinidine, procainamide, methyl lidocaine) slow conduction of extrasystoles at all coupling intervals (MAN and DRESEL 1979). These effects are consistent with the effects of "fast" and "slow" drugs on the recovery of excitability.

If the impulse circulates in a path around a functional barrier, the effects of local anesthetic antiarrhythmic drugs will depend crucially on the condition of the fibers that constitute the barrier. In the case of the leading circle model, prediction and observation agree as far as tests have been made (ALLESSIE et al. 1977). A decrease in the duration of the action potential and period of effective refractoriness increases the rate of the rhythm be decreasing the size of the leading circle. A decrease in the stimulating efficacy of the action potential as caused by partial blocking doses of TTX, has the opposite effect. Prolongation of the action potential or the effective refractory period slows the rhythm and increases the size of the leading circle. One would predict that a sufficient increase in the size of the leading circle might terminate the circus movement because cells that had constituted the barrier no longer would be maintained in an inexcitable state by electrotonus. Similarly, a sufficient decrease in action potential duration and length of the leading circle should terminate the circus movement because the degree to which conduction can slow is limited with this mechanism.

Because local anesthetic-type drugs can demonstrate both tonic and use-dependent block and because both effects vary according to the drug and drug concentration, one would anticipate some variability in effects of different drugs. With the leading circle model, the leading edge of the impulse travels in partially depolarized tissues; thus, tonic block of sodium channels might be apparent at a drug concentration too low to influence conduction in normal regions of the heart. If a drug decreased action potential duration and effective refractoriness sufficiently to permit a significant increase in rate, use-dependent block might become more intense and, by slowing conduction, limit that increase. The net effect of a given drug thus would be difficult to interpret. The same interplay between cycle length and degree of use-dependent block would be observed with drugs that, as an initial effect, were expected to slow the rate. Clearly drugs with known actions have to be tested in this model and effects correlated with data on kinetics and relative magnitudes of tonic and use-dependent block. Finally, the outcome of administration of a local anesthetic antiarrhythmic drug might be influenced to some degree by the extent to which the drug combined with open versus inactivated channels. One would expect that the leading circle type of circus movement to be relatively insensitive to drugs that combined only with open channels and quite sensitive to those that combine with inactivated channels.

In the case of different types of functional barriers, predictions about the mechanisms of action of local anesthetics depend upon a precise specification of the functional and anatomical properties of the barrier. Probably the most difficult case to consider is circus movement caused by infarction since the geometry and condition of the damaged area vary with the site and duration of the coronary artery occlusion as well as the age of the infarct. Convincing data demonstrating circus movement for experimental infarcts are sparse (Klein et al. 1979; Janse et al. 1980; Wit et al. 1982; El-Sherif et al. 1982). A number of studies have been based on the recording of so-called continuous activity through dispersed electrodes (Scherlag et al. 1974; El-Sherif et al. 1977a, b) and drug effects have been interpreted in terms of changes in the delayed or continous activity. No conclusions are possible here since a decrease in delayed activity could result either from improved conduction or enhanced block. Only a limited amount of data on drug effects is available for reentrant rhythms when the excitation sequence has been directly demonstrated by recording from a sufficient number of sites (Cardinal et al. 1981).

A premature impulse can cause reentrant excitation in tissue with nonhomogenous recovery of excitability. In such a case, it is likely that a properly timed premature impulse will block only in regions which have not fully recovered excitability, resulting in transient unidirectional block necessary for reentry (Han and Moe 1964; Moe 1965; Sasyniuk and Mendez 1971). If the timing and conduction velocity are such that the impulse returns to the site of transient block after excitability has been restored, the impulse might traverse the site of block to cause reentry. With such a mechanism only a limited range of coupled premature intervals would be capable of initiating reentrant excitation. Such conditions are likely in ischemic regions of myocardium where dispersion of refractoriness may be great and conduction impaired (Lazzara et al. 1973; see also Sasyniuk and McQuillan 1985).

The effects of local anesthetic agents in this model of reentry may be very complex. A drug could prevent reentry by preventing transient unidirectional block. This could be accomplished by reducing the differences in refractoriness between regions, through either preferential shortening of the more prolonged action potentials, or by prolongation of the shorter action potentials. A drug could prevent reentry by speeding conduction around the loop sufficiently such that the returning impulse would encounter refractory tissue. This could result if a drug shortened the action potential duration within the loop without slowing voltage-dependent reactivation, thereby allowing greater recovery of excitability prior to the arrival of the premature impulse. A drug also could prevent reentry by depressing conduction around the loop to cause block. This effect could result from tonic block (if fibers around the loop were partially depolarized), use-dependent block (thus reducing the effective stimulus invading the region of impaired conduction) or depression of membrane responsiveness (causing further slowing of conduction of the premature impulse).

The effects of local anesthetic-type drugs on reentry due to reflection are complex and depend largely on the initial conditions. If an impulse is marginally sufficient to elicit an active response across the inexcitable segment, a decrease in either depolarizing electrotonic current or the excitability of the distal active region could prevent reflection. Alternatively, the further impairment of conduction across the inexcitable segment could provide sufficient delay to cause reflection in regions where conduction previously was minimally impaired (LAMANNA et al. 1982; ANTZELEVITCH et al. 1985). Reflection could also be prevented by preferentially prolonging the action potential duration or recovery of excitability on the proximal side of the inexcitable segment.

E. Conclusion

Although much information has been gathered on the possible mechanisms responsible for the genesis of arrhythmias, we do not yet know with certainty which mechanisms are responsible for most types of arrhythmias. Similarly, although much information has been gathered on the effects of local anesthetic antiarrhythmic agents on arrhythmic models and on cardiac fibers representing different physiological and pathological states, we do not yet fully understand the effects of these agents on cardiac fibers, or which effects are responsible for modifying any specific arrhythmic mechanism. As a consequence, the approach to antiarrhythmic drug therapy is still largely empirical. The challenge of the future is to link the growing knowledge of cardiac pathophysiology, electrophysiology, and pharmacology towards a rational basis for the identification and treatment of the different types of cardiac arrhythmias observed clinically.

Acknowledgments. The authors would like to thank Dr. M. R. Rosen for critical comments, Dr. I. S. Cohen for stimulating discussions and hospitality, and Maryann Gintant for secretarial assistance.
Grant Support. Supported in part by an N. R. S. A. (G. G.) and grants HL-08508 and HL-12738-15 from the National Heart, Lung, and Blood Institute, National Institutes of Health, Bethesda, Maryland.

References

Allen JD, Brennan FJ, Wit AL (1978) Actions of lidocaine on transmembrane potentials of subendocardial Purkinje fibers surviving in infarcted canine hearts. Circ Res 43:470–481

Allessie MA, Bonke FIM, Schopman FJG (1976) Circus movement in rabbit atrial muscle as a mechanism of tachycardia: II. The role of nonuniform recovery of excitability in the occurrence of unidirectional block as studied with multiple microelectrodes. Circ Res 39:168–177

Allessie MA, Bonke FIM, Schopman FJG (1977) Circus movement in rabbit atrial muscle as a mechanism of tachycardia. III. The "leading circle" concept: a new model of circus movement in cardiac tissue without the involvement of an anatomical obstacle. Circ Res 41:9–18

Allessie MA, Lammers WJEP, Bonke IM, Hollen J (1984) Intra-atrial reentry as a mechanism for atrial flutter induced by acetylcholine and rapid pacing in the dog. Circulation 70:123–135

Antzelevitch C, Moe GK (1981) Electrotonically mediated delayed conduction and reentry in relation to "slow responses" in mammalian ventricular conducting tissue. Circ Res 49:1129–1139

Antzelevitch C, Jalife J, Moe GK (1980) Characteristics of reflection as a mechanism of reentrant arrhythmias and its relationship to parasystole. Circulation 61:182–191

Antzelevitch C, Davidenko JM, Shen X, Moe GK (1985) Reflected reentry: electrophysiology and pharmacology. In: Zipes DP, Jalife J (eds), Cardiac electrophysiology and arrhythmias. Grune and Stratton, Orlando, Florida, pp 253–264

Arhem P, Frankenhaeuser B (1974) Local anesthetics: effects on permeability properties of nodal membrane in myelinated nerve fibres from Xenopus. Potential clamp experiments. Acta Physiol Scand 91:11–21

Arnsdorf MF (1977) The effect of antiarrhythmic drugs on triggered sustained rhythmic activity in cardiac Purkinje fibers. J Pharmacol Exp Ther 201:689–700

Aronson RS, Cranefield PF (1973) The electrical activity of canine cardiac Purkinje fibers in sodium-free, calcium-rich solutions. J Gen Physiol 61:786–808

Aronson RS, Cranefield PF (1974) The effect of resting potential on the electrical activity of canine cardiac Purkinje fibers exposed to Na-free solutions or to ouabain. Pflügers Arch 347:101–116

Attwell D, Cohen I (1977) The voltage clamp of multicellular preparations. Prog Biophys Mol Biol 31:201–245

Attwell D, Cohen I, Eisner D, Ohba M, Ojeda C (1979) The steady-state TTX-sensitive ("window") sodium current in cardiac Purkinje fibers. Pflügers Arch 379:137–142

Ban T, Sada S, Takahashi Y, Sada H, Fujita T (1985) Effects of para-substituted beta-adrenoceptor blocking agents and methyl-substituted phenoxypropanolamine derivatives on maximum upstroke velocity of action potentials in guinea-pig papillary muscles. Naunyn-Schmiedebergs Arch Pharmacol 329:77–85

Bean BP, Cohen CJ, Tsien RW (1983) Lidocaine block of cardiac sodium channels. J Gen Physiol 81:613–642

Beeler GW, McGuigan JAS (1978) Voltage clamping of multicellular myocardial preparations: capabilities and limitations of existing methods. Prog Biophys Mol Biol 34:219–254

Bigger JT, Jr (1980) Management of arrhythmias. In: Braunwald E (ed) Heart disease: a textbook of cardiovascular Medicine. Saunders, Baltimore, pp 691–743

Bigger JT, Jr, Hoffman BF (1980) Antiarrhythmic drugs. In: Gilman AG, Goodman LS, Gilman A (eds) The pharmacological basis of therapeutics, 6th edn. Macmillan, New York, pp 761–792

Bigger JT, Jr, Mandel WJ (1970) Effect of lidocaine on the electrophysiological properties of ventricular muscle and Purkinje fibers. J Clin Invest 49:63–77

Brennan FJ, Cranefield PF, Wit AL (1978) Effects of lidocaine on slow response and depressed fast response action potentials of canine cardiac Purkinje fibers. J Pharmacol Exp Ther 204:312–324

Brooks C McC, Hoffman BF, Suckling EE, Orias O (1955) Excitability of the heart. Grune and Stratton, New York

Broughton A, Grant AS, Starmer CF, Klinger JK, Stambler BS, Strauss HC (1984) Lipid solubility modulates pH potentiation of local anesthetics block of V_{max} reduction in guinea-pig myocardium. Circ Res 55:513–523

Brown AM, Lee KS, Powell T (1981 a) Voltage clamp and internal perfusion of single rat heart muscle cells. J Physiol (Lond) 318:455–477

Brown AM, Lee KS, Powell T (1981 b) Sodium current in single rat heart muscle cells. J Physiol (Lond) 318:479–500

Bush HL, Jr, Gelband H, Hoffman BF, Malm Jr (1971) Electrophysiological basis for supraventricular arrhythmias. Arch Surg 103:620–625

Bustamante JO, McDonald TF (1983) Sodium current in segments of human heart cells. Science 220:320–321

Cachelin AB, de Peyer JE, Kokubun S, Reuter H (1983) Sodium channels in cultured cardiac cells. J Physiol (Lond) 340:389–401

Campbell TJ (1983) Importance of physico-chemical properties in determining the kinetics of the effects of Class I antiarrhythmic drugs on maximum rate of depolarization in guinea-pig ventricle. Br J Pharmacol 80:33–40

Cardinal R, Janse MJ, Eeden IV, Werner G, D'Alloncourt CN, Durrer D (1981) The effects of lidocaine on intracellular and extracellular potentials, activation, and ventricular arrhythmias during acute regional ischemia in the isolated porcine heart. Circ Res 49:792–806

Carmeliet E, Saikawa T (1982) Shortening of the action potential and reduction of pacemaker activity by lidocaine, quinidine, and procainamide in sheep cardiac Purkine fibers: an effect on Na or K currents. Circ Res 50:257–272

Carmeliet E, Vereecke JL (1969) Adrenaline and the plateau phase of the cardiac action potential. Pflügers Arch 313:300–315

Carmeliet E, Vereecke J (1979) Electrogenesis of the action potential and automaticity. In: Berne RB, Sperelakis N, Geiger SR (eds) The heart. American Physiological Society, Bethesda, Maryland, pp 269–334 (Handbook of physiology, sect 2, vol 1)

Carson DL, Dresel PE (1981) Effects of lidocaine on conduction of extrasystoles in the normal heart. J Cardiovasc Pharmacol 31:924–935

Carson DL, Dresel PE (1983) Effect of lidocaine on ventricular conduction in acutely ischemic dog hearts. J Cardiovasc Pharmacol 5:357–363

Chen CM, Gettes LS, Katzung BG (1975) Effect of lidocaine and quinidine on steady-state characteristics and recovery kinetics of $(dV/dt)_{max}$ in guinea-pig ventricular myocardium. Circ Res 37:20–29

Clarkson CW, Hondeghem LH (1985) Evidence for a specific receptor site for lidocaine, quinidine, and bupicavaine associated with cardiac sodium channels in guinea pig ventricular myocardium. Circ Res 56:496–506

Cohen CJ, Bean BP, Colatsky TJ, Tsien RW (1981) Tetrodotoxin block of sodium channels in rabbit Purkinje fibers: interactions between toxin binding and channel gating. J Gen Physiol 78:383–411

Cohen CJ, Bean BP, Tsien RW (1984) Maximum upstroke velocity as an index of available sodium conductance. Comparison of maximal upstroke velocity and voltage clamp measurements of sodium current in rabbit Purkinje fibers. Circ Res 54:636–651

Cohen IS, Strichartz GR (1977) On the voltage-dependent action of tetrodotoxin. Biophys J 275:279–283

Cohen IS, Attwell D, Strichartz G (1981) The dependence of the rate of rise of the action potential on membrane parameters. Proc R Soc Lond [Biol] 214:85–98

Cohen IS, Datyner NB, Gintant GA, Kline RP (1986) Time-dependent outward currents in the heart. In: Fozzard HM, Haber E, Jennings RB, Katz AM, Morgan HE (eds) Handbook of experimental cardiology, Raven Press, NY

Colatsky TJ (1982) Mechanisms of action of lidocaine and quinidine on action potential duration in rabbit cardiac Purkinje fibers: an effect on steady-state sodium currents? Circ Res 50:17–27

Colatsky TJ, Gadsby DC (1980) Is tetrodotoxin block of background sodium channels in canine cardiac Purkinje fibers voltage-dependent? J Physiol (Lond) 306:20P

Colatsky TJ, Tsien RW (1979) Sodium channels in rabbit cardiac Purkinje fibers. Nature 278:265–268

Colquhoun D, Neher E, Reuter H, Stevens CF (1981) Inward current channels activated by intracellular Ca in cultured cardiac cells. Nature 294(24):752–754

Coraboeuf E (1980) Voltage clamp studies of the slow inward current. In: Zipes DP, Bailey JC, Elharrar V (eds) The slow inward current and cardiac arrhythmias. Nijhoff, The Hague

Coraboeuf E, Weidmann S (1954) Temperature effects on the electrical activity of Purkinje fibers. Helv Physiol Pharmacol Acta 12:32–41

Coraboeuf E, Deroubaix E, Coulombe A (1979) Effect of tetrodotoxin on action potentials of the conducting system in the dog heart. Am J Physiol 236:H561–567

Courtney KR (1975) Mechanism of frequency-dependent inhibition of sodium currents in frog myelinated nerve by the lidocaine derivative GEA-968. J Pharmacol Exp Ther 195:225–236

Courtney KR (1980) Interval-dependent effects of small antiarrhythmic drugs on excitability of guinea-pig myocardium. J Mol Cell Cardiol 12:1273–1286

Courtney KR (1983 a) Quantifying antiarrhythmic drug blocking during action potentials in guinea-pig papillary muscle. J Mol Cell Cardiol 15:749–757

Courtney KR (1983 b) Tests of the size/solubility hypothesis. Circulation 68:296a

Cranefield PF (1975) The conduction of the cardiac impulse. Future, Mt Kisco, NY

Cranefield PF (1977) Action potentials, afterpotentials, and arrhythmias. Circ Res 41:415–423

Cranefield PF, Aronson RS (1974) Initiation of sustained rhythmic activity by single propagated action potentials in canine cardiac Purkinje fibers exposed to sodium-free solution or to ouabain. Circ Res 34:477–481

Cranefield PF, Dodge FA (1980) Slow conduction in the heart. In: Zipes DP, Bailey JC, Elharrar V (eds) The slow inward current and cardiac arrhythmias. Nijhoff, The Hague, pp 149–171

Cranefield PF, Hoffman BF (1971) Conduction of the cardiac impulse: II. Summation and inhibition. Circ Res 28:220–233

Cranefield PF, Klein HO, Hoffman BF (1971) Conduction of the cardiac impulse: I. Delay, block, and one-way block in depressed Purkinje fibers. Circ Res 28:199–219

Cranefield PF, Wit AL, Hoffman BF (1972) Conduction of the cardiac impulse: III. Characteristics of very slow conduction. J Gen Physiol 59:227–246

Dangman KH (1984) Cardiac effects of cibenzoline. J Cardiovasc Pharmacol 6:300–311

Dangman KH, Hoffman BF (1980) Effects of nifedipine on electrical activity of cardiac cells. Am J Cardiol 46:1059–1067

Dangman KH, Hoffman BF (1981) In vivo and in vitro anti-arrhythmic and arrhythmogenic effects of N-acetyl procainamide. J Pharmacol Exp Ther 217:851–862

Dangman KH, Hoffman BF (1983) Antiarrhythmic effects of ethmozin in cardiac Purkinje fibers: suppression of automaticity and abolition of triggering. J Pharmacol Exp Ther 227:578–586

Davis LD, Temte JV (1969) Electrophysiological action of lidocaine on canine ventricular muscle and Purkinje fibers. Circ Res 24:639–655

DiFrancesco D (1981) A new interpretation of the pacemaker current in calf Purkinje fibers. J Physiol (Lond) 314:359–376

DiFrancesco D, Ojeda C (1980) Properties of the current i_f in the sino-atrial node of the rabbit compared with those of the current $i_{K,2}$ in Purkinje fibers. J Physiol (Lond) 308:353–367

Downar E, Janse MJ, Durrer D (1977) The effect of acute coronary artery occlusion on subepicardial transmembrane potentials in the intact porcine heart. Circulation 56:217–224

Dudel J, Peper K, Rudel R, Trautwein W (1967) The effect of tetrodotoxin on the membrane current in cardiac muscle (Purkinje fibers). Pflügers Arch 295:213–226

Eisner DA, Lederer WJ (1979) A cellular basis for lidocaine's antiarrhythmic action. J Physiol (Lond) 295:25P

El-Sherif N, Hope RR, Scherlag BJ, Lazzara R (1977a) Reentrant ventricular arrhythmias in the late myocardial infarction period: 1. Conduction characteristics in the infarction zone. Circulation 55:686–702

El-Sherif N, Hope RR, Scherlag BJ, Lazzara R (1977b) Reentrant ventricular arrhythmias in the late myocardial infarction period: 2. Patterns of initiation and termination of reentry. Circulation 55:702–718

El-Sherif N, Scherlag BJ, Lazzara R, Hope RR (1977c) Reentrant ventricular arrhythmias in the late myocardial infarction period: 4. Mechanism of action of lidocaine. Circulation 56:395–402

El-Sherif N, Mehra R, Gough WB, Zeiler RH (1982) Ventricular activation patterns of spontaneous and induced ventricular rhythms in canine one-day-old myocardial infarction. Evidence for focal and reentrant mechanism. Circ Res 51:152–166

Falk R, Cohen IS (1984) Membrane current following activity in canine cardiac Purkinje fibers. J Gen Physiol 83:771–799

Fenoglio JJ, Jr, Karagueuzian HS, Friedman PL, Albala A, Wit AL (1979) Time course of infarct growth toward the endocardium after coronary occlusion. Am J Physiol 236:H356–H370

Ferrier GR (1976) The effects of tension on acetylstrophanthidin-induced transient depolarizations and aftercontractions in canine myocardium and Purkinje tissues. Circ Res 38:156–162

Ferrier GR, Moe G (1973) Effect of calcium on acetylstrophanthidin-induced transient depolarizations in the canine Purkinje tissue. Circ Res 33:508:515

Ferrier GR, Rosenthal JE (1980) Automaticity and entrance block induced by focal depolarization of mammalian ventricular tissues. Circ Res 47:238–248

Ferrier GR, Moffat MP, Lukas A (1985) Possible mechanisms of ventricular arrhythmias elicited by ischemia followed by reperfusion. Circ Res 56:184–194

Fishman MC, Spector I (1981) Potassium current suppression by quinidine reveals additional calcium currents in neuroblastoma cells. Proc Natl Acad Sci USA 78:5245–5249

Fozzard Ha, January CT, Makielski JC (1985) New studies of the excitatory sodium currents in heart muscle. Circ Res 56:475–485

Frame LH, Hoffman BF (1981) Disopyramide's effects are enhanced by fast pacing rates in depolarized tissue. Circulation 64 [Suppl 4]:272

Frame LH, Gintant GA, Hoffman BF (1981) Site of action of local anesthetics on heart fibers. Am J Cardiol 47:475

Frazier DT, Narahashi T, Yamada M (1970) The site of action and active form of local anesthetics. II. Experiments with quaternary compounds. J Pharmacol Exp Ther 171:45–51

Friedman PL, Stewart Jr, Fenoglio JJ, Jr, Wit AL (1973a) Survival of subendocardial Purkinje fibers after extensive myocardial infarction in dogs: In vitro and in vivo correlations. Circ Res 33:597–611

Friedman PF, Stewart JR, Wit AL (1973b) Spontaneous and induced cardiac arrhythmias in subendocardial Purkinje fibers surviving extensive myocardial infarction in dogs. Circ Res 33:612–626

Gadsby DC, Cranefield PF (1977) Two levels of resting membrane potential in cardiac Purkinje fibers. J Gen Physiol 79:725–746

Gadsby DC, Cranefield PF (1979) Electrogenic sodium extrusion in cardiac Purkinje fibers. J Gen Physiol 73:819–837

Gadsby DC, Wit AL (1980) Normal and abnormal electrophysiology of cardiac cells. In: Mandel WJ (ed) Cardiac arrhythmias. Lippincott, Philadelphia, pp 55–82

Garlick PB, Radda GK, Seeley PJ (1979) Studies of acidosis in the ischaemic heart by phosphorus nuclear magnetic resonance. Biochem J 184:547–554

Garrey WE (1924) Auricular fibrillation. Physiol Rev 4:215–250

Gerbert G, Benzig H, Strohm M (1971) Changes in interstitial pH of dog myocardium in response to local ischaemia, hypoxia, hyper- and hypocapnia, measured continously by means of glass microelectrodes. Pflügers Arch 329:72–81

Gettes LS, Reuter H (1974) Slow recovery from inactivation of inward currents in mammalian myocardial fibers. J Physiol (Lond) 240:703–724

Giardina EGV, Bigger JT, Jr (1973) Procaine amide against reentrant ventricular arrhythmias: lengthening R–V intervals of coupled ventricular premature depolarizations as an insight into the mechanism of action of procainamide. Circulation 48:959–970

Gintant GA, Hoffman BF (1984) Use-dependent block of cardiac sodium channels by quaternary derivatives of lidocaine. Pflügers Arch 400:121–129

Gintant GA, Hoffman BF, Naylor RE (1983) The influence of molecular form of local anesthetic-type antiarrhythmic agents on reduction of the maximum upstroke velocity of canine cardiac Purkinje fibers. Circ Res 52:735–746

Gintant GA, Datyner NB, Cohen IS (1984) Slow inactivation of a tetrodotoxin-sensitive current in cardiac fibers. Biophys J 45:509–512

Gliklich JI, Hoffman BF (1978) Sites of action and active forms of lidocaine and some derivatives on cardiac Purkinje fibers. Circ Res 43:638–651

Grant AO, Katzung BG (1976) The effects of quinidine and verapamil on electrically-induced automaticity in the ventricular myocardium of guinea-pig. J Pharmacol Exp Ther 196:407–419

Grant AO, Strauss LJ, Wallace AG, Strauss HC (1980) The influence of pH on the electrophysiological effects of lidocaine in guinea pig ventricular myocardium. Circ Res 47:542–550

Grant AO, Trantham JL, Brown KK, Strauss HC (1982) pH-Dependent effects of quinidine on the kinetics of dV/dt_{max} in guinea pig ventricular myocardium. Circ Res 50:210–217

Grant AO, Starmer CF, Strauss HC (1983) Unitary sodium channels in isolated cardiac myocytes of rabbit. Circ Res 53:823–829

Grant AO, Starmer CF, Strauss HC (1984) Antiarrhythmic drug action: Blockade of the inward sodium current. Circ Res 55:427–439

Han J, Moe GK (1964) Nonuniform recovery of excitability in ventricular muscle. Circ Res 14:44–60

Hauswirth A, Noble D, Tsien RW (1969) The mechanism of oscillatory activity at low membrane potentials in cardiac Purkinje fibers. J Physiol (Lond) 200:255–265

Heissenbüttel RH, Bigger Jt, Jr (1970) The effect of oral quinidine on intraventricular conduction in man: correlation of plasma quinidine with changes in QRS duration. Am Heart J 80(4):453–462

Heistracher P (1971) Mechanism of action of antifibrillatory drugs. Naunyn-Schmiedebergs Arch Pharmacol 269:199–212

Henning B, Wit AL (1984) The time course of action potential repolarization affects delayed afterdepolarization amplitude in atrial fibers of the canine coronary sinus. Circ Res 55:110–115

Hess P, Lansman JB, Tsien RW (1984) Different modes of Ca channel gating behaviour favoured by dihydropyridine Ca agonists and antagonists. Nature 311:538–544

Hewett KH, Gessman L, Rosen MR (1983) Effects of ethmozin, procainamide and quinidine on digitalis-induced afterdepolarizations. Eur J Pharmacol 96(1–2):21–28

Hille B (1966) Common mode of action of three agents that decrease the transient change in sodium permeability in nerves. Nature 210:1220–1222

Hille B (1977) Local anesthetics: hydrophilic and hydrophobic pathways for the drug-receptor reaction. J Gen Physiol 69:497–515

Hille B (1978) Local anesthetic action on inactivation of the Na channel in nerve and skeletal muscle: possible mechanisms for antiarrhythmic agents. In: Morad M (ed) Biophysical aspects of cardiac muscle. Academic, New York, pp 55–74

Hille B (1984) Ionic channels of excitable membranes. Sinauer, Sunderland

Hoffman BF (1960) Physiological basis of disturbances of cardiac rhythm and conduction. Prog Cardiovasc Dis 2: 319–333

Hoffman BF, Bigger Jt, Jr (1971) Antiarrhythmic drugs. In: DiPalma JR (ed) Drill's pharmacology in medicine. McGraw-Hill, New York, pp 824–852

Hoffman BF, Cranefield PF (1960) Electrophysiology of the Heart. McGraw-Hill, New York

Hoffman BF, Cranefield PF (1964) The physiological basis of cardiac arrhythmias. Am J Med 37:670–684

Hoffman BF, Rosen MR (1981) Cellular mechanisms for cardiac arrhythmias. Circ Res 49:1–15

Hondeghem LM, Katzung BG (1977) Time- and voltage-dependent interactions of antiarrhythmic drugs with cardiac sodium channels. Biochim Biophys Acta 472:373–398

Hondeghem LM, Katzung BG (1980) Test of a model of antiarrhythmic drug action. Effects of quinidine and lidocaine on myocardial conduction. Circulation 61:1217–1224

Hondeghem LM, Katzung BG (1984) Antiarrhythmic agents: the modulated receptor mechanisms of action of sodium and calcium channel-blocking drugs. Annu Rev Pharmacol Toxicol 24:387–423

Hordof A, Edie R, Malm J, Hoffman B, Rosen M (1976) Electrophysiological properties and response to pharmacologic agents of fibers from diseased human atria. Circulation 54:774–779

Hunter PJ, McNaughton PA, Noble D (1975) Analytical models of propagation in excitable cells. Prog Biophys Mol Biol 30:99–144

Imanishi S (1971) Calcium-sensitive discharges in canine Purkinje fibers. Jpn J Physiol 21:443–463

Imanishi S, Surawicz B (1976) Automatic activity in depolarized guinea-pig ventricular myocardium: characteristics and mechanisms. Circ Res 39:751–759

Imanishi S, McAllister RG, Jr, Surawicz B (1978) The effects of verapamil and lidocaine on the automatic depolarization in guinea-pig ventricular myocardium. J Pharmacol Exp Ther 207:294–303

Isenberg G, Klockner U (1982) Calcium currents of isolated bovine ventricular myocytes are fast and of large amplitude. Pflügers Arch 395:30–41

Janse MJ, Kleber AG (1981) Electrophysiological changes and ventricular arrhythmias in the early phase of regional myocardial ischemia. Circ Res 49:1069–1081

Janse MJ, van Cepelle FJL, Morsink H, Kleber AG, Wilms-Schopman F, Cardinal R, d'Alloncourt CN, Durrer D (1980) Flow of "injury" current and patterns of excitation during early ventricular arrhythmias in acute regional myocardial ischemia in isolated porcine and canine hearts. Evidence for two different arrhythmogenic mechanisms. Circ Res 47:151–165

Johnson EA, Lieberman M (1971) Heart: excitation and contraction. Annu Rev Physiol 33:479–532

Johnson EA, McKinnon MC (1957) The differential effect of quinidine and pyrilamine on the myocardial action potential at various rates of stimulation. J Pharmacol Exp Ther 120:460–468

Josephson I, Sperelakis N (1976) Local anesthetic blockade of Ca^{2+} mediated action potentials in cardiac muscle. Eur J Pharmacol 40:201–208

Kao CY, Hoffman BF (1958) Graded and decremental response in heart muscle fibers. Am J Physiol 194:187–196

Kass RS, Tsien RW (1975) Multiple effects of calcium antagonists on plateau currents in cardiac Purkinje fibers. J Gen Physiol 66:169–192

Kass RS, Lederer WJ, Tsien RW, Weingart R (1978a) Role of calcium ions in transient inward currents and aftercontractions induced by strophanthidin in cardiac Purkinje fibers. J Physiol (Lond) 281:187–208

Kass RS, Tsien RW, Weingart R (1978b) Ionic basis of transient inward current induced by strophanthidin in cardiac Purkinje fibers. J Physiol (Lond) 281:209–226

Katzung B (1975) Effects of extracellular calcium and sodium on depolarization-induced automaticity in guinea-pig papillary muscle. Circ Res 37:118–127

Katzung BG, Morgenstern JA (1977) Effects of extracellular potassium on ventricular automaticity and evidence for a pacemaker current in mammalian ventricular myocardium. Circ Res 40:105–111

Klein GJ, Ideker RE, Smith WM, Harrison LA, Kasell J, Wallace AG, Gallagher JJ (1979) Epicardial mapping of the onset of ventricular tachycardia initiated by programmed stimulation in the canine heart with chronic infarction. Circulation 60:1375–1384

Kohlhardt M, Seifert C (1980) Inhibition of $\dot{V}_{max}$ of the action potential by propafenone and its voltage-, time-, and pH-dependence in mammalian ventricular myocardium. Naunyn-Schmiedebergs Arch Pharmacol 315:55–62

Kohlhardt M, Bauer B, Krause H, Fleckenstein A (1972) Differentiation of the transmembrane Na and Ca channels in mammalian cardiac fibers by the use of specific inhibitors. Pflügers Arch 335:309–322

Kohlhardt M, Bauer B, Krause H, Fleckenstein A (1973) Selective inhibition of the transmembrane Ca conductivity of mammalian cardiac fibers by the use of specific inhibitors. Pflügers Arch 338:115–123

Kojima M (1981) Effects of disopyramide on transmembrane action potentials in guinea-pig papillary muscle. Eur J Pharmacol 69:11–24

Kupersmith J, Antman EM, Hoffman BF (1975) In vivo electrophysiological effects of lidocaine in canine acute myocardial infarction Circ Res 36:84–91

Lamanna V, Antzelevitch C, Moe GK (1982) Effects of lidocaine on conduction through depolarized canine false tendons and on a model of reflected reentry. J Pharmacol Exp Ther 221:353–361

Lazzara R, El-Sherif N, Scherlag BJ (1973) Electrophysiological properties of canine Purkinje cells in one-day-old myocardial infarction. Circ Res 33:722–734

Lazzara R, El-Sherif N, Sherlag BJ (1974) Early and late effects of coronary artery occlusion on canine Purkinje fibers. Circ Res 35:391–399

Lazzara R, El-Sherif N, Scherlag BJ (1975) Disorders of cellular electrophysiology produced by ischemia of the canine His bundle. Circ Res 36:444–454

Lederer WJ, Tsien RW (1976) Transient inward current underlying arrhythmogenic effects of cardiotonic steroids in Purkinje fibers. J Physiol (Lond) 263:73–100

Lee KS, Hume JR, Giles W, Brown AM (1981) Sodium current depression by lidocaine and quinidine in isolated ventricular cells. Nature 291:325–327

Lewis T, Drury AN (1926) Revised views of the refractory period in relation to drugs reputed to prolong it, and in relation to circus movement. Heart 13:95–100

Lipsius SL, Gibbons WR (1982) Membrane currents, contractions, and aftercontractions in cardiac Purkinje fibers. Am J Physiol 243:H77–86

Man RYK, Dresel PE (1979) A specific effect of lidocaine and tocainide on ventricular conduction of mid-range extrasystoles. J Cardiovasc Pharmacol 1:329–342

Mary-Rabine L, Hordof AJ, Danilo P, Jr, Malm JR, Rosen MR (1980) Mechanisms for impulse initiation in isolated human atrial fibers. Circ Res 47(2):267–277

Mason JW, Hondeghem LM, Katzung BG (1983) Amiodarone blocks inactivated cardiac sodium channels. Pflügers Arch 396:79–81

Matsuda K, Hoshi T, Kameyama S (1959) Effects of aconitine on the cardiac membrane potential of the dog. Jpn J Physiol 9:419–429

Matsuda H, Noam A, Kurachi Y, Irisawa H (1982) Transient depolarization and spontaneous voltage fluctuations in isolated single cells from guinea pig ventricles: calcium-mediated membrane potential fluctuations. Circ Res 51:142–151

Mines GR (1914) On circulating excitations in heart muscles and their possible relation to tachycardia and fibrillation. Trans R Soc Can Ser 3 (Sect IV) 8:43–52

Mitchell MR, Powell T, Terrar DA, Twist VW (1983) Characteristics of the second inward current in cells isolated from rat ventricular muscle. Proc R Soc Lond [Biol] 219:447–469

Moe GK, Mendez C, Han J (1965) Aberrant AV impulse propagation in the dog heart: a study of functional bundle branch block. Circ Res 16:261–286

Morikawa Y, Rosen MR (1984) Developmental changes in the effects of lidocaine on the electrophysiological properties of cardiac Purkinje fibers. Circ Res 55:633–641

Narahashi T, Frazier DT, Yamada M (1970) The site of action and active form of local anesthetics. I. Theory and pH experiments with tertiary compounds. J Pharmacol Exp Ther 171:32–44

Noble D (1984) The surprising heart: a review of recent progress in cardiac electrophysiology. J Physiol (Lond) 353:1–50

Noble D, Tsien RW (1968) The kinetics and rectifier properties of the slow potassium current in cardiac Purkinje fibers. J Physiol (Lond) 195:185–214

Oshita S, Sada H, Kojima J, Ban T (1980) Effects of tocainide and lidocaine on the transmembrane action potential as related to external potassium and calcium concentrations in guinea-pig papillary muscle. Naunyn-Schmiedebergs Arch Pharmacol 316:67–82

Pappano AJ (1970) Calcium-dependent action potentials produced by catecholamines in guinea pig atrial muscle fibers depolarized by potassium. Circ Res 27:379–390

Pappano AJ, Carmeliet EE (1979) Epinephrine and the pacemaking mechanism at plateau potentials in sheep cardiac Purkinje fibers. Pflügers Arch 382:17–26

Reder RF, Rosen MR (1982) Delayed afterdepolarizations and clinical arrhythmogenesis. In: Paes de Carvalho A, Hoffman BF, Lieberman M (eds) Normal and abnormal conduction in the heart, Futura, Mount Kisco, NY, pp 449–460

Reid JA, Hecht HH (1967) Barium-induced automaticity in right ventricular muscle in the dog. Circ Res 21:849–855

Reuter H (1983) Calcium channel modulation by neurotransmitters, enzymes and drugs. Nature 301:569–574

Reuter H, Scholz H (1968) Über den Einfluß der extrazellulären Ca-Konzentration auf Membranpotential und Kontraktion isolierter Herzpräparate bei graduierter Depolarisation. Pflügers Arch 300:87–107

Reuter H, Scholz H (1977) A study of the ion selectivity and the kinetic properties of the calcium-dependent slow inward current in mammalian cardiac muscle. J Physiol (Lond) 264:17–47

Reuter H, Baer M, Best PM (1978) Voltage dependence of TTX action in mammalian cardiac muscle. In: Morad M (ed) Biophysical aspects of cardiac muscle. Academic, New York, pp 129–142

Reuter H, Cahelin AB, de Peyer JE and Kokubun S (1985) Whole-cell Na^+ current and single Na^+ channel measurements in cultured cardiac cells. In: Zipes Dp, Jalife J (eds) Cardiac electrophysiology and arrhythmias. Grune and Stratton, Orlando

Roden DM, Hoffman BF (1985) Action potential prolongation and induction of abnormal automaticity by low quinidine concentrations in canine Purkinje fibers: relation to potassium and cycle length. Circ Res 56:857–867

Rosen MR, Danilo P, Jr (1980) Effects of tetrodotoxin, lidocaine, verapamil, and AHR-2666 on ouabain-induced delayed afterdepolarization in canine Purkinje fibers. Circ Res 46:117–124

Rosen MR, Gelband H, Hoffman BF (1973a) Correlation between effects of ouabain on the canine electrogram and transmembrane potentials of isolated Purkinje fibers. Circulation 47:65–72

Rosen MR, Merker C, Gelband H, Hoffman BF (1973b) Effects of procaine amide on the electrophysiologic properties of the canine ventricular conducting system. J Pharmacol Exp Ther 185:438–446

Rosen MR, Wit AL, Hoffman BF (1975) Electrophysiology and pharmacology of cardiac arrhythmias: IV. Cardiac antiarrhythmic and toxic effects of digitalis. Am Heart J 89(3):391–399

Rosen MR, Danilo P, Jr, Alonson MB, Pippenger CE (1976) Effect of therapeutic concentrations of diphenylhydantoin on transmembrane potentials of normal and depolarized Purkinje fibers. J Pharmacol Exp Ther 197:594–604

Rosen MR, Fisch C, Hoffman BF, Danilo P, Jr, Lovelace DE, Knoebel SB (1980) Can accelerated atrioventricular junctional escape rhythms be explained by delayed afterdepolarizations? Am J Cardiol 45:1272–1284

Rosenblueth A, Garcia-Ramos J (1947) Studies on flutter and fibrillation. II. The influence of artificial obstacles on experimental auricular flutter. Am Heart J 33:677–684

Rougier O, Vassort G, Garnier D, Gargouil YM, Coraboeuf E (1969) Existence and role of a slow inward current during the frog atrial action potential. Pflügers Arch 308:91–110

Sada H, Ban T (1981) Effects of various structurally related beta-adrenoceptor blocking agents on maximum upstroke velocity of action potentials of guinea-pig papillary muscles. Naunyn Schmiedebergs Arch Pharmacol 317:245–251

Sada H, Kojima M, Ban T (1979) Effect of procainamide on transmembrane action potentials in guinea-pig papillary muscles as affected by external potassium concentrations. Naunyn Schmiedebergs Arch Pharmacol 309:179–190

Saito S, Chen CM, Buchanan J, Jr, Gettes LS, Lynch MR (1978) Steady state and time-dependent slowing of conduction in canine hearts. Effects of potassium and lidocaine. Circ Res 42:246–254

Sanchez-Chapula J, Tsuda Y, Josephson I (1983) Voltage- and use-dependent effects of lidocaine on sodium current in rat single ventricular cells. Circ Res 52:557–565

Sasyniuk BI, McQuillan J (1985) Mechanisms by which antiarrhythmic drugs influence induction of reentrant responses in the subendocardial Purkinje network of 1-day-old infarcted canine ventricle. In: Zipes DP, Jalife J (eds) Cardiac electrophysiology and arrhythmias. Grune and Stratton, Orlando, pp 389–396

Sasyniuk BI, Mendez C (1971) A mechanism for reentry in canine ventricular tissue. Circ Res 28:3–15

Scherlag BJ, El-Sherif N, Hope R, Lazzara R (1974) Characterization and localization of ventricular arrhythmias resulting from myocardial ischemia and infarction. Circ Res 35:372–383

Schramm M, Thomas G, Towart R, Franckowiak G (1983) Novel dihydropyridines with positive inotropic action through activation of Ca^{2+} channels. Nature 303:535–537

Schmitt FO, Erlanger J (1928) Directional differences in the conduction of the impulse through heart muscle and their possible relation to extrasystolic and fibrillary contractions. Am J Physiol 87:326–347

Schwarz W, Palade PT, Hille B (1977) Local anesthetics: Effect of pH on use-dependent block of sodium channels in frog muscle. Biophys J 20:343–368

Singer DH, Ten Eick RE (1969) Pharmacology of cardiac arrhythmias. Prog Cardiovasc Dis 11:488–514

Singh BN, Vaghan-Williams EM (1970) The effect of amiodarone, a new anti-anginal drug, on cardiac muscle. Br J Pharmacol 39:657–667

Spach MS, Miller WT III, Dolber PC, Kootsey JM, Sommer JR, Mosher CE, Jr (1982) The functional role of structural complexities in the propagation of depolarization in the atrium of the dog: cardiac conduction disturbances due to discontinuities of effective axial resistivity. Circ Res 50:175–191

Spear JF, Michelson EL, Moore EN (1983) Cellular electrophysiologic characteristics of chronically infarcted myocardium in dogs susceptible to sustained ventricular tachyarrhythmias. J Am Coll Cardiol 1:1099–1110

Sperelakis N, Schneider MF, Harris EJ (1967) Decreased K^+ conductance produced by Ba^{2+} in frog sartorius fibers. J Gen Physiol 50:1565–1583

Starmer CF, Grant AO, Strauss HC (1984) Mechanism of use-dependent block of sodium channels in excitable membranes by local anesthetics. Biophys J 46:15–27

Strauss HC, Bigger JT, Jr (1972) Electrophysiologic properties of the rabbit sino-atrial perinodal fibers. Circ Res 31:490–509

Strauss HC, Bigger JT, Jr, Hoffman BF (1970) Electrophysiological and β-receptor blocking effects of MJ 1999 on dog and rabbit cardiac tissues. Circ Res 26:661–678

Strichartz GR (1973) The inhibition of sodium currents in myelinated nerve by quaternary derivatives of lidocaine. J Gen Physiol 62:37–57

Sugimoto T, Schaal SF, Dunn NM, Wallace AG (1969) Electrophysiological effects of lidocaine in awake dogs. J Pharmacol Exp Ther 166:146–150

Tait GA, Young RB, Wilson GJ, Steward DJ, MacGregor DC (1982) Myocardial pH during regional ischemia: evaluation of a fiber-optic photometric probe. Am J Physiol 243:H1027–H1031

Ten Eick R, Yeh J, Matsuki N (1984) Two types of voltage dependent Na channels suggested by differential sensitivity of single channels to tetrodotoxin. Biophys J 45:70–73

Tsien RW, Carpenter DO (1978) Ionic mechanisms of pacemaker activity in cardiac Purkinje fibers. Fed Proc 37:2127–2131

Vassalle M (1966) Analysis of cardiac pacemaker potential using a "voltage clamp" technique. Am J Physiol 210:1335–1341

Wald RW, Waxman MB, Downar E (1980) The effect of antiarrhythmic drugs on depressed conduction and unidirectional block in sheep Purkinje fibers. Circ Res 46:612–619

Walton M, Fozzard H (1979) The relation of $\dot{V}_{max}$ to I_{Na}, $\bar{G}_{Na}$ and h_∞ in a model of the cardiac Purkinje fiber. Biophys J 25:407–420

Wang CM, James CA, Maxwell RA (1979) Effects of lidocaine on the electrophysiological properties of subendocardial Purkinje fibers surviving acute myocardial infarction. J Mol Cell Cardiol 11:669–681

Wasserstrom JA, Ferrier GR (1982) Effects of phenytoin and quinidine on digitalis-induced oscillatory afterpotentials, aftercontractions, and inotropy in canine ventricular tissues. J Mol Cell Cardiol 14:725–736

Weidmann S (1955 a) The effect of the cardiac membrane potential on the rapid availability of the sodium carrying system. J Physiol (Lond) 127:213–224

Weidmann S (1955 b) Effects of calcium ions and local anesthetics on electrical properties of Purkinje fibers. J Physiol (Lond) 129:568–582

Weidmann S (1956) Elektrophysiologie der Herzmuskelfaser. Huber, Bern

Weld FM, Bigger JT, Jr (1975) Effect of lidocaine on the early inward transient current in sheep cardiac Purkinje fibers. Circ Res 37:630–639

Weld FM, Coromilas J, Rottman JN, Bigger JT, Jr (1982) Mechanisms of quinidine-induced depression of maximum upstroke velocity in ovine cardiac Purkinje fibers. Circ Res 50:369–376

Wellens HJJ (1976) The electrophysiologic properties of the accessory pathway in the Wolff-Parkinson-White syndrome. In: Wellens HJJ, Lie KI, Janse MJ (eds) The conduction system of the heart. Stenfert Kroese, Leiden, pp 613–632

Wennemark JR, Ruesta VJ, Brody DA (1968) Microelectrode study of delayed conduction in the canine right bundle branch. Circ Res 23:753–769

Wit AL, Cranefield PF (1977) Triggered and automatic activity in the canine coronary sinus. Circ Res 41:435–445

Wit AL, Cranefield PF (1978) Reentrant excitation as a cause of cardiac arrhythmias. Am J Physiol 235(1):H1–H17

Wit AL, Hoffman BF, Cranefield PF (1972 a) Slow conduction and reentry in the ventricular conducting system. I. Return extrasystoles in canine Purkinje fibers. Circ Res 30:1–10

Wit AL, Cranefield PF, Hoffman BF (1972 b) Slow conduction and reentry in the ventricular conducting system. II. Single and sustained circus movement in networks of canine and bovine Purkinje fibers. Circ Res 30:11–22

Wit AL, Allessie MA, Bonke FIM, Lammers W, Smeets J, Fenoglio JJ, Jr (1982) Electrophysiologic mapping to determine the mechanism of experimental ventricular tachycardia initiated by premature impulses: experimental approach and initial results demonstrating reentrant excitation. Am J Cardiol 49:166–185

Wittig J, Harrison LA, Wallace AG (1973) Electrophysiological effects of lidocaine on distal Purkinje fibers of canine heart. Am Heart J 86:69–78

Woodbury LA, Hecht HH, Christopherson AR (1951) Membrane resting and action potentials of single cardiac muscle fibers of the frog ventricle. Am J Physiol 164:307–318

Yeh JZ (1980) Blockage of sodium channels by stereoisomers of local anesthetics. In: Raymond Fink B (ed) Molecular Mechanisms of Anesthesiology. Progress in Anesthesiology, vol 2, Raven Press, NY, pp 35–44

Yeh JZ, Narahashi T (1976) Mechanism of action of quinidine on squid axon membranes. J Pharmacol Exp Ther 196:62–70

Zipes DP, Arbel F, Knope RF, Moe GK (1974) Accelerated ventricular escape rhythms caused by ouabain intoxication. Am J Cardiol 33:248–253

. . . .

CHAPTER 8

Central Effects of Local Anesthetic Agents

J. M. Garfield and L. Gugino

A. Introduction

The term "local anesthetic", as used clinically, implies a substance that blocks sensory and motor innervation of a discrete, peripheral area or region of the body, as opposed to the state of central narcosis induced by general anesthetic agents. Despite this clinical distinction, local anesthetics are potent drugs, affecting cell membranes, neurotransmitter function, and neuronal excitability. When these agents enter the central nervous system (CNS), a myriad of excitatory and inhibitory behavioral effects can occur, including somnolence, confusion, agitation, excitation and, ultimately, frank seizure activity. In this chapter, we will first consider routes by which the local anesthetics gain access to the CNS, then discuss their behavioral and neuropharmacologic effects, and, finally, their effects on neuronal excitability at regional CNS sites.

B. Routes of Entry of Local Anesthetic Agents into the CNS

There are several routes by which local anesthetics can gain entry to the CNS, as outlined in Table 1. Most local anesthetic agents are largely unionised at normal body pH (Covino and Vasallo 1976). Because it is the unionised form that crosses cell membranes, local anesthetic agents are readily absorbed into the bloodstream when injected into tissues. Cocaine, a local anesthetic with potent central effects on mood and behavior, is rapidly absorbed through respiratory mucous membranes and thus is effective when applied to the nasal mucosa, i.e., "sniffed." Once in the bloodstream, local anesthetics readily penetrate the blood-brain barrier owing to their lipid solubility. The blood-brain barrier functions as a selective filtration system by virtue of the relative continuity of the endothelial basement membrane of the cerebral capillaries and the presence of tight sheaths of glial cells which surround the cerebral blood vessels (Cooper et al. 1978). Local anesthetics, owing to their lipid solubility, readily pass through the pores in the capillary basement membranes as well as the fatty glial cells to gain entry into the brain parenchyma itself. Usubiaga and colleagues studied the transfer of procaine and lidocaine from blood to cerebrospinal fluid (CSF) in a series of 6 neurosurgical patients (Usubiaga et al. 1967). The lateral cerebral ventricle was cannulated during surgery for tumor removal and procaine or lidocaine administered intravenously over a 5–10 min interval. The doses used were within the range used in intravenous general anesthesia (Usubiaga and Wikinski 1964). Samples of

Table 1. Routes of entry of local anesthetics into the CNS

Route	Comments
1. Direct application to surface of brain or spinal cord.	Usually reduces amplitude of ongoing EEG-activity in animals; topical application of lidocaine to human cerebral cortex ineffective in evoking seizures; i.v. or intra-carotid injection reliably produces seizures
2. Microinjection into brain parenchyma	Produces localized effects; hippocampal injection in monkeys produces focal epileptiform discharges; artifacts relating to concentration, toxicity, and diffusion of agent can occur
3. Introduction of agent into cerebrospinal fluid (CFS)	Perfusion of procaine in cerebral ventricles of conscious dogs rapidly produces diffuse behavioral and autonomic effects. Spinal anesthesia accrues from uptake of agent from CFS into spinal nerves and neural elements of spinal cord; entry into brain is very unlikely
4. Absorption from tissue via bloodstream; access to CNS via blood-brain barrier	Highly perfused tissues apt to take up large quantities of local anesthetics; CNS toxicity can result from injection given into a highly perfused area. I.v. administration leads to rapid entry into CNS; nonionised form readily penetrates blood-brain barrier

Table 2. Local anesthetic concentrations in arterial blood and CSF 5 min following the intravenous administration of procaine or lidocaine to 6 neurosurgical patients

	Local anesthetic injection (mg/kg)	Arterial blood concentration (µg/ml)	Cerebrospinal fluid concentration (µg/ml)
Procaine	10	12.5	7.2
	15	16.0	9.5
	20	28.0	16.5
Lidocaine	5	5.2	3.8
	8	6.1	5.0
	10	15.0	11.5

Data of Usubiaga et al. (1967). Reprinted (modified) with permission from The Macmillam Press

CSF and arterial blood were taken both before the administration of the local anesthetics and at intervals thereafter. As shown in Table 2, 5 min after the intravenous infusion was completed, procaine and lidocaine were noted in the CSF of all 6 patients studied. In the patients receiving procaine, para-aminobenzoic acid (PABA), its principal metabolite owing to rapid enzymatic hydrolysis by plasma pseudocholinesterase, was also present in blood and CSF samples. In a parallel experiment in dogs, procaine concentrations in CSF were about 0.9 times that of venous blood in 20 min, attesting to its rapid CNS uptake and equilibration.

C. Behavioral Pharmacology of Local Anesthetic Agents

As stated earlier, when significant concentrations of local anesthetics enter the CNS, a myriad of behavioral effects occur. These accrue from 2 sources: 1) Effects on neuronal excitability; 2) effects on neurotransmitter systems. In the intact organism, the electrical and neurochemical properties of the neuronal populations of the brain are interdependent, and it is somewhat arbitrary to consider the two as separate entities. However, for organizational purposes, we will sort out effects owing to changes in neuronal excitability from the neurochemical and behavioral effects of the local anesthetic agents. This will allow us to discuss taxonomically discrete phenomona such as analgesia, sedation, and behavioral stimulation produced by local anesthetic agents. When we discuss effects on neuronal excitability, we will try to relate them to their neurochemical and behavioral counterparts as much as possible.

I. Animal Studies of Locomotor Activity, Behavior and Correlative Neural Activity

1. Cocaine

Of all the compounds possessing local anesthetic activity, cocaine has the most potent behavioral effects. When inhaled nasally as a powder, as little as 10 or 20 mg induces feelings of euphoria and a sense of clarity or power of thought for approximately 30 min (VAN DYKE and BYCK 1982). These properties have made the recreational use of cocaine widespread throughout the United States and Europe and given rise to a huge, illicit network involving the growth, sale and distribution of the drug. VAN DYKE and BYCK (1982) document the economic impact of cocaine in the following quote: "If the cocaine trade were included by *Fortune* in its list of the 500 largest industrial corporations, cocaine would rank 7 th in volume of domestic sales, between the Ford Motor Company and the Gulf Oil Corporation. Based on U.S. estimates, the monetary value of Bolivia's cocaine exports may now surpass the value of the country's largest legal industry, tin. Columbia's more highly refined cocaine exports total about $1 billion annually, half the value of the coffee crop".

In view of the pervasive social, and political implications of the cocaine trade, it is of compelling interest to examine the pharmacologic bases for its behavioral effects.

a) Peripheral Effects

Cocaine is a potent local anesthetic, effective when applied topically as well as regionally by injection. The mechanism by which impulse conduction in peripheral nerves is blocked by this agent, i.e., blockage of sodium channels resulting in a reduction in the rate of rise of the depolarization phase of the action potential, is similar to the other local anesthetic agents. However, cocaine has a unique property shared by no other local anesthetic, its ability to block the re-uptake of norepinephrine at sympathetic nerve terminals. AXELROD et al. (1959) first showed that most of the norepinephrine released at sympathetic nerve endings is reabsorbed into these same endings, with only a very small percentage undergoing oxidation. Hertting et al. (1961), Muscholl (1961) and MacMillan (1959) demonstrated that cocaine interferes with this re-uptake process, thereby resulting in higher concentrations of norepinephrine and epinephrine near the receptors of the effector organs and accounting for the significant vasoconstriction resulting when cocaine is applied topically to the nasal mucosa. Consequently, the elevated catecholamine levels can produce elevated pulse rates, myocardial irritability, and ventricular arrythmias when certain volatile inhalational anesthetics, i.e., halothane, trichloroethylene, cyclopropane and chloroform are administered (Dripps et al. 1982). These 4 agents sensitize the myocardium to the effects of endogenous and exogenous catecholamines, and, on occasion, ventricular fibrillation has resulted when cocaine was administered concurrently.

b) Central Behavioral and Neural Effects

Cocaine stimulates both behavioral output and the electrical activity of the brain. When administered to laboratory animals, i.e., mice, rats, cats, monkeys, a marked stimulant effect on behavior results (Stripling and Ellinwood 1977). At low to moderate doses, spontaneous locomotor activity is increased in mice (Dews 1953). At higher doses, sterotyped behavior, resembling that seen with amphetamine, occurs in rats and monkeys (Stripling et al. 1977). Stereotypy refers to the onset of exaggerated repetitive motor movements and posturing including sniffing, grooming and chewing behaviors. It is felt that this may relate to schizophrenia in man, especially the catatonic form (Iverson and Iverson 1981). On repeated dosing of the drug, its locomotor and sterotypic effects become accentuated. With chronic administration of cocaine, these effects often persist well beyond the termination of the drug treatment (Post and Rose 1976). Post and colleagues, using Rhesus monkeys in whom cocaine was administered chronically for up to 6 months, found a progression of behavioral effects beginning with hyperactive, stereotypic responses during the first 2 months. Thereafter, the animals began to display what was termed "inhibitory behavior," consisting of catalepsy, motor inhibition, visual tracking and staring (Post and Rose 1976; Post et al. 1976; Post 1977). These effects are similar to those following repeated administration of amphetamine in monkeys, and are thought to represent a general response to sustained psychomotor stimulation (Segal and Janowsky 1978).

Stripling and Ellinwood (1977) studied the behavioral and electrophysiologic effects of repeated cocaine administration in male Sprague Dawly rats implanted with electrodes in the amygdala. The 3 treatment groups received, respectively, saline, 20 mg/kg cocaine and 40 mg/kg cocaine intraperitoneally (IP) once daily for 13 days. The 2 cocaine groups each had highly significant increases in locomotor activity compared to saline controls over a 15 min period following injection. In the saline group, locomotor output was unchanged. Moderate longitudinal enhancement of the locomotor effect over the 13 day period was also seen in the cocaine groups in that locomotor effects increased with successive treatments. Following the initial 13 days of drug administration, animals in each treatment group then received daily electrical stimulation of the left amygdala for up to 13 additional days. Behavioral responses to the stimulation were scored according to the following stages: 1) chewing movements; 2) forelimb clonus;

3) rearing and 4) falling. The electrical stimulation each day was continued until a stage 3 or 4 response occurred on 2 consecutive days. This paradigm was employed in order to determine whether cocaine influenced the latency period to electrical "kindling" in the limbic system. Kindling is defined as follows: GODDARD (1967) showed that when certain areas of the brain, particularly the limbic system, are stimulated repeatedly, usually at daily intervals, the behavioral and electrical effects of such stimulation become progressively increased. In fact, brief daily periods of stimulation initially without observable effect can eventually elicit both prolonged after-discharges and clonic convulsive activity, sometimes persisting for months after the last stimulation. This phenomenon is known as "kindling." STRIPLING and ELLINWOOD (1977) feel that it represents local neuronal reactions at the site of stimulation as well as enhanced propagation of neuronal activity from the site. Because cocaine has electrophysiologic effects in areas which are quite susceptible to kindling, including the amygdala, olfactory bulb and prepyriform cortex, where large amplitude spindles at 20–60 Hz occur in response to the drug, Stripling and Ellinwood felt that cocaine might well induce this phenomenon. With saline, no significant changes in electrical activity from the amygdala occurred over the 13 day treatment session. However, the animals receiving 20 mg/kg cocaine showed progressive increased activity in the left amygdala, but no spindling was observed. In the 40 mg/kg group, both amygdala showed progressive increases in mean maximum amplitude as well as the onset of spingling. However, the latency period to kindling was not significantly decreased by either dose of cocaine. Moreover, afterdischarges were not reliably observed, so that classical kindling, per se, did not occur in this experiment. Thus, the mechanism of enhancement of the behavioral and electrical amplitude effects of repeated administration remains unclear. The authors considered 2 hypotheses. The first was that the physiologic responses became conditioned by the pairing of the drug treatment, i.e., saline or cocaine, with the electrical stimulation somewhat in the manner of a classical, or Type I conditioned response. This was rejected because the saline controls showed no evidence of progressive effects and also because the development of stereotypy is difficult to explain in terms of a conditioned response. In addition, the drug treatments were not temporally concurrent with the electrical stimulation, so that classical conditioning is very doubtful in this paradigm. The second hypothesis, i.e., with repeated administrations more drug reaches critical sites of actions in the CNS, is also largely unsupported because the half-life of cocaine is shortened by repeated administrations (HO et al. 1977). The authors conclude that the behavioral and electrophysiologic enhancement with chronic cocaine administration may accrue from changes in CNS function owing perhaps to such mechanisms as altered receptor sensitivity and depletion of critical but as yet unidentified inhibitory neurotransmitter systems.

2. Effects of Lidocaine on Animal Behavior and Latency to Seizures

In a related study, POST et al. (1975) studied the effects of chronic lidocaine administration on behavior and seizure threshold in the rat. The anesthetic potency of lidocaine approximates that of cocaine. However, lidocaine is considered devoid of psychomotor stimulant effects at subtoxic dosages and does not affect catecholamine re-uptake (Covino and Vasallo 1976; Aberg et al. 1973). Male Sprague-Dawley rats were given IP lidocaine, 60 mg/kg once daily with control rats receiving saline, over an 8 week period. The lidocaine dose was previously determined to be near, but below the seizure threshold. The rats receiving lidocaine had a significantly greater weight gain than controls (72% vs. 45%) after 8 weeks and, in addition, developed abnormal eating patterns manifested by the ingestion of significantly more feces, straw, and gauze than saline controls. The lidocaine-treated animals also developed increases in convulsive activity after daily dosing, the average being after 16 prior lidocaine injections. The seizures increased both in frequency and duration with the number of daily injections and the latency period to seizure activity also progressively decreased (1–2 min following injection after 8 weeks of treatment as opposed to the 10–15 min latency seen initially). In addition, in those animals who developed multiple lidocaine-induced seizures, some showed typical stereotypic and hyperactive behavior resembling that seen after amphetamine administration. Thus, a drug with no known catecholamine-potentiating effects was shown to produce progressive behavioral and convulsive effects resembling those of cocaine, amphetamine and apomorphine, agents which increase central catecholamine levels by various mechanisms. The authors attributed these effects of lidocaine to a true pharmacologic kindling action of the drug, whereby the limbic system became progressively disrupted. Possible mechanisms will be discussed further in the section dealing with effects on electrical activity of the brain.

II. Effects of Local Anesthetics on Conditioned Behavior

Local anesthetics also affect performance on behavioral schedules. When a naïve, moderately food-deprived laboratory animal, i.e., a mouse, rat, or monkey, is placed in a novel environment such as a cage fitted with a lever, it will usually exhibit exploratory activity. If a particular behavior, such as randomly touching the lever in the course of exploring is rewarded, i.e., reinforced by food, the response desired will soon be associated with the reward and the frequency of the response will increase until it is emitted almost exclusively. Thus, a desired response can be brought under the control of a behavioral schedule which governs the frequency of reinforcement. In a fixed-ratio (FR) schedule, every n[th] response is reinforced. Thus, in an FR-30 schedule, every 30th response is rewarded. An FR schedule tends to generate a very high, sustained response rate and is useful to test drug effects on high baseline rates of responding. In a fixed-interval schedule (FI), the first response occurring after n minutes have elapsed is reinforced. In an FI-5 min schedule, the first response after 5 min have elapsed is rewarded. The rate of baseline responding on an FI-schedule, once the animal has been trained, is quite slow at the beginning of the interval, then gradually accelerates. By the end of the interval, the response rate becomes quite rapid as the animal anticipates the reward. The FI is widely utilized in behavioral pharmacology studies because of the initial slow response rate it engenders. Thus, rate-increasing effects of drugs, which would tend not to be apparent on an FR-schedule, are often manifest on the FI-schedule. FR- and FI-schedules are often combined into a multiple schedule. For example, the FR-30 and FR-5 min components are combined into a multiple, alternating FR-30, FI-5 min. Thus, a drug's effects on 2 diverse schedule components can be studied concurrently over a single session, thereby saving considerable training time on the part of the experimenter (GARFIELD and VIVALDI 1983).

1. Effects of Cocaine on Behavioral Schedules

Cocaine has been widely studied under various schedules of reinforcement. Because of its pronounced stimulant activity and inhibition of catecholamine re-uptake, this drug would be expected to have major effects on conditioned responding and, indeed, this is the case. When administered as a pre-treatment, cocaine significantly increases response rates in a fixed-interval schedule in pigeons (SMITH 1964) and in monkeys (BYRD 1975). On an FR-schedule, however, where response rates are high under control conditions, cocaine typically decreases responding in rats, pigeons, and monkeys (BYRD 1980). These effects also occur with amphetamine. CLARK and STEELE (1966) studied effects of amphetamine on FR- and FI-responding in rats. They felt that the low baseline response roles typical of an FI-schedule become accelerated to a point owing to the stimulatory action of amphetamine. High baseline response rates, on the other hand, can not increase much beyond their control values. Thus, the FR-component shows progressive decreases in responding with increasing amphetamine doses owing to motor incoordination. This is also the probable mechanism with cocaine as well. Its counterpart in man will be discussed in a following section.

To our knowledge, the effects of other local anesthetics, i.e., procaine, lidocaine, bupivicaine, on behavioral schedules have not been reported. We are beginning a study of these agents in our laboratory to determine whether lidocaine, in particular, will enhance low rates of responding on an FI-schedule, and will report our data as soon as it is available.

2. Local Anesthetics as Self-Reinforcers

Cocaine and amphetamine are themselves potent reinforcers in rats and monkeys, i.e., these species will lever-press on behavioral schedules to receive intravenous injections of these drugs given though indwelling cannulae (DENEAU et al. 1969; PICKENS and HARRIS 1968; PICKENS and THOMPSON 1968). The patterns of responding closely resemble those produced by food. There is considerable evidence that operant reinforcement may be mediated by catecholamine systems, in particular norepinephrine, which Stein believes to "guide response selection via a knowledge of response consequences" (STEIN 1978). One of the most important pieces of evidence supporting this hypothesis is the observation that intracranial selfstimulation behavior (ICSS) is selectively augmented by drugs that affect central catecholamine transmission. If electrodes are implanted in certain discrete "reward areas" of the brain, predominantly the lateral hypothalamus and Medical Forebrain Bundle (MFB) and a short microamperage burst of current delivered to the electrodes as a consequence of a behavioral schedule of lever-pressing, the current functions as a potent reinforcer. The mechanism is thought to be mobilization of norepinephrine and/or dopamine in response to the electrical stimulation. Thus, as Stein points out, drugs that rapidly release catecholamines from functional stores, (amphetamine, α-methyl-m-tyrosine) or increase central catecholamine levels though inhibition of re-uptake, (cocaine and imipramine), facilitate ICSS. On the other hand, central catecholamine depleters (reserpine), catecholamine receptor blockers (chlorpromazine, haloperidol) and catecholamine synthesis inhibitors (α-methyl-p-tyrosine) all inhibit ICSS responding (Stein 1978). Waugier and Niemegeers (1974) studied the effects of cocaine on ICSS in rats using subcutaneous doses ranging between 0.63–10.0 mg/kg. Monopolar electrodes were implanted in the MFB in 6 rats and stimulation provided by biphasic square waves produced a constant-current stimulator. They found dose-related increases in ICSS rates except at the lowest dose of 0.63 mg/kg. The increases were greatest when the control rate of responding was lowest.

This data is consistent with Stein's theory of catecholamine mediation in operant reinforcement as discussed. There have been no published studies of the effects of any other local anesthetic agents on ICSS to our knowledge. We conducted some preliminary investigations in our laboratory where effects of lidocaine, 10, 20, and 40 mg/kg IP, were studied on thresholds for ICSS in rats implanted with bipolar electrodes in the MFB (Garfield 1982). The data suggested that lidocaine moderately increased ICSS thresholds ath the higher doses, implying a depressant effect of the anesthetic. No significant effects were noted at 10 mg/kg. Thus, lidocaine appears not to have any facilitating effect on reward pathways. However, this data is preliminary and further studies must be performed in order to make any definitive statements relative to effects of lidocaine on ICSS.

On the other hand, Ford and Balster (1977) found intravenous procaine to be a primary reinforcer in rhesus monkeys, in that these animals worked on behavioral schedules to receive injections of the drug as reinforcement. This is direct evidence that the drug may have euphorogenic or stimulant qualitites. This will be discussed further in the next section.

III. Behavioral Effects of Local Anesthetics in Man

Having outlined the behavioral pharmacology of the local anesthetics in animals, we will now discuss their behavioral effects in man. Cocaine, procaine and lidocaine will be discussed since these are prototypical agents. Cocaine, as mentioned earlier, is the only local anesthetic that inhibits norepinephrine uptake in man. Lidocaine is the most widely used local anesthetic in clinical practice and is employed systemically for analgesia and treatment of ventricular arrhythmias. Procaine, although its use today has fallen off owing to the popularity of lidocaine and bupivicaine, has been utilized extensively for systemic analgesia and sedation. Consequently, there have been many studies of its behavioral effects.

1. Cocaine

As pointed out earlier, cocaine increases locomotor activity and behavioral output in laboratory animals. This occurs in man as well. In the laboratory setting, the euphoric effects of cocaine resemble those of amphetamine very closely. Jaffee (1980) points out that cocaine-experienced subjects cannot differentiate between the subjective effects of 8–10 mg of cocaine and 10 mg D-amphetamine if both are administered intravenously, according to a study by FISCHMAN et al. (1976). In the U.S., most cocaine is taken intranasally or smoked, but an appreciable number also administer it intravenously as well. Cocaine powder, as sold in the illicit drug market, is usually marketed as the hydrochloride, which is more susceptible to heat decomposition than the free-base. Hence, a procedure called "free-basing" has arisen among users. The hydrochloride is incubated with an organic solvent, such as ether, in which the free-base concentrates. The ether is than evaporated, and the remaining free-base is harvested and vaporized for inhalation through a device called a "base pipe."

On ingestion, the overall behavioral effects of cocaine are those of brief, but intense behavioral stimulation. There is marked euphoria, feelings of elevation and alertness. VAN DYKE and BYCK (1982) found that 25–100 mg of intra-nasal cocaine in experienced users reliably produced reports of euphoria in 15–30 min. At 45–60 min, anxiety, fatigue and a desire for more drug tend to appear. They also found that euphoria is most pronounced shortly before the plasma concentration has begun to fall. They also observed that the euphoric effects disappeared several hours before the plasma concentration returned to zero. They felt, then, that these observations suggest that the psychologic effects of cocaine may be related to the rate of change of plasma concentration rather than to its absolute level. Additional evidence for this hypothesis is provided by the observation that more pronounced psychologic effects accrue from smoking or injecting cocaine than from intranasal or oral administration. Despite the fact that cocaine is well absorbed orally, plasma concentrations change much more abruptly following smoking or intravenous use than after oral ingestion or intranasal administration, thus supporting their hypothesis.

The question arises to what mechanisms are responsible for these euphoric effects. Are they simply the consequence of cocaine's ability to block norepinephrine re-uptake in the CNS? This is probably not the case, for certain tricylic antidepressants, i.e., nortriptyline, which block re-uptake of norepinephrine at central sites do not induce euphoria. Nor do monoamine oxidase inhibitors, i.e., tranylcypramine, when administered to normal or depressed patients (COOPER et al. 1978).

On the other hand, VAN DYKE and colleagues found that cocaine and lidocaine have similar psychological effects after intranasal application (VAN DYKE et al. 1979). 6 adult males with previous experience in using intranasal cocaine were given 3 matched doses of intranasal cocaine and lidocaine, both as solutions, i.e., 10% cocaine vs. 4% lidocaine. For each of the three doses, 0.19 mg/kg, 0.38 mg/kg, 0.75 mg/kg, psychological ratings did not differ significantly between drugs, although a saline placebo produced peak "high" ratings similar to those observed after the 0.19 mg dose of each drug. The authors concluded that the differences between cocaine and lidocaine may be subtle and perhaps indistinguishable. They also hypothesized that "euphoria may be an ordinary effect of local anesthetics rather than an extraordinary effect of cocaine." Nonetheless, the underlying mechanisms for the euphoroganic properties of cocaine, and the question of to what extent this occurs with other local anesthetic, are far from clear.

2. Behavioral and Analgesic Effects of Procaine and Lidocaine

Cocaine was discussed separately because its potent behavioral stimulatory actions and inhibition of norepinephrine re-uptake at sympathetic nerve endings render it unique among the local anesthetic agents. We shall now discuss several other prototypical agents: procaine, lidocaine and bupivicaine. Procaine is an ester, hydrolyzed by plasma pseudocholinesterase, whereas lidocaine is an amide, metabolized mainly by the liver. Nonetheless, these 2 compounds are quite similar in their behavioral and analgesic effects, and so will be discussed together.

a) Clinical Effects of Systemic Administration of Local Anesthetics

The initial effect of local anesthetics on the CNS is to produce signs of CNS excitation. Human volunteers receiving intravenous infusions of these agents first report feelings of lightheadedness, giddiness, and dizziness. On occasion, one sees a garrulous affect, similar to that often seen following alcoholic ingestion. At this stage, systemic analgesia occurs, which has been utilized as an adjunct to general anesthesia and for treatment of pain status. This is discussed separately. At higher concentrations, patients report difficulty in focusing their eyes, tinnitus and circumoral numbness and tingling. At this point, shivering, muscle tremors, and disorientation attest to CNS-excitation, although some patients become drowsy. At still higher levels, Jacksonian twitching movements and tremors occur, giving way to tonic-clonic grandmal seizure activity. At grossly toxic dosages, generalized CNS depression follows these excitatory phenomena and respiratory and even cardiac arrest can occur as seizure activity ceases. Later in the chapter we discuss in detail the electrical and convulsant properties of the local anesthetics. The reader is also referred to Covino's Chapter: "Toxicity and Systemic Effects of Local Anesthetic Agents," in this volume.

b) Systemic Analgesic Effects of Local Anesthetic Agents

α) *Procaine.* Well before the introduction of lidocaine and other amide agents, procaine was known to produce systemic analgesia when administered in high doses (Koppany 1962). Bigelow and Harrison (1944) studied the systemic analgesic effect of subcutaneously administered procaine, comparing it with saline placebo using the Hardy, Wolff and Goodell method for measuring pain thresholds. They found that 800 mg of procaine, a dose near the clinical limit of 1000 mg, produced a 35% increase in cutaneous pain threshold, equivalent to that produced by 600 mg of aspirin. The procaine effect lasted approximately 1 h, whereas the aspirin's duration was 4 h. The procaine group, however, had occasional members reporting giddiness, lightheadedness, and faintness, indicative of incipient CNS toxicity. Other investigators and clinicians used the drug intravenously with better success. Keats, D'Alessandro, and Beecher (1950) studied the effects of a bolus of intravenous procaine as compared to saline placebo and morphine, on relief of postoperative pain. They found that the incidence of pain relief with procaine was 40%. Although significantly higher than placebo (20%), it was still well below the incidence of postoperative pain relief with morphine, i.e., 70% vs. 40%. The authors concluded that procaine had a definite analgetic effect on intravenous administration, but not enough to warrant its clinical use. Relative to side effects, some found the procaine injections subjectively pleasant, whereas other reported dysphoria. At any rate, procaine as a systemic analgesic agent is largely of historical interest, owing to its rapid metabolism and relatively high incidence of allergic phenomena as contrasted to lidocaine.

β) Lidocaine. Lidocaine is, today, the most widely clinically employed local anesthetic agent, owing to its extremely slow incidence of allergic reactions, relatively low toxicity, longer duration of effect than procaine, and its suppressant actions on ventricular cardiac arrhythmias. Lidocaine has also been used for systemic analgesia to supplement general anesthetic agents, to provide postoperative analgesia and to suppress coughing and reflex responses prior to insertion and removal of endotracheal tubes. DE CLIVE-LOWE and colleagues (1958) reported on the use of intravenous lidocaine as a supplement to surgical anesthesia in a study of 400 patients. Following a bolus dose of thiopental (500 mg) and succinylcholine to facilitate endotracheal intubation, the patients were ventilated with a mixture of nitrous oxide-oxygen (5:2 L per min). During the 1st hour of surgery, 40 mg (2 ml of a 2% solution) of lidocaine were administered iv every 5 min, giving a total dosage of 480 mg over the 1st hour. If surgery extended over the 2nd h, the dosage was reduced to 20 mg every 5 min, giving a total of 720 mg for the 2-h period. If the procedure carried over to the 3rd h, the dosage was reduced to 20 mg every 10 min, giving a maximum of 840 mg. The authors did not use a ratio scale for calculating their lidocaine dosage, but they encountered no toxic symptoms. Intraoperative lidocaine conferred a high incidence of postoperative analgesia, i.e., 89% of the group had analgesia of some duration postoperatively, and 43% had analgesia up to 18 h duration. Those patients receiving a total lidocaine dosage of 0–251–mg had the highest incidence of satisfactory and prolonged analgesia. Patients in this 1st sub-group tended to have procedures of shorter length, and hernia repairs and hemorrhoidectomics were associated with the most marked postoperative analgesia. Those patients requiring larger doses, i.e., 252–501 mg and 502–750 mg, had a lower incidence of satisfactory pain relief. The authors found that the magnitude of the surgery and degree of surgical stimulation tended to be higher in these two sub-groups and postulated that the lidocaine dosage was not adequate for severe postoperative pain.

The incidence of side effects reported, including postoperative nausea, vomiting, and respiratory complications, was low. Although the authors state that no seizures occurred, they do not give data relative to other signs of CNS-toxicity, such as confusion, change in affect, numbness about the lips, tinnitus, etc. Accordingly, we cannot draw any definitive conclusions from this study relative to minor or moderate toxic signs, nor do they report on the patients' perceptions of the experience. On the other hand, systemic lidocaine administered according to the authors' protocol appears to be relatively effective and apparently free of serious problems. However, as the authors state, the dosages must be exact and the patients very carefully monitored.

Today however, the majority of institutions do not use this technique for postoperative pain relief, feeling that the potential for toxicity is too great in relation to its moderate efficacy. Rather, they advocate use of systemic narcotics and epidural analgesia in the immediate post-operative period.

D. Effects of Local Anesthetics on Electrical Activity of the Brain

I. The Convulsant Properties of Local Anesthesia

1. Signs and Symptoms

When local anesthetics are used clinically, a variety of systemic toxic effects can occur, and, on occasion, frank convulsions are seen. Accordingly, many research efforts have been directed toward elucidating the mechanisms underlying the central nervous system (CNS) effects of local anesthetics.

With respect to the convulsant properties of local agents, a number of investigators have published on the incidence of seizures secondary to their clinical use. Moore and co-workers reviewed their experience with regional blocks from 1948–1979 (MOORE et al. 1980). The incidence of untoward CNS reactions in this series was 1.5%, with 98% of this figure, i.e., 1.47% secondary to nonallergic toxic reactions. The seizure incidence with the use of the potent local anesthetics, i.e., bupivicaine and etidocaine was 0.1% and 0.07% respectively (MOORE 1980). In a review of toxic CNS reactions seen with the use of regional anesthesia in obstetrical patients, an incidence of 4.1/1000 blocks was reported (BERGER et al. 1974). Seizures have been reported to occur with the use of lidocaine during cardiac surgery (AMDUROUX et al. 1975). de Jong cites an incidence of 6.2/1000 lidocaine treatments in medical patients for cardiac arrhythmias (DE JONG 1977).

Local anesthetics have been found to cause seizures not only in man, but cats, rabbits, dogs, monkeys, rats, and mice as well (DE JONG 1977; MUNSON et al. 1975; HOFFMAN et al. 1977). Even fetal and newborn lambs, as well as human newborns have been reported to experience local anesthetic induced seizures (STEIN and MICHENFELDER 1979).

→

[a] The doses given under CD_{100} for man represent the threshold dose for producing preconvulsive behavior and/or overt seizures. For all other 100 species, the CD_{100} represents the threshold dose for convulsions in 100% of the population. The values are given as mg/kg.

[b] The CD_{50} represents the threshold dose in mg/kg for which 50% of the studied population convulse.

[c] The infusion rate is given as mg/kg/min.

[d] The blood level is given as µg/ml.

[e] Sources

1. SMITH and DUCE (1971)
2. MUNSON and WAGMAN (1972)
3. KRENIS et al. (1971)
4. WESSELING et al. (1971)
5. BLUMER et al. (1973)
6. ÄKERMAN et al. (1966)
7. SOREL and LEJEUNE (1955)
8. DE JONG and HAEVNER (1974)
9. DE JONG and HAEVNER (1971)
10. ENGLESSON and MATAUSEK (1975)
11. MAEKAWA et al. (1974)
12. SEO et al. (1982)
13. LIU et al. (1983)
14. MUNSON et al. (1970)
15. MUNSON et al. (1975)
16. USUBIAGA et al. (1966)
17. MORISHIMA et al. (1981)
18. SANDERS (1967)
19. EIDELBERG et al. (1965)
20. MARK et al. (1964)
21. GOLDBERG and GOLDBERG (1970)
22. DE JONG and BONIN (1981)
23. DE JONG et al. (1980)
24. MORISHIMA et al. (1983)
25. ENGLESSON (1973)
26. FOLDES et al. (1965)
27. SCOTT (1975)

Table 3. Central nervous system toxic doses of local anesthetics

Agent	Specy	Route	CD[b]50	CD[b]100	Infusion rate[c]	Blood level[d]	Source[e]
Cocaine	Mouse	IP	47.5	–	–	–	3
	Rat	IP	–	60	–	–	19
Chloro-procaine	Man[a]	IV	–	22.8	–	–	26
Procaine	Mouse	IP	–	200	–	–	18
	Rabbit	IV	–	15	–	–	7
	Cat	IV	–	35	–	–	25
	Dog	IV	–	100	–	–	20
	Man[a]	IV	–	19.2–27.8	–	–	16, 26
Prilocaine	Rat	IP	–	200	–	–	6
	Cat	IV	–	22	–	–	25
	Monkey	IV	–	18.1	4	20.5	14, 15
	Man[a]	IV	–	76	–	–	27
Mepivacaine	Mouse	IP	–	100	–	–	21
	Cat	IV	–	18	–	–	25
	Monkey	IV	–	18.8	4	22.5	14, 15
	Man[a]	IV	–	9.8	–	–	26
Lidocaine	Mouse	Oral	256	–	–	–	1
	Mouse	IP	82.9–100	–	–	–	2, 3
	Mouse	IV	21.5	–	–	–	4
	Rat	IP	52	100	–	–	5, 6
	Rabbit	IV	5.3–6.0	–	–	–	2, 7
	Cat	IV	8.4	15–27.5	–	–	8–10, 12
	Dog	IV		22–23.3	–	–	11,13
	Lamb fetus	IV		41.9	2	16.4	17
	Lamb new born	IV		18.4	2	16.6	17
	Lamb adult	IV		5.8	2	11.7	17
	Monkey	IV	12.8	14.2–22.5	4	18.2–24.5	14, 15, 8
Lidocaine	Man[a]	IV		>4–7.3	–	–	26, 27, 16
Etidocaine	Mouse	IP	54.9	–	–	–	22
	Cat	IV	–	6.5	1	6.57	23
	Dog	IV	–	8	–	–	13
	Lamb fetus	IV	–	2.2	0.5	3	24
	Lamb new born	IV	–	5.7	0.5	3.2	24
	Lamb adult	IV	–	15.6	0.5	1.4	24
	Monkey	IV	–	5.4	1	4.3	14, 15
	Man[a]	IV	–	1.6	–	–	32
Tetracaine	Mouse	IV	3	–	–	–	34
	Rabbit	IV	–	3	–	–	7
	Dog	IV	–	5	–	–	13
	Man[a]	IV	–	2.5	–	–	31
Bupivacaine	Mouse	IP	57.7	–	–	–	22
	Cat	IV	–	5.4	1	3.05	23
	Dog	IV	–	4	–	–	13
	Monkey	IV	–	4.4	1	4.5	14, 15
	Man[a]	IV	–	3.4	–	74.0	27

Most investigators agree that some local anesthetic-induced seizures are preceeded by one or a combination of the following subjective symptoms in the nonpremedicated patient; restlessness, a dizzy sensation, nervousness, apprehension, numbness, visual and/or auditory hallucinations, nausea, lightheadedness, a sensation of twitching before actual twitches are seen, tinnitis or roaring in the ears, and a metallic taste (DE JONG 1977; STEIN and MICHENFELDER 1979; MOORE 1980). Objective signs premonitary to local anesthetic induced seizures include, euphoria, dysarthria, nystagmus, sweating, vomiting, pugnaciousness, loquaciousness, failure to follow commands or to be reasoned with, disorientation, periodic loss of consciousness, headaches, and a generalized loss of response to painful stimuli. In man, an intravenous (I.V.) bolus of 1 mg/kg of lidocaine which corresponded to a blood level of 4.5 µg/ml (KLEIN et al. 1968) produced lightheadedness in less than 10% of the group of patients. When the dose was increased to 1.5 mg/kg, more than 80% experienced slurred speech and lightheadedness. The lidocaine blood-level was 5.4 µg/ml. When 5 mg/kg of lidocaine or mepivicaine were given I.V. over a 20-min period, slightly higher blood levels, i.e., 5–6 µg/ml, resulted, but euphoria and muscle twitching were now noted (JORFELDT et al. 1968), and at 6 mg/ml I.V., fasiculations of all 4 extremities were noted, but no generalized seizure activity occurred (SJÖGREN and WRIGHT 1972). At still higher blood levels, generalized seizures did occur after these premonitary signs and symptoms. Table 3, derived from a number of investigations, shows the arterial blood levels obtained at the onset of generalized seizures. The generalized seizure can take the form of tonic and/or tonic-clonic seizure (DE JONG 1977). Moore has pointed out that these premonitary warnings may be blunted or absent in the premedicated patient (MOORE 1980).

Of particular interest is the observation that many of the toxic systemic premonitary signs and symptoms mimick the presentation of temporal-lobe epilepsy (DE JONG 1977). Thus, de Jong and Walts studied 8 patients with longstanding temporal-lobe seizures in which stereotaxically placed electrodes were present for diagnostic purposes. When given lidocaine I.V., typical seizure activity resulted in the limbic system. This was seen at a blood level of 4–10 µg/ml and corresponded with typical temporal lobe seizure symptoms (DE JONG et al. 1966). 5 of the 8 patients at this blood level progressed from temporal lobe seizure activity to fully developed grand mal seizures. Other investigators have shown that subconvulsant doses of procaine can also produce limbic system seizure manifestations (STARK et al. 1982). By analyzing the facial displays and verbal reports of patients with temporal lobe epilepsy, and comparing the results to the type of hallucinations, emotions and alimentary sensations seen with electrical stimulation, they concluded that procaine could serve as a noninvasive method for detecting limbic system pathology, i.e., foci.

2. Factors Affecting the CNS Toxic Dose of Local Anesthetics

A number of investigators have determined the doses of various local anesthetics necessary to produce generalized convulsions in laboratory animals, and through clinical observation, in man. Table 3 is a compilation of their data with respect to the species studied, route of administration, and type of local anesthetic employed. A number of considerations in interpreting these data arise. First, local anesthetic seizure-producing doses are given only at 2 points on the continuum, i.e., the CD_{50} and CD_{100}. CD_{50} is defined as that dose necessary to produce seizures in 50% of the population studied, whereas, the CD_{100} defines the dose producing seizures in 100% of the population. [1]

Another difficulty arises because of the fact that local anesthetics have different protein binding characteristics (WOOD and WOOD 1981). Protein-binding can vary, depending on the growth and development of the animal, its nutritional status, and a host of other variables. For example, alpha-1-acid glycoprotein (A-1-A glycoprt) is a major protein which binds lidocaine in the blood (ROUTLEDGE et al. 1981). Its concentration varies as a function of sex, in that females have lower concentrations than males. Others have shown that A-1-A-glycoprt is also reduced in pregnant females to a greater extent than females taking birth control pills (BCP's), who in turn have lower concentrations than females not taking BCP's (WOOD and WOOD 1981). The newborn infant was shown to have lower values than their mothers in this study. The lower A-1-A glycoprt concentrations correlated with higher free lidocaine plasma levels. Estrogen has been implicated in decreasing the level of this carrier protein. Finally, patients with renal disease have been shown to have higher free lidocaine plasma levels secondary to lower A-1-A-glycoprt plasma concentrations (GROSSMAN et al. 1982). Because of protein binding competition, meperidine has been shown to raise the free lidocaine plasma levels (LAMPE et al. 1976), as has phenytoin, quinidine and desipramine (STEIN and MICHENFELDER 1979). Thus, patients taking these drugs concurrently with lidocaine may experience toxic effects at lower doses.

The speed of infusion of a local anesthetic has also been shown to be important in determining the toxic dose. Thus, when increasing the infusion rate of etidocaine from 0.5–2 mg/kg, the incidence of seizures increased (MALAGODI et al. 1977). Bupivicaine's seizure incidence was not affected in this infusion range. The authors explained this discrepancy in the monkey by showing that the volume of distribution for etidocaine was greater than for bupivicaine. The dependance of the toxic dose on infusion rate has been shown for other local anesthetics as well (DE JONG 1977; STEIN and MICHENER 1979).

When comparing the toxic dose for lidocaine in cats, monkeys, and man, de Jong points out that the volume of distribution, for lidocaine as a function of species is an important factor (DE JONG 1977). The cat's volume of distribution for lidocaine is 10 times smaller than the monkey's and tends more closely to approximate that of man, resulting in a toxic dose closer to man's.

As mentioned above, local anesthetic induced seizures have also been described in the fetus, newborn as well as the mother (DE JONG 1977, STEIN and MICHENER 1979). In fetal lambs, (fetal age 126 days to 145 days; gestation length 148 days) seizures were produced with I.V. lidocaine administered to the mother, as well as in 1–5 day old newborns (MORISHIMA et al. 1981). An identical sequence

---

[1] With only one point on a dose-response curve, estimations, of relative toxicity among agents is hazardous because their curves may not be parallel. Note, in Table 3, that the CD_{50} and CD_{100} values together, are known only for lidocaine and even they differ significantly among different species.

of events of seizures, respiratory arrest, hypotension and cardiovascular arrest was noted in the fetus, newborn and adult. The seizure-threshold dose in the fetus was 41.9 mg/kg, whereas the newborn seized at a dose of 18.4 mg/kg and the adult at a dose of 5.8 mg/kg. The plasma concentrations noted in the fetus, newborn and adult, however, were not significantly different. The higher dose in the fetus was felt to be related to the efficient placental clearence of lidocaine into the mother's plasma, and better fetal maintenance of arterial oxygenation during respiratory arrest (but not with maternal hypotension and cariovascular arrest) because of the fetal dependance on the placenta for its blood gas maintenance.

On the other hand, other investigators have shown that the lamb fetus has an increasing susceptibility to local anesthetic induced seizures as the CNS develops. Thus, the toxic doses necessary for inducing seizures in a 138 day old fetus was less than in a 116 day old fetus (8 mg/kg as compared to 34 mg/kg with arterial lidocaine concentrations of 6.9 µg/ml and 40 µg/ml respectively). The increased susceptability of the mature fetus was attributed to the increased permeability of local anesthetics in the more mature CNS.

Another difficulty in comparing toxic doses for local anesthetic induced seizures relates to the site of administration of local anesthetics (DE JONG 1977; STEIN et al. 1979). Thus, intraperitoneal injections (i.p.) require larger doses than intravenous (i.v.) injections for producing seizures (see Table 3). Moore points out that if a seizure occurs within a minute of an injection, an inadvertant i.v. injection has taken place as opposed to a toxic reaction occuring after a latency of 5 min, where absorption into the intravascular compartment is responsible for toxic reactions (MOORE 1981).

Another important variable affecting the CD_{50} is the acid-base status of the patient (ENGLESSON and MATAUSEK 1975). Thus, an elevation of PCO_2 from 25–40 Torr decreases the toxic dose of procaine from 35 mg/kg–17 mg/kg. A metabolic acidosis potentiates this effect whereas a metabolic alkalosis will antagonize this effect. Differing pH and PCO_2 values have been shown to affect seizure-thresholds for prilocaine, lidocaine, mepivicaine, bupivicaine and etidocaine in both cats and dogs (DE JONG 1977). An increasing PCO_2 increases cerebral blood flow by inducing cerebral vasodilation, and therefore, increases the delivery of local anesthetics to the brain. On the other hand, a more acidic pH favors a higher concentration of charged molecules in the vascular compartment which would decrease the diffusion of local anesthetic across the blood/brain barrier, an effect which should increase the toxic dose. Englesson has helped to resolve this dilemma by noting that a high brain/blood partition coefficient for local anesthetics will tend to maintain the brain concentration of local anesthetics irrespective of pH effects on the ionic component of local anesthetics in the intravascular compartment. Thus, with elevated intracerebral PCO_2 diffusing intraneuronally, more local anesthetic will be in its active charged form intracellularly. This effect will favor toxic reactions taking place at lower doses (DE JONG 1977).

Temperature also is a factor in determining the toxic doses for local anesthetics (PETERSON and HARDINGE 1967). A rise in temperature from 26–34 °C doubles the incidence of seizures secondary to cocaine. Finally, circadian rhythms have been evoked as a causal factor in determining the toxic dose in mice for lidocaine seizures (DE JONG 1977).

With so many variables affecting the CD_{50} for local anesthetic induced seizures, it is little wonder that some investigators have resorted to plasma levels for defining more precisely the toxic doses for local anesthetics. In this regard, arterial levels are probably superior to venous levels because of the effect of volume of distribution and metabolism on local anesthetic intravascular concentrations.

Covino and Vassallo have demonstrated a direct relationship between the dose of a local anesthetic necessary for producing seizures in animals and the intrinsic anesthetic potency of the local anesthetic (COVINO and VASSALLO 1976). Thus, procaine a weak local anesthetic has a much higher CD_{50} than the more potent bupivacaine. This relationship has been confirmed recently for lidocaine, etidocaine and bupivacaine in the dog (LIU et al. 1983).

E. Anticonvulsant Properties of Local Anesthetics

Procaine, lidocaine, cocaine, dibucaine, tetracaine, prilocaine, and mepivicaine have all been shown to possess anticonvulsant properties at doses below the convulsive threshold (DE JONG 1977). In man, lidocaine has been used effectively to abort grand mal seizures from a variety of causes (LEMMEN et al. 1978). These investigators used either 2–3 mg/kg I.V. boluses or 6–10 mg/kg/h continuous infusions in conjunction with other antiepileptogenic drugs. The lidocaine blood levels ranged from 1.4–2.8 µg/ml. Lidocaine and procaine have both been shown to elevate seizure foci thresholds to electrical stimulation, when infiltrated along the scalp wound margins during neurosurgical procedures for epilepsy (JULIAN 1973). Recently, lidocaine, in doses typical for control of ventricular extopy, has been shown to raise the convulsive threshold in patients undergoing electroconvulsive therapy (HOOD and MECCA 1983).

With respect to experimental epilepsy in animals, local anesthetics have also been shown to abort seizures. In mice, seizures induced with hyperbaric oxygen were prevented with lidocaine doses of 25 mg/kg (i.p.) or cocaine 27.5–40 mg/kg (i.p.). All doses were in the subconvulsant dose range (KRENIS et al. 1971). Alcohol withdrawal seizures in mice while resistance to phenytoin, succumbed to subcutaneous dose of licodaine of 20 mg/kg (FREUND 1973). Mice specifically bred for the trait of low thresholds to audiogenic seizures also had threshold elevations for this type of seizure in the presence of a local anesthetic (ESSMAN 1966). In cats, whose seizure foci were produced with penicillin, lidocaine blood levels of 0.5–4 µg/ml have also been shown to depress seizure activity (JULIAN 1973). Beyond this level, one sees signs and symptoms of increased central nervous system excitability, which progresses to seizures. Thus, in both man and animals, local anesthetics in subconvulsant dosages protect against seizure activity.

F. Temporal and Spatial Effects of Local Anesthetics at Regional CNS Sites

I. The Amygdaloid Complex as the Initial CNS Target of Local Anesthetics

A number of investigators, using a variety of experimental protocols, have attempted to find the locus of action of local anesthetics in the central nervous system (DE JONG 1977). In man, the surface electroencephalogram (EEG) has been unrewarding in this regard. In human volunteers exposed to increasing doses of local anesthetics, the EEG showed little alteration until overt motor seizures were seen (STEIN and MICHENFELDER 1979). There was however, loss of the normal alpha activity, and an increase in their delta and theta activity. A failure of EEG desynchronization with painful stimuli was also seen in some patients.

In monkeys given intravenous lidocaine (MUNSON et al. 1975), the cortical EEG also showed a generalized loss of alpha rhythm. This converted to a typical seizure pattern with the onset of motor seizures. With lidocaine, there were pre-ictal irregular large amplitude spike and slow wave complexes seen, but pre-seizure electrical changes were absent with bupivicaine and etidocaine. The discrepancy between the pre-ictal cortical EEG activity seen with lidocaine but not with the more potent local anesthetics has been confirmed by others. Englesson and coworkers analyzed the power spectrum of the pre-ictal EEG. Only lidocaine caused a significant difference in the first third of the local anesthetic induced preseizure cortical electrical activity (ENGLESSON and MATAUSEK 1975). When applied directly to the cortical surface, both procaine and lidocaine have been shown to depress spontaneous electrical activity and to suppress cortical seizure foci, but without eliciting seizure activity (ELLIOT et al. 1960; STEIN and MICHENFELDER 1979; DE JONG 1977). These depressant effects on the cortex were further shown in the cats' pericruciate cortical neurons (CRAWFORD 1970). In this case, Crawford showed that procaine, electrophoretically injected near cholinceptive neurons, decreased their acetylcholine and dl-homocysteic acid induced electrical activity. While the pre-seizure depression of cortical activity may help to explain, in part, the anticonvulsant properties of local anesthetics, this evidence suggests that a CNS focus located somewhere other than the cortex serves as the trigger area for seizures.

Cerebral ventricular infusion of procaine, while producing a change in ventilatory pattern, nystagmus, urination, defacation and muscle weakness, failed to elicit motor seizures (HARANATH et al. 1969). Seizure activity was also absent with micro injection of local anesthetics into the reticular formation (TUTTLE and ELLIOT 1969), as well as vertebral artery injection in the vascularly isolated rabbit brain (JOLLY and STEINHAUS 1956; DE JONG 1977).

Seizures are elicited, however, when local anesthetics are injected in the carotid arteries (JOLLY and STEINHAUS 1956). All of the above experimental data discussed to this point, would suggest a subcortical seizure focus, above the brain stem, as the local anesthetic trigger area (DE JONG 1977). That this focus lies within the limbic system has been demonstrated by a number of investigators. One study, in which stereotaxically placed electrodes were inserted in the temporal lobes of patients having a history of temporal lobe seizures, showed activation of electrical seizure activity in response to i.v. lidocaine. The patients reported behavioral and emotional sensations typical of their seizures experienced in the past (DE JONG and WALTS 1966). Another study in the monkey showed hippocampal seizure foci, produced by alumina, to be activated by i.v. procaine, although the behavioral manifestations of temporal lobe seizures were not seen (BABB et al. 1979).

WAGMAN and coworkers recorded from stereotaxically placed electrodes in a number of cat and rabbit CNS structures (WAGMAN et al. 1967). Bolus subconvulsant as well as convulsant doses of i.v. lidocaine were given. At subconvulsant doses the most striking and consistant electrical activity was seen in the amygdala. Rhythmic high voltage discharges (spindling) with or without brief high frequency superimposed bursts were recorded in this structure. The rhythmic spindling activity was found to correlate with the nasal air flow during respiration. At times episodic synchronous but lower voltage activity was recorded from other subcortical structures, i.e., the reticular formation, hippocampus, the medial dorsalis nuclei as well as the orbito-frontal cortex. Recordings from the reticular formation and cortex usually showed a drepression of electrical activity which began after the onset of amygdaloid activation. The animals showed a depression of motor activity, decreased response to sensory stimuli, dilated pupils and a vacant stare, suggesting a decrease in level of consciousness.

Convulsant doses of lidocaine produced a focal rhythmic discharge of augmenting voltage in the amygdala with concommittant arrest of activity and staring behavior. This activity was followed by a generalized electrical seizure activity in all recording sites with tonic and tonic-clonic seizure activity at the behavioral level. Thus, Lidocaine induces increased electrical activity in the cat and rabbit amygdala at a time when other central neural sites are depressed. Only with higher doses does one observe motor seizure behavior.

II. Anatomy and Function of the Amygdaloid Complex

At this point in the discussion, an overview of amygdaloid anatomy and its functional role will help put the experimental data in perspective (see Fig. 1). The amygdaloid nuclear complex is related to the limbic system and is located anterior to and partly superior to the tips of the inferior horn of the lateral ventricle (TRUEX and CARPENTER 1971). It is usually divided into a basolateral and a corticomedial nuclear group, of which the former is highly developed in man. Well-defined afferents to the amygdala are the olfactory fibers which, by way of the lateral olfactory tract, project onto cells of the corticomedial nuclear group (see Fig. 1). Indirect olfactory input to the amygdala requires synaptic relays in the prepyriform cortex (that part of the cortex which extends from the lateral olfactory stria to the rostral amygdaloid area). Thus, this dual olfactory sensory pathway can in part explain the respiratory variation of the amygdaloid spindling noted by Wagman. As would be expected, this variation disappears when cocaine is applied to the nasal mucosa or in animals ventilated via a tracheostomy (STEIN et al. 1979).

The efferent paths from the amygdala are via the stria terminalis and the ventral amygdalofugal fibers. The stria terminalis projects to the hypothalamus,

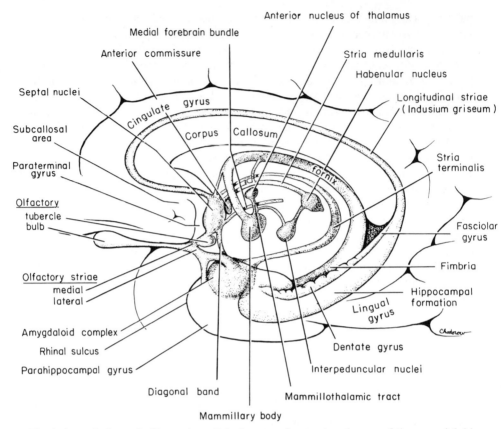

Fig. 1. A semischematic illustration of the input and output pathways of the amygdaloid complex as seen in a medial view of the right hemisphere. With permission from TRUEX and CARPENTER (1971)

whereas the ventral amygdalofugal fibers terminate in the septal nuclei, hypothalamus, the diagonal band, olfactory tubercle, the rostral cingulate cortex and the thalamus via the thalamic peduncle. Efferent fibers from the septal nuclei in turn project to the midbrain via the medial forebrain bundle and the habinular complex via stria medularis, thereby allowing amygdaloid input to the reticular formation. Additionally, there are numerous synaptic interconnections between the amygdaloid complex and both ispilateral and contralateral limbic system structures. Further details of these pathways can be found in Truex's anatomical description of the limbic system (TRUEX and CARPENTER 1971).

The amygdaloid complex's function has also been studied in both man and animals. Ablation of the amygdaloid complex in cats and monkeys result in a placid appearence, and a loss of their typical pre-ablative reactions to fear threats, or molestations (POIRIER 1952; PRIBRAM and BAGSHAW 1953; GLOOR 1960; NARABAYASHI et al. 1963; GREEN et al. 1951). Likewise, amygdaloid complex ablation in man result in a decrease in aggressive and assaultive type behavior (GREEN et al. 1951; POOL 1954).

Electrical stimulation of the amygdaloid complex in animals result in changes in visceral and autonomic function. Additionally, the animals turn their head and eyes to the contralateral side and demonstrate chewing, licking and swallowing movements, as well as reactions of attention, rage, and fear (MACLEAN and DEL-GADO 1953; GLOOR 1960). In man, amygdaloid stimulation results in confusional states and amnesia (FEINDEL and PENFIELD 1954).

Thus, both ablative and electrical stimulation studies relate the amygdaloid complex's function to the regulation and mediation of emotional behavior.

III. Other CNS Structures Affected by Local Anesthetics

We are now prepared to discuss a further refinement of Wagmen's work accomplished by Seo and colleagues (SEO et al. 1982). Chronic recording electrodes were implanted in the cat's medial amygdala, dorsal hippocampus and mid brain reticular formation (MRF), along with surface EEG recording from the anterior suprasylvian gyrus. Instead of an i.v. bolus injection, a continuous i.v. infusion of lidocaine was used. With this approach 4 distinct phases of lidocaine effects on these areas were noted (see Fig. 2).

The first phase was one of behavioral depression. An arrest of ongoing activity occurred with the animals lying on the floor with forelimbs extended and hindlimbs flexed. The eyes remained open. Control cortical low-voltage fast wave and hippocampal theta waves were replaced by irregular high-voltage slow waves. Amygdaloid recordings demonstrated the typical lidocaine spindling activity in synchrony with respiration. The mid brain reticular formation (MRF) showed a 19% decrease in spike activity from control, as measured by a summated record of neuronal action potentials.

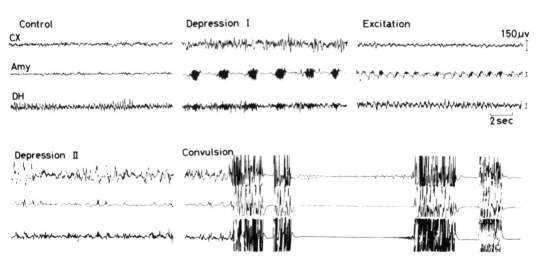

Fig. 2. Lidocaine induced effects on the cat EEG at an infusion rate of $1 \text{ mg} \cdot \text{kg}^{-1} \cdot \text{min}^{-1}$. Recording sites are the anterior suprasylvian gyrus (*CX*), the medial amygdaloid nucleus (*Amy*), and the dorsal hippocampal formation (*DH*). Note the 4 stages of electrical activity. See text for further explanation. With permission from SEO et al. (1982)

The second phase was one of behavioral excitation, characterized by head extension, panting respirations, urinary and fecal incontinence, dilated pupils and loss of behavioral responses to painful stimuli. The cats vocalized during this stage. The neurophysiological correlates of this behavior was cortical EEG low-voltage fast wave activity, spindling in the amygdala and now the hippocampus, again in synchrony with respiration. The MRF spike activity was increased 54% over control values.

The third phase of CNS electrical changes was called the late depression phase. Behaviorally, the cats vocalized less, while demonstrating episodic head swinging as well as an overall quiet demeaner. The animals showed no response to external stimuli. This stage was characterized electrically by cortical EEG irregular high-voltage slow waves, and a loss of spindling in the amygdala. Irregular spike and slow waves now predominated in the amygdala as well as decreased MRF activity. The convulsant stage was characterized by typical electrical seizure activity alternating with 2–8 s quiesent periods seen in all recorded areas. Typical tonic-clonic motor seizures were correlated with this electrical activity. The post-ictal period was essentially a reversal of the above first 3 phases.

With increased infusion rates, the same sequence of events were noted, but a compression of the depression phases appeared to highlight the early excitation and convulsion phase. This finding helps to explain why Wagman's groups, who used I.V. boluses, were not able to discern these 4 distinct phases. Seo also reviewed Munson's cortical EEG recordings from the monkey and was able to discern comparable changes in this species. Thus, the data from the cat and rabbit both demonstrate an initial local anesthetic-induced excitatory effect in the amygdala, with concomittant depression in other CNS structures in subconvulsant doses. As the pre-ictal phase develops, changes in the cortical EEG, when viewed as an isolated entity, can be confused with typical EEG changes of wakefulness. Therefore, the cortical EEG, by itself, is not useful as a monitor of impending lidocaine motor seizures. Finally, both the cat and rabbit demonstrate stereotyped behaviorial patterns which in part could represent the auras of temporal lobe seizures in these species (SEO et al. 1982; DE JONG 1977). This behavior is accompanied by marked fluctuations in subcortical electrical activity, and eventually culminates in overt motor seizures.

While most data point to the amygdala as the main focus for local anesthetic-induced seizures, other workers have demonstrated the hippocampus to be a secondary focus. Microinjection of dibucaine into the hippocampus as well as the amygdala of the monkey leads to initial depression of the electrical activity of both structures. With hippocampal injections, however, electrical excitation was seen to follow the initial depression phase (DELGADO and KITAHATA 1967). As spindling seems to occur normally in monkey hippocampus, the initial depression phase may correlate with the phase of initial depression in the cat and rabbit. Behavior reminescent of temporal lobe auras or overt motor seizures were not noted in this report. In one monkey, hippocompal injections resulted in a delayed excitation in both the amygdala and hippocampus. The amygdaloid excitation subsided after 6 days, whereas the hippocampus required a month to return to a control level activity. The fact that amygdaloid injection of dibucaine failed to elicit an excitatory focus may have been due to the fact that the parental route of local anesthetic may be necessary for amygdaloid excitation (DE JONG 1977). The supplementary role of the hippocampus as a focus for local anesthetic-induced seizures, was also demonstrated by Ingvar and coworkers in the cat (INGVAR and SHAPIRO 1981). Using a quantitative autoradiographic technique, these workers demonstrated a selective uptake in the hippocampus of C14 labeled 2-deoxy glucose during the i.v. infusion of preconvulsant lidocaine doses. This would imply a selective excitation of this structure (COLLINS et al. 1976). These experiments were done under nitrous oxide anesthesia which may have raised the amygdala's threshold to lidocaine excitation (DE JONG 1977). The amygdala, however, appears to be necessary for local anesthesia-induced seizures, as they fail to develop in cocaine-challenged rats whose amygdala have been ablated (EIDELBERG et al. 1963).

The evidence seems incontrovertible that local anesthetics can activate limbic system seizure activity in both man and animals. The amygdala seems to be the initial limbic system structure activated through the intravenous route of local anesthetic administration, and seizure activity both electrically and behaviorally mimics temporal lobe epilepsy, with subsequent progression to generalized seizures (DE JONG 1977; STEIN et al. 1979; MOORE 1980).

We have seen that the afferent and efferent connections of the amygdala (see above) help to explain the electrical and behavioral responses of animals challenged with local anesthetics, i.e., olfactory driving of amygdaloid spindles, and the progression of seizure activity to structures distant to the amygdala. Another important efferent pathway from the amygdala is the amygdalofugal paths to the hypothalamus (TRUEX and CARPENTER 1971; DE JONG 1977). This affords the amygdala an important influence on the autonomic nervous system. Rosenbaum and coworkers recorded from isolated fibers teased out from strands of cervical preganglionic sympathetic fibers in cats (ROSENBAUM et al. 1978). This activity was correlated with the parietal EEG, peripheral blood pressure and heart rate. They found, upon giving repeated i.v. boluses of lidocaine until the cats convulsed, that the sympathetic preganglionic firing ratio changed to bursts which correlated with the EEG bursts of seizure activity. The overall mean rate of sympathetic activity remained unchanged from control, or that seen with preconvulsive doses of lidocaine. These effects were not influenced by the barostatic reflexes (as judged by the effects of epinephrene on blood pressure and heart rate), which appeared to be depressed. Blood pressure was maintained in these experiments. Whether these effects were due to direct amygdalo-hypothalamic pathways or more complex system relays to the sympathetic system was not shown in these experiments. That the effects were supraspinal in origin was shown by Kao and Jolan, who showed a drop in blood pressure and cardiac output in decerebrate dogs (KAO and JOLAN et al. 1959). More experimental work is needed in order to better define the supraspinal autonomic influence of local anesthetics.

G. The Mechanisms Underlying
Local Anesthetic-Induced Seizures

I. Local Anesthetic Induced Disinhibition of Neuronal Pathways

The mechanisms underlying local anesthetic effects on the central nervous system have also been studied with a number of different approaches. As we will see, most investigators agree that these effects can be explained by the membrane-stabilizing properties of local anesthetics, although some investigators have hypothesized a receptor blocking action. Crawford electrophoretically injected procaine near intracortical cat neurons. These neurons were excited by both d/-homocysteic acid (DH) and acetylcholine (ACH). Procaine injections depressed the sensitivity of these neurons to these purported neurotransmitters. Procaine also reduced the amplitude of the action potentials suggesting that procaine either had a blocking action of neurotransmitters at their receptor sites or that the postsynaptic membrane was unable to respond electrically to their action (CRAWFORD 1970). Curtis and coworkers demonstrated with procaine iontophoretic application (CURTIS and ECCLES 1958) a depression of spinal cord Renshaw cells to ACH. These investigators explained these events by hypothesizing that procaine blocked receptor access to ACH. Curtis and Phillis, however, reasoned that procaine could also cause Renshow cell inhibition by a direct action on its membrane (CURTIS and PHILLIS 1960). They analyzed the effects of iontophoretically applied procaine on spinal cord interneurons, Renshaw cells, and motoneurons. Again, procaine was shown to block the excitant affects of ACH and glutamic acid on Renshaw cells and interneurons. The question of whether procaine's depressive effect on spinal cord cells was due to receptor competition or to membrane stabilization was elegantly answered by motoneuron intracellular recordings. Using multibarrelled electrodes, CURTIS and colleagues were able to impale single motoneurons with one barrel used for stimulation and recording. Another barrel lay resting just outside the impaled cell and was used for iontophoretic application of procaine. Peripheral nerves were stimulated in order to activate the impaled motoneuron either antidromically or orthodromically. When procaine was applied to the motoneuron soma, the threshold for direct activation by stimulation through the recording electrode was increased and returned to baseline after the procaine injection was stopped. Both direct stimulation as well as antidromic activiation of the motoneuron were able to produce initial segment action potentials, but soma-dendritic action potentials were absent during procaine administration. It is known that the initial segment (I.S.) spike has the greatest margin of safety or lowest threshold for action potential formation when compared to action potential production of the soma and dendritic parts of the neuron (ECCLES 1957). These results were interpreted as a generalized membrane-stabilizing effect of procaine on the electrically excitable membranes of motoneurons. Due to this stabilizing influence, only the low threshold initial segment could generate on action potential. Orthodramic activation of the impaled motoneurons, however, produced normal EPSP's and IPSP's during procaine injection demonstrating that the involved neuronal transmitters and receptor site function were not influenced by the presence of procaine.

De Jong and coworkers studied the effects of lidocaine on spinal cord reflexes in decerebrate and spinal cats (DE JONG et al. 1969). They found that during i.v. lidocaine infusion, the amplitude of the monosynaptic reflex was increased whereas the activity in polysynaptic reflex pathways was depressed. Since inhibitory and polysynaptic pathways involved neurons of small caliber, they interpreted their results to indicate that a selective inhibition of small spinal neurons at the doses used resulted in loss of inhibitory influences on the monosynaptic reflex, as this inhibition depends on small caliber fibers.

The hypothesis that local anesthetics in subconvulsive doses depresses inhibitory pathways via membrane stabilization of these neurons (at least initially) is further substantiated by data from studies on supraspinal centers (DE JONG 1977). A number of supraspinal inhibitory pathways have been studied with regard to local anesthetic affects. Thus, it was shown that the inhibitory effect of cerebellar stimulation on vestibular nuclear activity was depressed by i.v. lidocaine to a much greater extent than the excitatory effect on these nuclei from vestibular nerve stimulation (SINCLAIR and YIM 1969). Likewise, lidocaine reduced the inhibitory effect of darkness on the visual cortex excitation induced with optic nerve stimulation (HAZRA 1970). Warnick and collegues have shown that i.v. lidocaine in cats will also decrease transcallosal inhibition of the L-glutamate induced contralateral cortical neuron excitation (WARNICK et al. 1971). This disinhibition did not involve a direct effect of lidocaine on the inhibitory transmitter GABA or its receptor sites. Thus, local anesthetics appear initially to depress inhibitory pathways in both the spinal cord and brain. Most authorities then reason that this disinhibition allows increased electrical activity to take place in the limbic system. At the same time, a concomittant depression of cortical activity is seen. With increasing plasma levels of local anesthetics, this depression is overcome as subcortical seizure activity spreads to involve the cortex. The specific reason for local anesthetic initial disinhibition of limbic system structures is unknown.

II. The Interplay of Local Anesthetics and Putative Neurotransmitters and Neuromodulators

Some investigators have reasoned that local anesthetics may alter excitability in specific inhibitory (but non-GABA) pathways. It is known that serotonin (5-HT) dopamine (DA) and norepinephrine (NE) may serve as either neuromodulators or neurotransmitters in the central nervous system. All 3 amines have been implicated in an inhibitory function (HAIGLER and ADHAYANIAN 1977). 5-HT and NE have been shown to be highly concentrated in the limbic system (EIDELBERG and WOODBURY 1972). Depending on its site of iontophoretic application 5-HT has been shown either to increase or decrease neuronal activity. Investigators have therefore studied the interplay of these substances with local anesthetics, particularly with respect to seizures. Thus, it has been shown that prior treatment of rats with parachlorophenylalanine resulted in both a depletion of brain serotonin to 57% of control and an increase in the lidocaine plasma concentration necessary for motor seizures (NIEDERLEHNER et al. 1982). Increases in 5-HT and/or DA brain content had no effect on thresholds for lidocaine induced seizures. Others had shown that increases in 5-HT-content led to a decrease in lidocaine seizure thresholds, but these investigators did not check lidocaine-plasma concentrations (DE OLIVERA et al. 1974). It is known that manipulation of these amines can also lead to changes in the blood flow to the liver, where lidocaine is metabolized (NIEDERLEHNER et al. 1982). Therefore, changes in lidocaine metabolism may have accounted for this discrepancy. Ciarlone has shown that 5-HT-depletion decreased lidocaine, but not procaine seizure thresholds (CIARLONE 1981). Thus, since procaine has a nonhepatic route of metabolism, serotonin depletion may not have affected the procaine seizure threshold in his studies. Ciarlone also demonstrated that CNS-depletion of DA can also reduce the dose necessary for both lidocaine and procaine seizures (CIARLONE 1981). Plasma concentrations of these local anesthetic were not reported. Related to these results, however, are studies in which cocaine and lidocaine were compared with respect to the speed with which amygdala kindling in rats led to motor seizures (STRIPLING et al. 1919). These investigators reasoned that cocaine blocks the re-uptake of catacholamines, i.e., norpinephrine and dopamine. Thus, more of these compounds should be available in the brain, whereas lidocaine has no such effect. Thus, if DA is important as an agent in local anesthetic-induced seizures, its effects would be seen during the kindling process. When using i.p. subconvalsant doses of each drug, these investigators found a decreased latency to clonus during kindling compared to saline controls. Of interest is that the NE and DA CNS content was unchanged in these experiments, suggesting that both cocaine and lidocaine affected the amygdala in the same fashion with respect to latency to clonus, and that DA concentration was not an important factor in local anesthetic-induced seizures. Obviously, the effect of 5-HT-depletion should be studied with respect to the kindling phenemonon. Most investigators, however, believe that the experimental data presented above does support the postulate that local anesthetic's convulsive activity is secondary to inhibition of central inhibitory pathways (CIARLONE 1981). This disinhibition apparently involves the CNS-content of 5-HT. Hopefully, future research will help to clarify the role of this and other amines in local anesthetic seizures.

H. Central Nervous System Metabolic Effects of Local Anesthetics

Lidocaine, for the most part, has been used as a prototype for studying the metabolic effects of local anesthetics on the central nervous system (CNS). Maekawa and coworkers have shown that subconvulsant doses of lidocaine depress both the cerebral metabolic rate for oxygen (CMRO$_2$) and the cerebral blood flow (CBF) in the dog (MAEKAWA et al. 1974). When convulsant doses were given, however, the CMRO$_2$ and CBF increased to 112% of control and 157% of control respectively. That the increase in CBF was sufficient to meet the increased oxygen demands of the seizure without conversion from aerobic to anerobic metabolism was demonstrated by stable cerebral venous oxygen tensions and oxygen-glucose indices. These values represent a CNS global state of affairs and may not apply to local changes, i.e., in the amygdala or hippocampus. Ingvar and colleagues demonstrated an increase of 23% over control of the cerebral metabolic rate for glucose (CMR_g) in the hippocampus during preconvulsant levels of lidocaine (INGVAR and SHAPIRO 1981). The corresponding values of local $CMRO_2$ or CBF were not available in their study. They did demonstrate that 19 out of 26 regions of the brain, including the cerebral cortex, had a depressed CMR_g during preconvulsant lidocaine doses.

The fact that CBF more than compensates for the increased oxygen demands in the cortex during lidocaine seizures was further substantiated by Maekawa and coworkers (MAEKAWA et al. 1981). Rats were infused with 0.75 mg/ml/min of lidocaine. The cortices of the rats were analyzed for lactate, pyruvate, ATP, ADP, and phosphocreatine. These results, taken as a measure of the cerebral energy state (CES), were compared during preseizure activity, seizures and during the recovery period. There were no significant changes in CES, except for a small increase in phosphocreatines PCr in the seizure group and a small decrease in ADP in the preseizure groups. The increase in PCr was attributed to a pH dependant shift in the phosphocreatine kinase equilibrium. Bicuculline induced seizures on the other hand reduced the CES of the rats cortex. Again, only the cortex was studied, and studies of the CES in the limbic system would be valuable, as it is known that the hippocampus, in particular, is very sensitive to ischemic injury (MEYER 1963).

There is animal behavioral data available which shows that if a local anesthetic seizure is brief, no permanent neurologic or behavioral sequalae are produced post-ictally (DE JONG and HEAVNER 1971; WAGMAN et al. 1967). This data implies that local anesthetic seizures of short duration do not produce ischemic CNS damage.

I. Summary

In this chapter, we have discussed aspects of the behavioral physiological, pharmacological and biochemical effects of local anesthetics on the central nervous system (CNS). As noted in this discussion, many questions concerning the mechanism of local anesthetic CNS-effects remain unanswered. Hopefully, new research strategies in the next few years will provide answers to these fascinating questions. For a discussion of the clinical aspects of local anesthetic toxicity the reader is referred to Covino's chapter: "Toxicity and Systemic Effects of Local Anesthetic Agents," in this volume.

References

Aberg G, Morck E, Waldeck B (1973) Studies on the effects of some local anesthetics on the uptake of ^{3}H-2-noradrenaline into vascular and cardiac tissue in vitro. Acta Pharmacol Toxicol 33:476

Akerman B, Aström A, Roes S, Teli A (1966) Studies on the absorption, distribution, and metabolism of labelled prilocaine and lidocaine in some animal species. Acta Pharmacol Toxicol 24:389–403

Amduroux C, DuCres B, Estanove S (1975) Complications of lignocaine. Anesth Analg 16(1):8–19

Axelrod J, Weil-Malherbe H, Tomchick R (1959) The physiological disposition of H^3-epinephrine and its metabolite metanephrine. J Pharmacol Exp Ther 127:251–256

Babb TL, Perryman KM, Lieb JP, Finch DM, Crandall PH (1979) Procaine induced seizures in epileptic monkeys with bilateral hippocampal foci. Electroencephalogr Clin Neurophysiol 47(6):725–737

Berger GS, Tyler CW, Harrod EK (1974) Maternal deaths associated with paracervical block anesthesia. Am J Obstet Gynecol 118:1142–1143

Bigelow N, Harrison I (1944) General analgesic effects of procaine. J Pharmacol Exp Ther 81:368

Blumer J, Strong JM, Atkinson AJ (1973) The convulsant potency of lidocaine and its N-dealkylated metabolites. J Pharmacol Exp Ther 186:31–36

Byrd LD (1979) The behavioral effects of cocaine: rate dependency or rate constancy. Eur J Pharmacol 56:355–362

Byrd LD (1980) Magnitude and duration of the effects of cocaine on conditioned and adjunctive behaviors in the chimpanzee. J Exp Anal Behav 33(1):131–140

Ciarlone AE (1981) Alteration of lidocaine or procaine induced convulsions by manipulation of brain amines. J Dent Res 60(2):182–186

Clark FC, Steele BJ (1966) Effects of D-amphetamine on performance under a multiple scheudle in the rat. Psychopharmacologia 9:157–169

Collins RC, Kennedy C, Sakoloff L, Plum F (1976) Metabolic anatomy of focal motor seizures. Arch Neurol 33:536–542

Cooper JR, Bloom FG, Roth RH (1978) The biochemical basis of neuropharmacology, 3rd edn. Oxford University Press, New York, pp 18–20

Covino BG, Vassallo HG (1976) General pharmacological and toxicological aspects of local anesthetic agents. Local anesthetics: mechanisms of action and clinical use. Grune and Stratton, New York, pp 129–161

Crawford JM (1970) Anaesthetic agents and the chemical sensitivity of cortical neurones. Neuropharmacology 9:31–46

Curtis DR, Eccles RM (1958) The affect of diffusional barriers upon the pharmacology of cells within the central nervous system. J Physiol (Lond) 141:446–463

Curtis DR, Phillis JW (1960) The action of procaine and atropine on spinal neurones. J Physiol (Lond) 153:17–34

De Clive-Lowe SG, Desmond J, North J (1958) Intravenous lignocaine anaesthesia. Anaesthesia 13:138

De Jong RH (1969) Local anesthetic seizures. Anesthesiology 30:5–6

De Jong RH (1977) Central nervous system effects. In: Local anesthetics, 2nd edn. Thomas, Springfield, Ill, pp 84–114

De Jong RH, Bonin JD (1981) Benzadiazepines protect mice from local anesthetic convulsions and death. Anesth Analg 60:385–389

De Jong RH, Heavner JE (1971) Diazepam prevents local anesthetic seizures. Anesthesiology 34:523–531

De Jong RH, Heavner JE (1974) Diazepam prevents and aborts lidocaine convulsions in monkeys. Anesthesiology 41:226–230

De Jong RH, Robles R, Corbin RW (1969) Central actions of lidocaine on synaptic transmission. Anesthesiology 30:19–23

De Jong RH, Walts LF (1966) Lidocaine-induced psychomotor seizures in man. Acta Anesthesiol Scand [Suppl] 23:598–604

De Jong RH, De Rosa R, Bonin JD, Gamble C (1980) Cerebral and circulatory effects of high dose bupivicaine and etidocaine. Anesthesiology 535:Abstract S224

De Oliveira LF, Heavner JE, de Jong RH (1974) 5-hydroxytryptophan intensifies local anesthetic-induced convulsions. Arch Int Pharmacodyn Ther 207:333–339

Delgado JMR, Kitahata LM (1967) Reversible depression of hippocampus by local injections of anesthetics in monkeys. Electroencephalogr Clin Neurophysiol 22:453–464

Deneau G, Yanagito T, Seevers MH (1969) Self-administration of psychoactive substances by the monkey. Psychopharmacologia 16:30–48

Dews PB (1953) The measurement of the influence of drugs on voluntary activity in mice. Br J Pharmacol 8:46–48

Dripps RD, Eckenhoff JE, Vandam LD (1983) Introduction to anesthesia – the principles of safe practice, 6th edn. Saunders, Philadelphia

Eccles JC (1957) The physiology of nerve cells. Jophn Hopkins, Baltimore

Eidelberg E, Woodbury LM (1972) Electrical activity in the amygdala and its modifications by drugs. Possible nature of synaptic transmitters, a review. In: Eleftherion BE (ed) The neurobiology of the amygdala. Plenum, New York, pp 609–622

Eidelberg E, Lesse H, Gault FP (1963) An experimental model of temporal lobe epilepsy. Studies of the convulsant properties of cocaine. In: Glaser GH (ed) EEG and behavior. Basic Books, New York, chap 10

Eidelberg E, Neer HN, Miller MK (1965) Anticonvulsant properties of some benzodiazepane derivatives. Neurology 15:223–230

Elliot HW, Quilici GC, Elison C (1960) Central effects of local anesthetics. Fed Proc 19:274

Englesson S (1973) The influence of acid-base changes on central nervous system toxicity of local anaesthetics agents. Dissertation, Faculty of Medicine, University of Uppsala

Englesson S, Matausek M (1975) Central nervous system effects of local anaesthetic agents. Br J Anaesth 47:241–246

Essman WB (1966) Anticonvulsive properties of xylocaine in mice susceptable to audiogenic seizures. Arch Int Pharmacodyn 164:376

Feindel W, Penfield W (1954) Localization of discharge in temporal lobe automatism. Arch Neurol Psychiatry 72:605–630

Fischman MW, Schuster CR, Resnekov L, Shick JFE, Krasnegor NA, Fennel W, Freedman DX (1976) Cardio-vascular and subjective effects of intravenous cocaine administration in humans. Arch Gen Psychiatr 33:983–989

Foldes FF, Davidson GW, Duncalf D, Kuwabara J (1965) The intravenous toxicity of local anaesthetic agents in man. Clin Pharmacol Ther 6:328–335

Ford RD, Balster RL (1977) Reinforcing properties of intravenous procaine in rhesus monkeys. Pharmacol Biochem Behavior 6:289–296

Freund G (1973) The prevention of ethanol withdrawal seizures in mice by lidocaine. Neurology 23:91–94

Garfield JM, Vivaldi E (1983) Effects of halothane and enflurane on schedule-controlled behavior in the rat. Anesthesiology 59:207–214

Gloor P (1960) Amygdala. Field J (ed) Handbook of physiology, sect 1, vol 11, chap 57. American Physiological Society, Washington, pp 1395–1420

Goddard GV (1967) Development of epileptic seizures through brain stimulation at low intensity. Nature 214:1020–1021

Goldberg WB, Goldberg AF (1970) Mepivacaine toxicity – the effect of ambient PO_2 variation. Pharmacolog Ther Dent 1:56–58

Green JD, Duisberg REH, McGrath WB (1951) Focal epilepsy of psychomotor type. A preliminary report of observations on effects of surgical therapy. J Neurosurg 8:157–172

Grossman SH, Davis SD, Kitchell BB, Shand PG, Routledge PA (1982) Diazepam and lidocaine plasma protein binding in renal disease. Clin Pharmacol Ther 31(3):350–357

Haigler HJ, Adhayanian GK (1977) Serotonin receptors in the brain. Fed Proc 36:2159–2164

Hanna MK, Blackbaum JG, Ogiloie RW, Campbell SL (1978) The effects of lidocaine on hyperoxic seizure activity in the rat. J Exp Neurol 58(3):562–565

Haranath PSRK, Ven Katakriesna Bhatt H (1968) Procaine perfused into cerebral ventricles and subarachnoid space in conscious and anaesthetized dogs. Br J Pharmacol 34:408–416

Hazra J (1970) Disinhibition of the inhibitary effect of darkness on optic evoked potentials by lidocaine. Fed Proc 29:256

Hertting G, Axelrod J, Witby LG (1961) Effect of drugs on the uptake and metabolism of H^3-norepinephrine. J Pharmacol Exp Ther 134:146–153

Ho BT (1977) Behavioral effects of cocaine: metabolic and neurochemical approach. In: Ellinwood EH, Kilbey MM (eds) Cocaine and other stimulants. Plenum, New York

Hoffman WF, Jerram DC, Gangarosa CP (1977) Cardiorespiratory and behavioral reactions to the lidocaine induced convulsions in the dog. Res Commun Chem Pathol Pharmacol 16(4):581–591

Hood D, Mecca R (1983) Failure to initiate electroconvulsive seizures in a patient pretreated with lidocaine. Anesthesiology 58:379–381

Ingvar M, Shapiro HM (1981) Selective metabolic activation of the hippocampus during lidocaine induced pre-seizure activity. Anesthesiology 54(1):33–37

Iverson S, Iverson LL (1981) Behavioral pharmacology, 2nd edn. Oxford University Press, New York

Jaffe J (1980) Drug Addiction and drug abuse. In: Goodman Gilman (eds) The pharmacological basis of therapeutics, Chap 23. MacMillan, New York, pp 535–584

Jain PD, Pandey K, Chandra HK (1975) Diazepam prophylaxis for lignocaine induced convulsions. Anesth Intensive Care 3(4):331–333

Jolly ER, Steinhaus JE (1956) The effect of drugs injected into limited portions of the cerebral circulation. J Pharmacol Exp Ther 116:273–281

Jorfeldt L, Löfstrom B, Persson B, Wahren J, Widmar B (1968) The effect of local anesthetics or the central circulation and respiration in man and dog. Acta Anaesthesiol Scand 12:153–169

Julian RM (1973) Lidocaine in experimental epilepsy. J Life Sci 4:27–30

Kao FF, Jolan VH (1959) The central action of lignocaine and its effect on cardiac output. Br J Pharmacol 14:522

Keats A, D'Alessandro GL, Beecher HK (1950) Pain Relief with hypnotic doses of barbiturates and a hypothesis. J Pharmacol Exp Ther 100:1

Kilbey MM, Ellinwood EH, Essler ME (1979) The effects of chronic cocaine pretreatment on kindled seizures and behavioral sterotypsies. Exp Neurol 64:306–314

Klein SW, Sutherland RK, Worth JE (1969) Hemodynamic effects of intravenous lidocaine in man. J Can Med Assoc 99:472–475

Koppanyl T (1962) The sedative, central analgesic and anticonvulsant actions of local anesthetics. Am J Med Sci 654:150–158

Krenis LJ, Liu PL, Ngai SH (1971) The effect of local anesthetics on the central nervous system toxicity of hyperbaric oxygen. Neuropharmacology 10:637–641

Lampe D, Mai I, Lange B (1976) Our additive increase of the toxicity of lidocaine by pethidine. Z Gesamte Inn Med 31:178–180, Abstract in English

Lemmen LJ, Klassen M, Duiser B (1978) Intravenous lidocaine in the treatment of convulsions. Jama 239(19):22025

Liu PL, Feldman HS, Giasi R, Patterson MK, Covino BG (1983) Comparative CNS toxicity of lidocaine, etidocaine, bupivacaine, and tetracaine in awake dogs following rapid I.V. administration. Anesth Analg 62:375–379

MacLean PD, Delgado JMR (1952) Electrical and chemical stimulation of fronto-temporal portion of limbic system in the waking animal. Electroencephalogr Clin Neurophysiol 5:91–100

MacMillan WH (1959) A hypothesis concerning the effect of cocaine on the action of sympathomimetic amines. Br J Pharmacol Chemother 14:385

Maekawa T, Sakabe T, Takeshita H (1974) Diazepam blocks cerebral metabolic and circulatory response to local anesthetic-induced seizures. Anesthesiology 41:389–391

Maekawa T, Oshibuchi T, Takao, Takeshita H, Imamura A, Akihisa (1981) Cerebral energy state and glycolytic metabolism during lidocaine infusion in the rat. Anesthesiology 54:278–283

Malagodi MH, Munson ES, Embro WJ (1977) Relation of etidocaine and bupivicaine toxicity to rate of infusion in rhesus monkeys. Br J Anaesth 49:121–125

Mark CC, Brand L, Goldensakn ES (1964) Recovery after procaine-induced seizures in dogs. Electroencephalogr Clin Neurophysiol 16:280

Meyer A (1963) Intoxications. In: Blackwood WH, McMenemey W, Meyer A et al. (eds) Greenfield's neuropathology. Williams and Wilkins, Baltimore, pp 255–261

Moore DC (1980) Administer oxygen first in the treatment of local anesthetic-induced convulsions. Anesthesiology 53:346–347

Moore DC (1981) Local anesthetic drugs: tissue and systemic toxicity. Acta Anaesthesiol Scand 4:283–300

Moore DC, Crawford RD, Scurlack JE (1980) Severe hypoxia and acidosis following local anesthetic-induced convulsions. Anesthesiology 53:259–260

Morishima HO, Pederson H, Tinister K, Sakema SC, Bruce BB, Gutschke RI, Stark, Covino BG (1981) Toxicity of lidocaine in adult, newborn, and fetal sheep. Anesthesiology 55:57–61

Morishima HO, Pederson H, Mieczyslaw F, Feldman H, Covino BG (1983) Etidocaine toxicity in adult, newborn, and fetal sheep. Anesthesiology 58:347–352

Munson ES, Wagman IH (1972) Diazepam treatment of local anesthetic induced seizures. Anesthesiology 37:523–528

Munson ES, Gutnick MJ, Wagman IH (1970) Local anesthetic drug-induced seizures in rhesus monkeys. Anesth Analg 49:986–994

Munson ES, Tucker W, Ausinsch B, Malagodi M (1975) Etidocaine, bupivacaine, lidocaine seizures thresholds in monkeys. Anesthesiology 42(4):471–478

Muscholl E (1961) Effect of cocaine and related drugs on the uptake of norodvenaline by heart and spleen. Br J Pharmacol Chemother 16:352–359

Narabayashi H, Nagao T, Saito Y, Yoshida M, Nagahata M (1963) Sterotoxic amygdalotomy for behavior disorders. Arch Neurol 9:1–16

Niederlehner J, Cosmo A, Di Zazio Foster J, Westfall T (1982) Cerebral monoamines and lidocaine toxicity in rats. Anesthesiology 56:184–187

Peterson DI, Hardinge MG (1967) The effect of various environmental factors on cocaine and ephedrine toxicity. J Pharm Pharmacol 19:810–814

Pickens R, Harris WC (1968) Self-administration of d-amphetamine by rats. Psychopharmacologia 12:158–163

Pickens R, Thompson T (1968) Cocaine-reinforced behavior in rats: effects of reinforcement magnitude and fixed ratio size. J Pharmacol Exp Ther 161:122–129

Poirier LJ (1952) Anatomical and experimental studies on the temporal pale of the macague. J Comp Neurology 96:209–248

Pool JL (1954) Neurophysiological symposium: visceral brain in man. J Neurosurg 11:45–63

Post RM (1977) Progressive changes in behavior and seizures following chronic cocaine administration: relationship to kindling and psychosis. In: Ellinwood EH, Kilbey MM (eds) Cocaine and other stimulants. Plenum, New York, pp 353–372

Post RM, Rose H (1976) Increasing effects of repetitive cocaine administration in the rat. Nature 260:731–732

Post RM, Kopanda RT, Lee A (1975) Progressive behavioral changes during lidocaine administration: relationship to kindling. Life Sci 17:943–950

Post RM, Kopanda RT, Black KE (1976) Progressive effects of cocaine on behavior and centralamine metabolism in rhesus monkeys: Relationship to kindling and psychosis. Biol Psychiatry 11:403–419

Pribram KH, Bagshaw M (1953) Further analysis of the temporal lobe syndrome utilizing fronto-temporal ablations. J Comp Neurol 99:347–375

Robinson WM, Jenkins LC (1975) Central nervous system effects of bupivicaine. Can Anaesth Soc J 22:358–369

Rosenbaum KJ, Sapthavichaikeel, Skovsted P (1978) Nervous system response to lidocaine induced seizures in cats. Acta Anaesthesiol Scand 23:548–555

Routledge PA, Stargel WW, Kitchqel BB, Barchawsky A, Shand DE (1981) Sex Related Differences in the plasma protein binding of lignocaine and diazepam. Br J Clin Pharmacol (3):245–250

Sanders HD (1967) A comparison of the convulsant activity of procaine and pentydenetetranzal. Arch Int Pharmacodyn Ther 170:165–177

Scott DB (1975) Evaluation of the toxicity of local anesthetic agents in man. Br J Anesth 47:56–61

Segal DS, Janowsky DS (1978) Psychostimulant – induced behavioral effects: possible models of schizophrenia. In: Lipton MA, DiMascio A, Killam KF (eds) Psychopharmacology: a generation of progress, 2nd edn. Raven, New York, pp 1113–1123

Seo N, Oshima E, Stevens J, Marc K (1982) The tetraphasic action of lidocaine on CNS electrical activity and behavior in cats. Anesthesiology 57:451–457

Sinclair TG, Yim GKW (1969) Effects of diphenylaminoethylene and lidocaine on cerebellar inhibition of Deiter's neurons. Fed Proc 28:476

Sjögren S, Wright B (1972) Circulation respiration and lidocaine concentration during continuous epidural blockage. Acta Anaesthesiol Scand 46:5–56

Smith CB (1964) Effects of d-amphetamine upon operant behavior in pigeons: enhancement by reserpine. J Pharmacol Exp Ther 146:167–174

Smith ER, Duce BR (1971) The acute anti-arrhythmic and toxic effects in mice and dogs of 2-ethylamine-2 '6' acetoxylidene (L-86), a metabolite of lidocaine. J Pharmacol Exp Ther 179:580–585

Sorel L, Lejeune R (1955) Modifications de l'EEG du Lapen sous l'action de divers succedanes de la cocaine injectes par voie intraveinese. Arch Int Pharmacodn Ther 102:314–334

Stark AC, Adeno R, Graham JM, Braun-Myer SE, Perrin RG, Pallock D, Livingston EG (1982) Analysis of Facial displays and verbral report to assess subjective state in the non-invasive detection of limbic system activation by procaine hydrochloride. Behav Brain Res 4(1):77–94

Stein L (1978) Reward transmitters: catecholamines and opioid peptides. In: Lipton MA, DiMaseio A, Killam KF (eds) Psychopharmacology, a generation of progress. 2nd edn. Raven, New York, pp 569–581

Stein PA, Michenfelder JD (1979) Neurotoxicity of anesthetics. Anesthesiology 50:437–453

Stripling JS, Ellinwood EH, Jr (1977) Augmentation of the behavioral and electrophysiologic response to cocaine by chronic administration in the rat. Exp Neurol 54:546–554

Stripling JS, Hendricks C (1981) Effect of cocaine and lidocaine on the expression of kindled seizures in the rat. Pharmacol Biochem Behav 14:397–403

Teramo MD, Benowitz N, Hagman MA, Rudolph MD (1976) Gestational differences in lidocaine toxicity in the fetal lamb. Anesthesiology 44(2):133–138

Truex RC, Carpenter MB (1971) The basal ganglia and rhinencephal, olfactory and limbic system pathways. Human neuroanatomy, 6th edn, chap 20, chap 21. Williams and Wilkins, Baltimore, pp 498–542

Tuttle WW, Elliot HW (1969) Electrographic and behavioral study of convulsants in the cat. Anesthesiology 30:48–64

Usubiaga JE, Wikinski RL (1964) Uso da procaina intravenosa en anestesia general. Rev Bras Anest 14:400

Usubiaga JE, Wininski JA, Zerrero R, Usubiaga LEJ, Wininski R (1966) Local anesthetic-induced convulsions in man, an electroencephalography study. Anesth Analg 45:611–620

Usubiaga JE et al. (1967) Relationship between the passage of local anesthetics across the blood-brain barrier and their effects on the central nervous system. Br J Anesth 39:943–946

Van Dyke C, Byck R (1982) Cocaine. Sci Am 246(3):128–141

Van Dyke C, Jatlow P, Ungever J, Barash P, Byck R (1979) Cocaine and lidocaine have similar psychological effects after intra-nasal application. Life Sci 24:271–274

Wagman J, de Jong R, Prince D (1967) Effects of lidocaine on the central nervous system. Anesthesiology 28:155–167

Warnick J, Kee R, Yim (1971) The effects of lidocaine on inhibition in the cerebral cortex. Anesthesiology 34:327–332

Waugier A, Niemegeers (1974) Intra-cranial self-stimulation in rats as a function of various stimulus parameter: V. Influence of cocaine on medical forebrain bundle stimulation with monopolar electrodes. Psychopharmacologia 38:201–210

Wesseling H, Bovenharst GH, Wiers JW (1971) Effects of diazepam and pentobarbital on convulsions induced by local anesthetics in mice. Eur J Pharmacol 13:150–154

Wood M, Wood AJ (1981) Changes in plasma drug binding and alpha-1-acid glycoprotein in mother and newborn infant. Clin Pharmacol Ther 29(4):522–526

Subject Index

Abbreviations used in this index are: AP, action potential; BTX, batrachotoxin; CNS, central nervous system; LA, local anesthetic; Na channels, sodium channels

Handbook of Experimental Pharmacology

Continuation of
"Handbuch der
experimentellen
Pharmakologie"

Editorial Board
G. V. R. Born, A. Farah,
H. Herken, A. D. Welch

Springer-Verlag
Berlin Heidelberg New York
London Paris Tokyo

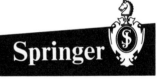

Springer

Handbook of Experimental Pharmacology

Continuation of
"Handbuch der
experimentellen
Pharmakologie"

Editorial Board
G. V. R. Born, A. Farah,
H. Herken, A. D. Welch

Springer-Verlag
Berlin Heidelberg New York
London Paris Tokyo

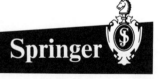

Springer